History and Hope

IHA BOOK SERIES

The International Humanitarian Affairs book series, edited by Kevin M. Cahill, M.D., is devoted to improving the effectiveness of humanitarian relief programs. With contributions by leading professionals, the books are practical guides to responding to the many different effects of civil strife, natural disasters, epidemics, and other crises. All books are available online at www.fordhampress.com. Books marked with an asterisk are available in French translation from Robert Laffont of Paris; books marked with a double asterisk are available in Spanish, German, Arabic, and French.

Preventive Diplomacy: Stopping Wars Before They Start, 2000*
Basics of International Humanitarian Missions, 2003*
Emergency Relief Operations, 2003*
Traditions, Values, and Humanitarian Action, 2003*
Human Security for All: A Tribute to Sergio Vieira de Mello, 2004
Technology for Humanitarian Action, 2004
To Bear Witness: A Journey of Healing and Solidarity, 2005*
Tropical Medicine: A Clinical Text, 7th edition, 2006
The Pulse of Humanitarian Assistance, 2007
Even in Chaos: Education in Times of Emergency, 2010
Sudan at the Brink: Self-Determination and National Unity, F. D. Deng, 2010**
Tropical Medicine: A Clinical Text, 8th edition (Jubilee Edition), 2011*
More with Less: Disasters in an Era of Diminishing Resources, 2012

IIHA OCCASIONAL PAPERS

Kevin M. Cahill, M.D., Abdulrahim Abby Farah, Abdirazak Haji Hussen, and David Shinn, *The Future of Somalia: Stateless and Tragic*, 2004
Mark Malloch Brown, *International Diploma in Humanitarian Assistance*, 2006
Francis Deng, *Sudan: From Genocidal Wars to Frontiers of Peace and Unity*, 2006
Kevin M. Cahill, M.D., *The University and Humanitarian Action*, 2008
Kevin M. Cahill, M.D., *Romance and Reality in Humanitarian Action*, 2008
Kevin M. Cahill, M.D., *Gaza: Destruction and Hope*, 2009
Daithi O'Ceallaigh, *The Tale Towards a Treaty—A Ban on Cluster Munition*, 2010

History and Hope

THE INTERNATIONAL HUMANITARIAN READER

Edited by **KEVIN M. CAHILL, M.D.**

A JOINT PUBLICATION OF **FORDHAM UNIVERSITY PRESS** AND
THE CENTER FOR INTERNATIONAL HUMANITARIAN COOPERATION
NEW YORK   2013

Fordham University Press has no responsibility for the persistence or accuracy of URLs for external or third-party Internet websites referred to in this publication and does not guarantee that any content on such websites is, or will remain, accurate or appropriate.

Fordham University Press also publishes its books in a variety of electronic formats. Some content that appears in print may not be available in electronic books.

Library of Congress Cataloging-in-Publication Data

History and hope : the international humanitarian reader / edited by Kevin M. Cahill, M.D. — First edition.
     pages cm. — (International humanitarian affairs)
  Includes bibliographical references and index.
  ISBN 978-0-8232-5196-4 (cloth : alk. paper) — ISBN 978-0-8232-5197-1 (pbk. : alk. paper)
  1. Humanitarian assistance. 2. International relief. 3. Humanitarianism. I. Cahill, Kevin M.
  HV544.5.H57 2013
  361.2—dc23

                              2012046488

Printed in the United States of America
15 14 13   5 4 3 2 1
First edition

All royalties from this book go to the training of humanitarian workers.

For Herbert Allen, whose steady, generous support of my clinical programs, research, and academic initiatives has changed dreams and visions into realities

Contents

CONTENTS

PART VII. EPILOGUE

Foreword

The pursuit of the goals of humanitarianism, whether through assistance or intervention, has no single way, follows no preconceived pattern. Almost by definition, each experience is different. This means, more perhaps than in any other human activity, that practitioners have to be ready to learn from experience and adapt to circumstance.

As the editor of, contributor to, and inspiration of this much-needed book, Kevin Cahill brings the insights of a clinician in tropical medicine and public health, as well as those of an academic in humanitarian studies. Standing behind the book are twelve volumes still with much relevance to present issues into which readers can delve. The Introduction warns that humanitarian professionals have to "tread softly, to offer change with great care. Attempts to introduce new methods and replace timeworn approaches can be devastating, especially in times of crises, when a society is extremely vulnerable and utterly dependent on strangers for the essentials of life."

In the summer of 2012, the world watched as a horrendous civil war developed in Syria with appalling humanitarian consequences, and international diplomacy, hopefully only for a short time, died with it. Yet even amidst these troubled times, this book is a testament to the humanitarian instinct which demands that we develop better policies and improve our techniques, our delivery, and above all our understanding. What it also demonstrates is that the structures of humanitarian activity are adjusting, evolving, and triumphing in many diverse and challenging surroundings.

The era of unbridled humanitarian intervention in support of human rights, which began with saving the Kurds in Iraq in 1991, looks as if it has had its day and that what happened over Libya could not be repeated over Syria. The circumstances were very different, but the months-long deadlock in the Security Council carries a warning, particularly for the five veto-carrying permanent members, that diplomacy must never die.

An adjustment to the sweeping delegation of "all necessary powers," in the language of Chapter 7 of the UN charter, was anyhow coming in the light of the mixed success rates associated with the many interventions over the past twenty years.

Just as professional standards have been developed in the field and in academia for humanitarian workers, so the Security Council is imposing through its voting structures limits on UN-authorized humanitarian interventions. Frustration, locally and internationally, at these constraints abounds. But they are a natural and inevitable tension that is certain to develop within the new humanitarian interpretation of the Charter.

Kevin Cahill and his distinguished fellow authors have distilled in this book much wisdom of lasting value.

Acronyms and Abbreviations

AERC	Assistant Emergency Relief Coordination
BRICs	Brazil, Russia, India, and China
BWIs	Bretton Woods Institutions
CAP	Consolidated Appeals Process (OCHA)
CDC	Centers for Disease Control and Prevention
CEDAW	Convention On the Elimination of All Forms of Discrimination against Women
CERF	Central Emergency Response Fund
CFA	Comprehensive Framework for Action
CFR	Case Fatality Rates
CGD	Commission on Growth and Development
CHAP	Common Humanitarian Action Plan
CIHC	Center for International Humanitarian Cooperation
CIMIC	Civil-Military Cooperation Issue
CMOC	Civil-Military Operations Center
CMR	Crude Mortality Rate
CNDD-FDD	Conseil National pour la Defense de la Democratie/Forces pour la Defense de la Democratie
CNDP	Congres National Pour la Defense du Peuple
CPN-UML	Communist Party of Nepal—United Marxist-Leninist
CRC	Convention on the Rights of the Child
CRS	Catholic Relief Services
CSW	commercial sex worker
CWS	Church World Services
DAC	Development Assistance Committee
DARPA	Defense Advanced Research Policy Agency
DEC	Disaster Emergency Committee (UK)

DFID	Department for International Development
DMT	Disaster Management Team
DOP	Declaration of Principles of Interim Self-Government Arrangements
DRC	Danish Refugee Council
DRC	Democratic Republic of Congo
DVI	Disaster Victim Identification
ECHO	Humanitarian Aid and Civil Protection department of the European Commission
ECOSOC	Economic and Social Council
EG	Educate Girls (Rajastani NGO)
FNL	Forces Nationales pour la Liberation
G8	Group of Eight
GDACS	Global Disaster Alert and Coordination System
GDP	Gross Domestic Profit
GHD	Good Humanitarian Donorship initiative
GIS	Geographic Information System
GNI	Gross National Income
GSM	Global System for Mobile Communication
HC	Humanitarian Coordinator
HFA	Hyogo Framework for Action
HIC	Humanitarian Information Center
HLTF	High-Level Task Force
HPT	High Performance Teams
HR	Human Resources
HRW	Human Rights Watch
IAPTC	International Association of Peacekeeping Training Center
ICC	International Criminal Court
ICJ	International Court of Justice
ICRC	International Committee of the Red Cross
IDF	Israeli Defense Force
IDHA	International Diploma in Humanitarian Assistance (Fordham University)
IDLO	International Development Law Organization
IDP	Internally Displaced Person
IFI	International Financial Institutions
IFRC	International Federation of Red Cross and Red Crescent Societies
IFOR	NATO Implementation Force

IGO	Intergovernmental Organization
IHA	International Humanitarian Affairs (Fordham University)
IHL	International Humanitarian Law
IIHA	Institute of International Humanitarian Affairs (Fordham University)
ILO	International Labor Organization
IMF	International Monetary Fund
INSARAG	International Search and Rescue Advisory Group
IOC	Intergovernmental Oceanographic Commission
IPU	Inter-Parliamentary Union
IPI	International Peace Institute
IRA	Irish Republican Army
IRC	International Rescue Committee
IRIN	Integrated Regional Information Network
ISAC	Inter Agency Stand-by Committee
JDC	Joint Distribution Committee
LogFrame	Logistical Framework Analysis
LRA	Lord's Resistance Army
MCDU	Military and Civil Defense Unit
MDG	Millennium Development Goal
MDM	Medicins du Monde
MIHA	Masters in International Humanitarian Action (Fordham University)
MOE	measures of effectiveness
MONUC	United Nations Peacekeeping Mission to the Congo
MSF	Médecins Sans Frontières
MUAC	mid-upper arm circumference
NAM	Non-Aligned Movement
NATO	North Atlantic Treaty Organization
NCD	noncommunicable disease
NGO	nongovernmental organization
OAS	Organization of American States
OAV	Organization of African Unity
OCHA	Office for the Coordination of Humanitarian Affairs
ODA	Office for Development Assistance
OECD	Organization for Economic Co-operation and Development

OHCHR	Office of the United Nations High Commissioner for Human Rights
OIC	Organization of Islamic Cooperation
OPT	Occupied Palestinian Territory
OSCE	Organization for Security and Cooperation in Europe
OSF	Open Society Foundations
OSOCC	On-Site Operations Coordination Centre
PA	Palestinian Authority
PEM	protein energy malnutrition
PGA	President of the United Nations General Assembly
PHC	primary health care
PIH	Partners in Health
PKO	Peacekeeping Operation
PLO	Palestine Liberation Organization
POP	People-Oriented Planning
POTI	Peace Operations Training Institute
R2P	Responsibility to Protect
RENAMO	Mozambican National Resistance
RC	Resident Coordinator
RCD-G	Rassemblement Congolaise pour le Democratie—Goma
RDRA	OCHA Regional Disaster Response Advisor
R/HC	Resident Coordinator and Humanitarian Coordinator
RPF	Rwanda Patriotic Front
RUF	Revolutionary United Front
SAR	search and rescue
SBTF	Standby Task Force
SIDS	Small Island Developing States
SRC	Security Council Resolution
SRSG-CAC	Office of the Special Representative for Children and Armed Conflict
TEC	Tsunami Evaluation Coalition
TIMSS	Trends in International Mathematics and Science Survey
TPIM	Terrorism Prevention and Investigation Measures Act
TRC	Truth and Reconciliation Commission
U5MR	Under Age 5 Mortality Rate
UDHR	Universal Declaration of Human Rights

UN	United Nations
UNA-MIR	United Nations Assistance Mission in Rwanda
UNDAC	United Nations Disaster Assessment and Coordination
UNDHA	United Nations Department of Humanitarian Affairs
UNDP	United Nations Development Programme
UNDRO	United Nations Disaster Relief Organization
UNEP	United Nations Environmental Program
UNESCO	United Nations Educational, Scientific and Cultural Organization
UNGA	United Nations General Assembly
UNHCR	United Nations High Commissioner for Refugees
UNHRC	United Nations Human Rights Council
UNICEF	United Nations Children's Fund
UNISDR	United Nations International Strategy for Disaster Reduction
UNITA	National Union for the Total Independence of Angola
UNJCL	United Nations Joint Logistics Centers
UNPF	United Nations Peace Force
UNPREDEP	United Nations Preventive Deployment Force
UNPROFOR	United Nations Protection Force
UNRPR	United Nations Relief for Palestine Refugees
UNRRA	United Nations Relief and Rehabilitation Agency
UNRWA	United Nations Relief and Works Agency
UNWTO	United Nations World Tourism Organization
USAID	United States Agency for International Development
USG/ERC	Under-Secretary General for Humanitarian Affairs and Emergency Relief Coordinator
WEF	World Economic Forum
WFP	World Food Programme
WHO	World Health Organization
WTO	World Trade Organization

Acknowledgments

As I prepare this book for publication, selecting chapters from twelve volumes in the International Humanitarian Affairs book series, editing, deleting, and updating texts so that they will be useful to students and practitioners for years to come, I offer, once again, my gratitude to all the past contributors, to Fordham University, to the volunteers at the Institute of International Humanitarian Affairs, and to the Directors of the Center for International Humanitarian Cooperation. A number of people deserve special recognition for their assistance with this volume.

Each of the authors chosen to revise a chapter did so efficiently, with enthusiasm, and under a very tight schedule. Peter Hansen, a Diplomat in Residence at Fordham, and Jenna Felz carefully read all the chapters and participated in the selection process. Denis Cahill, Alexandra DeBlock, and Radha Desai helped with various aspects of the complex editing process. Larry Hollingworth and Brendan Cahill gave, as always, wise counsel throughout.

My dear friend Massimo Vignelli designed the cover. The image on the front is that of a sphere within a sphere, a cracked globe that seems a perfect symbol for this book. The bronze sculpture was created by Arnoldo Pomodoro and comes from the Vignelli Collection; copies of this iconic figure are also prominently displayed in the United Nations lobby and the Vatican Museum, among other sites.

The Fordham University family, particularly President Joseph M. McShane, S.J.; Provost Stephen Freedman; Dean Nancy Busch; and the director of the University Press, Fredric Nachbaur, provided exceptional and consistent support. They deserve my deepest thanks, for they provided the essential academic foundation for this reader.

Finally, I gratefully acknowledge the shared efforts of colleagues, co-workers, and our thousands of graduates around the world. Their influences are reflected in every page of this book, and in what I try to do in the challenging—and satisfying—world of international humanitarian assistance.

The original publication data for each chapter in *History and Hope* is listed in the Notes section. As with all the volumes in the International Humanitarian book series, this book follows the UN style, capitalizing, for example, terms such as President, Resolution, and Member States.

History and Hope

Introduction

Kevin M. Cahill, M.D.

History and Hope: The International Humanitarian Reader is a compendium drawn from some of the best chapters on various aspects of humanitarian assistance in a series that I have written or edited for Fordham University Press since 2001, numbering twelve volumes to date. Books in the series are used in universities and training courses around the world.

Many fine essays by outstanding contributors could not be included in this *Reader* because of the very real publishing restrictions of size and cost; nonetheless, this volume offers an unusually comprehensive overview of a complex and multifaceted discipline. Most of the original chapters chosen have been shortened, either by the authors or the editor, and much dated material was deleted. However, many examples from the past were retained so that the opinions and observations of the authors—all authorities who have worked in many of the great humanitarian crises of the past half-century—have that ring of truth that can be conveyed only by those with firsthand experience. Lessons learned from errors, and even failure, often provide the foundation for better approaches in the future. Some chapters have a brief addendum of two or three paragraphs to update the text, while several authors chose to provide internal edits to accomplish the same goal.

History and Hope also represents the completion of a phase in an academic program that was carefully conceived several decades ago. Didactic modules for classroom and field were developed and implemented by colleagues who believed we could distill our experiences from the harsh settings of humanitarian crises into solid, practical, field-oriented courses that would be of university level quality. Utilizing the book series, we have now trained more than two thousand candidates from 133 nations in the ever-evolving discipline of international humanitarian assistance.

The series began with *Preventive Diplomacy: Stopping Wars Before They Start*, a text that argued for recognition of the centrality of humanitarian action in foreign policy, too often peripheral afterthoughts overshadowed by other national interests. The contributors utilized the methodology of public health in addressing the softer discipline of diplomacy. The second volume in the series, *Traditions, Values and Humanitarian Action*, was also a philosophic book assessing what influences determine how both individuals and societies develop healthy—or destructive—policies and practices in international humanitarian assistance. Both those volumes provided solid foundations for the technical texts that followed.

The next two titles, *Emergency Relief Operations* and *Basics of Humanitarian Action*, are self-explanatory. These books were primers that were needed as our academic programs developed. The chapters reflect my strong conviction that the practical challenges of disaster zones and refugee camps were proper subjects for university study, and that our texts (and teachers) should be deeply grounded in the harsh realities that are standard in complex emergencies.

The next volume in the series is the most personal. *To Bear Witness: A Journey of Healing and Solidarity* is a compilation of some of my editorial pieces, unpublished lectures, short essays, and introductions to earlier books. I collected them, searching for meaning and continuity, as a tribute to my wife, who was my partner in a full life of humanitarian service. After she died, I reviewed our travels; at that time I had worked in sixty-five countries, mostly in troubled areas, and she had been with me on forty-five of those trips. We had a remarkably shared marriage for forty-four years. This book has been widely reviewed, reprinted and translated; it is an essential part of the series.

The following three books in the series provide more detailed information on specific problems in humanitarian assistance. *Human Security for All: A Tribute to Sergio Vieira de Mello* was conceived as a practical contribution to honor the memory of a good friend and colleague who had paid the ultimate price for attempting to help those in humanitarian distress. Having attended numerous memorial services for Sergio, I felt that something more lasting was needed. Sergio had taught on our courses and delivered an eloquent commencement address for our graduates. He was the ultimate activist, and he deserved more than repetitive platitudes. I organized an academic symposium that drew together many of his UN co-workers, in which the President of Fordham University conferred on Sergio the first posthumous honorary doctorate in its 175-year history. The book is a practical, lasting testament to a remarkable life.

Technology and Humanitarian Action evolved from my experience as Chief Medical Advisor for Counterterrorism in the New York City Police Department. Scientists associated with the Defense Advanced Research Policy Agency (DARPA) impressed me greatly with their imaginative technologic proposals as we faced serious biological, chemical, and radiation threats to our safety. As my contact with these men and women deepened, I quickly realized how the intellectual and financial resources devoted to defense concerns dwarfed the attention given to the overwhelming, often intractable, problems that faced humanitarian workers. The book is built on vignettes detailing practical challenges in complex emergencies, followed by full chapters by DARPA scientists, most of whom had never considered applying their talents and techniques to the humanitarian field. Unfortunately, a decade in technology is analogous to a century—or more—in the liberal arts, and most of the chapters are now quite dated. I am sad to report that the vignettes, on the other hand, have remained only too valid.

The seventh and eighth editions of *Tropical Medicine: A Clinical Text* reflect my own professional background, as well as the cruel fact that in war zones and after disasters more people usually die of the treatable—and usually preventable—diseases that are the subject of these textbooks. Although *Tropical Medicine* is primarily intended for doctors, nurses, and public health personnel, it has also been used by nonmedical humanitarian workers whose duties require an understanding of the basic life cycles and transmission patterns of epidemic diseases. The eighth edition of *Tropical Medicine* is a "Jubilee Edition," reflecting its use in medical education for fifty years.

The next title in the series, *The Pulse of Humanitarian Assistance*, derives from my medical training. Taking the pulse—a basic diagnostic tool in medicine—is an ancient and trusted clinical exercise. At the bedside the physician uses a gentle, tactile measurement to see if the patient has a strong and steady circulation or one that is weak, irregular, thready, or even terminal. Taking the pulse is often the initial test performed by a medical doctor trying to establish an objective record rather than depending merely on a patient's subjective complaints. The nature of the pulse may lead to more refined studies, gradually building a foundation for rational therapy. Trying to detect a pulse is often the final act for a physician in determining if life has passed into death.

So, too, one can measure the pulse of humanitarian action today. In attempts to diagnose some of the major current problems that afflict the humanitarian profession, it also offers prognoses—predicting a way forward. If one is to address human suffering in the confusion that characterizes early complex humanitarian crises, especially those in the developing world, then the etiologic significance of poverty and ignorance, corruption and incompetence, and the all too often evil effects of religion and politics are areas of study as valid as the life cycles of microbes. Professionals in humanitarian assistance must try to measure these factors constantly, just as one carefully records the pulse on the bedside chart of a sick patient.

Even in Chaos: Education in Times of Emergency and *More with Less: Disasters in an Era of Diminishing Resources* were books developed during my capacity as Chief Advisor for Humanitarian and Public Health Issues for three Presidents of the United Nations General Assembly (PGA). The PGA is the most senior position of the United Nations, and they reflect the interests of all 193 Member States. These books became important parts of the legacies of the PGAs, and, as with the others in the series, are used by policymakers, practitioners, and students in universities around the world.

Books in the series are listed at the beginning of this volume. The full table of contents of each book is available at www.fordham.edu/iiha. Seven of the texts are available in French translations. Bernard Kouchner, the co-founder of Médecins Sans Frontières and of Médecins du Monde and, later, Foreign Minister of France, wrote Forewords for several of the books.

History and Hope is also a personal and professional culmination. I began working among populations traumatized by conflict, natural or manmade disasters, more than fifty years ago. My dreams of and plans for how to do difficult tasks better and how to create solutions to seemingly insoluble problems began in refugee camps and slowly coalesced in the stimulating atmosphere of halls of higher education. Preparing this anthology has allowed me to take stock of this particular body of work and to assess the continuity of a struggle that will never be complete.

It is clear, at least to me, that there has been much progress in our efforts to rationalize responses to the extreme challenges of delivering aid in complex humanitarian crises. An essential step was to create flexible structures through which both field operations and teaching programs could be linked. Many decades ago, with the practical help of former U.S. Secretary of State Cyrus Vance's law firm, and with the unequivocal support of Father Joseph O'Hare, S.J., then President of Fordham University, we established both a charitable entity and an academic Institute. The Center for International Humanitarian Cooperation (CIHC) is a public charity founded by a small group of international diplomats and physicians who realized that health and other humanitarian endeavors sometimes provide the only common ground for initiating dialogue, understanding, and cooperation among people and nations shattered by war, civil conflicts, and ethnic violence. The Founders of the Center, some now deceased, included Secretary Vance, former UK Foreign Minister Lord David Owen, UN Secretary General Boutros Boutros-Ghali, Lord Paul Hamlyn, and John Cardinal O'Connor. We owe a great debt for their wise guidance and generous support. The CIHC has been afforded full Consultative Status by the Economic and Social Council (ECOSOC) at the United Nations. In the United States, it is a fully approved charity by the Internal Revenue Service.

The CIHC and its Directors have been deeply involved in trying to alleviate the wounds of war in many areas. A CIHC amputee center for landmine victims in Northern Somalia was developed to provide a simple, rapid, and inexpensive prosthetic program that could be replicated in other areas where there were almost no health services. The center is still functioning in Northern Somalia, and the model has been used in Mozambique and Afghanistan. In the former Yugoslavia, the CIHC was active in prisoner and hostage release, as well as in providing legal assistance for human and political rights violations. It facilitated discussions between combatants. The CIHC has provided staff support on the ground in crisis management in conflict zones in Iraq, East Timor, Indonesia, the Balkans, Palestine, Albania, Lebanon, Pakistan, Somalia, Kenya, and other trouble spots.

The need to establish educational programs, as well as universally recognized academic standards for humanitarian assistance workers, was early recognized as urgent, and it soon became our top priority. To address this challenge, the CIHC joined with Fordham University in New York City, creating an Institute for International Humanitarian Affairs (IIHA). The essential, indeed indispensable, links between academia and humanitarian field operations are obvious in this *Reader* and in the IIHA's regular symposia and Occasional Papers.

The links are possibly most evident in our flagship course, the International Diploma in Humanitarian Assistance (IDHA), which is offered three times a year in different locations around the world. This diploma program is offered under the joint auspices of the CIHC, Fordham University, The Royal College of Surgeons in Ireland, and the United Nations System Staff College. Other academic partners for the IDHA have included the City University of New York, University of Geneva, University of Liverpool, and the Liverpool School of Tropical Medicine. It is a highly intense, month-long residential course with twelve-hour days of lectures, scenario exercises, and debates. The course was devised to simulate a humanitarian emergency situation. Candidates are judged by strict academic criteria with weekly oral and written exams. The average age of our candidates is thirty-eight, and most of them have had significant field experience. They represent virtually every discipline working in humanitarian crises.

Today, our thousands of alumni work in almost every agency of the United Nations and in most major nongovernmental organizations (NGOs) around the world. In addition, the IIHA at Fordham University offers a master's degree in International Humanitarian Action (MIHA) and an undergraduate International Humanitarian Affairs minor program. The IIHA also offers many specialized training courses including, inter alia, humanitarian negotiations, international human rights, humanitarian law, ethics accountability, and mental health in war zones.

The IIHA is the sole academic center in the United States recognized as a full partner by NOHA, the consortium of universities coordinating teaching and research in humanitarian assistance in Europe.

Total emergency relief aid spending has increased significantly in the last forty odd years. In 1970 global emergency aid spending was less than $1 billion per year. This figure began to rise sharply in the 1990s, and by 2010 annual spending was more than $20 billion per year. The end of the Cold War, the subsequent proliferations of civil wars, and their consequent displacement crises in the 1990s certainly suggest that this increase in spending was driven in part by a concomitant increase in need. A decade into the twenty-first century, we are able to observe the "humanitarian international"—a vast complex of international organizations endeavoring to deliver humanitarian assistance—as a globally powerful entity, with capabilities and ambitions far beyond what existed in the early 1970s.

The rapid expansion of humanitarian aid has been accompanied by extensive commentary on the successes and failures of relief and aid operations; on the delivery of goods and services; on the need for minimum standards; and on the need for training and qualifications for aid workers. Professionalization and accountability have been suggested time and again as panaceas for the persistent, significant flaws in humanitarian responses to disasters and emergencies. Concerned individuals, departments, and institutions dedicated to promoting professionalization and accountability are clearly emerging. *History and Hope* provides them with a single volume that details the major topics faced during this evolution.

It is difficult to describe the moment at which a new profession is recognized. Historically, professions have emerged through a mixture of public and private interests, associations between practitioners and academics, state institutions and private ones. These processes are messy, time-consuming, and essential. At Fordham University's IIHA, our faculty has been engaged in this development for decades, attempting to shape humanitarian practice while avoiding the pitfalls of creating a system that benefits the professionals more than those it claims to serve.

Humanitarian assistance is a discipline that attracts men and women who, in often-terrible situations, continue to strive for a better world. They have dreams and visions, values and traditions, which have not been suppressed by many earlier challenges. In fact, improvements in disaster prevention and response have often come because of adversity. The improvements—the establishment of accepted standards for shelter, food, protection, human rights, education, a code of ethics for workers, and an emerging body of human rights and humanitarian law—have been accomplished without abandoning the noble principles of independence, neutrality, and impartiality that are the foundation for our work. One of the main dangers ahead, in my opinion, is that this very foundation may be destroyed because fiscal concerns are subordinating humanitarian work to the political and military activities that accompany complex humanitarian crises.

When the United Nations Charter was drafted in 1945, there was but a single mention of humanitarian affairs. Maybe understandably, in the horrifying afterglow of World War II, the UN Charter focused mainly on human rights and the prevention of conflict. The full history of the United Nations, however, is far more nuanced than the words of the Charter. While the Charter is almost silent on humanitarian assistance, the deeds of the Organization speak for themselves. United Nations–led relief operations actually predate the final signing of the Charter.

The United Nations Relief and Rehabilitation Agency (UNRRA) was its first major international operation, offering critical help across the destroyed landscape of Europe, addressing hunger and other needs of refugees as World War II was winding down. Shortly, other agencies, such as UNICEF, UNRWA, and UNHCR, became essential tools in the UN arsenal for disaster relief, and their mandates grew—and changed—in response to the realities of the Cold War, superpower politics, instant communications, and, later, the collapse of the Soviet Union. Only then was there a greater willingness on the part of the world community to identify disaster zones and demand access to suffering populations.

The Charter has, as its foundation, the sovereignty of Member States. But today, almost everyone recognizes that international humanitarian action often requires moving across national borders in order to offer relief to victims. For that very reason, humanitarians also contend that their work warrants respect for a neutral—as opposed to political—space in which they can provide impartial assistance to all in need. There seems to be an inherent conflict in these views on sovereignty and intervention, at least as understood at the birth of the United Nations. Since then there have been emerging concepts of the fundamental obligations of States toward individual citizens, especially when it becomes clear to the international community that a State is not providing necessary basic assistance to those in desperate need. This period of evolution in our understanding of the nature of sovereignty, and the tensions that exist between those who favor intervention over the absolute rights of the State, are ongoing. The Right to Protect (R2P) thesis has been used to justify various humanitarian interventions (as, for example, in Libya), but not without a growing concern about the limits and justifications for such actions.

A further development at the United Nations, namely that the Organization should deliver assistance "as one," has inevitably increased the involvement of political and military actors in what had previously been solely a traditional humanitarian domain. I believe there are serious dangers in such an approach, since the humanitarian actor is almost always a minor partner, especially in financial terms, when compared with the budgets of military and peacekeeping operations. The goal of complete coordination of U.N. activity under one head in a complex humanitarian crisis sounds desirable from a fiscal and administrative point of view. But it could well destroy the very freedom that made humanitarian assistance unique and effective. There is almost certain to be significant resistance to this approach in the international humanitarian community.

Humanitarian assistance is a noble undertaking. At an individual level it is as old as mankind, with tales of generosity and compassion being part of the myths, legends, and foundations of every society. As a formal discipline, however, the organized response to the chaos and suffering that is an inevitable part of armed conflicts, or extraordinary natural disasters, has very slowly evolved. In modern times there has been a growing realization that both innocent victims and injured combatants deserve protection. Henry Dunant's attempt to establish neutral, "universal" space for humanitarian aid in 1859 in the midst of the Battle of Solferino is often cited as the beginning of what we now accept as international humanitarian law. The Geneva Conventions were later established to codify humankind's rules for the treatment of civilians and the injured, as well as for the behavior of combatants. The implementation of the Conventions has, sadly, been a tale of constant exceptions and shameful interpretations.

At the close of the Cold War humanitarian assistance entered an era of enormous complexity, and it was ill prepared for the challenges that aid agencies faced. There were no universally accepted standards for providing care in such dire situations. There were few comprehensive training programs; in fact, there was not even a common vocabulary for guiding humanitarian workers. Academia was not part of the solution, and its absence added to the problems.

More than three decades ago I insisted on a last-minute change in the title of one of my books. I did not want the planned *Threads in a Tapestry*, but rather, *Threads for a Tapestry*. I had to convince the publisher that the original title implied that the tapestry was already completed, while I still see the tapestry of my life as an ever-evolving one. Now, as I collect these written strands from the past, they are offered not as a final compilation but as part of an ongoing effort to use the platform provided to an international physician, teacher, and humanitarian worker to bear witness, especially in our privileged nation, to the sufferings and inequities experienced by the downtrodden masses of the world. The plight of the poor, the rights of the oppressed, the anguish and chaos of epidemics, and complex humanitarian crises have been my chosen fields.

Emergency relief operations are the starting point for most international humanitarian assistance programs. Wanton killing and brutality within supposedly sovereign borders; ethnic and religious strife; millions of near-starving refugees; other millions of migrants fleeing their homes out of fear for their lives; human rights trampled down; appalling poverty in the shadows of extraordinary wealth; inhumanity on an incredible scale in what was supposed to be a peaceful dawn following the Cold War—these are the awesome challenges that face the world community, and are quite different from the nation-state rivalries and alliances that preoccupied statesmen during most of the last century. More and more, these humanitarian crises are immediately known to us in an era of instant communications. They demand a response, and that response, to be effective, cannot be mere compassion or sympathy but must reflect an emerging science and the strengths of multiple partners.

It is often a dangerous and deceptive exercise to indulge in a "humanitarian intervention," implying that supplying food, water, shelter, or medical relief satisfies obligations when, in reality, such activities are often only a convenient way for governments to avoid dealing with difficult underlying political problems. The awareness that humanitarian aid can be a "band-aid" approach—satisfying but ultimately futile—is a humbling but essential realization for those who accept leadership positions in the field.

Everything evolves and grows, or it stagnates and dies. This is clearly true in nature, where plants and animals need to adapt constantly in order for their species to survive. Our most profound thoughts also evolve, often very slowly, and sometimes coalesce into workable concepts only after prolonged gestation. It is also obvious that the philosophic, economic, and even religious bases of civilization change in response to unforeseen challenges, sometimes influenced by new technology and knowledge, often in reaction to failures. The semantic specificity that is expected in medicine is equally necessary in disaster management. "Humanitarian crises" are rarely the result of just a failure of the humanitarian system. Solutions, therefore, will not be found by merely addressing unmet humanitarian needs.

Slowly but steadily, such philosophic observations led me more and more deeply over time into the uncharted seas that influence complex humanitarian crises. Some factors—medical, demographic, epidemiologic, logistical—are easily measured, and an effective response can usually be formulated. Yet it is those less definable, more subjective forces that so often determine the course of events. As in human relations, it is usually the subtle, but utterly essential, influences of natural empathy and understanding; a respect for the diversity of humanity; an appreciation of others' values and customs; a willingness to cooperate, and share; and the courage to give and to love that most often provide the critical defining balance between success and failure.

Professionals in humanitarian assistance must approach those in pain in a non-judgmental manner. They learn to leave behind their pride and preconceptions and to sublimate their own interests and agendas in an act of solidarity with refugees and displaced persons who need their help. One learns to tread softly, to offer change with great care. One quickly finds that existing customs and practices in any community, even in the chaos of a refugee camp, must not be altered without consultation and deliberation. The ways of a people, sometimes quite incomprehensible to one trained in a Western scientific system, are ultimately that group's own precious heritage and protection. Attempts to introduce new methods and replace timeworn approaches can be devastating, especially in times of crises, when a society is extremely vulnerable and utterly dependent on strangers for the essentials of life.

These personal observations were the primary genesis of the International Humanitarian Book Series. For many decades I have been privileged to work in remote areas among people far removed from the effects, good and bad, of modernity. The more I traveled, read, and participated in the daily lives of isolated clans and communities, the more convinced I was that the richness of humanity lay in its incredible diversity. I do not share the belief that there is only one right way—whether that is how to rule, or how to worship, or court a mate, or establish a family, or express love, or even how to die. Any diminution in that diversity diminishes all of us. Attempts to homogenize the world, to impose uniform standards of behavior, to stifle differences of opinion and style, to impose restrictions on customs and practices because they are different from our own are regressive, usually destructive, acts. The biologic world thrives in its complexity, and artistic creativity flourishes best when there are multiple stimuli.

Humanitarian workers, if they are to be effective, must be realists. They deal every day with the cruel facts of human suffering, and no amount of rhetoric can alleviate pain or provide sustenance in times of widespread natural or manmade crises. The most indispensible resource in disaster preparedness and response is trained personnel. Education is a manifestation of society's belief that somehow, someday, somewhere there will be a life after the near death that is reality for so many innocent victims in conflict and postconflict situations.

Only the university can provide the legitimacy and credibility needed in a new world where globalization and international regulations guide all our actions, including the provision of disaster relief. Only a university, empowered by government departments of education, can confer degrees and diplomas. This is absolutely critical for a discipline such as humanitarian assistance, where multiple skills, mandates, and qualifications must be brought under the same umbrella. By its very nature, experts in humanitarian work must be recognized as such by many nations, since those afflicted by war and disaster flee across borders seeking safe havens in neighboring lands.

The university has become an essential partner in international humanitarian assistance. Untrained workers are now rarely accepted, even as volunteers, by major NGOs and reputable international organizations. An academic diploma in humanitarian assistance has become a *sine qua non* as relief workers increasingly move from the UN and national relief agencies to the private sector and back. The imprimatur offered by a highly respected, university diploma, based on practical experience, is now appreciated around the world. *History and Hope* is a result of the long struggle to link academia and humanitarian action.

Ultimately, preserving "humanitarian space" will be imperative. Only the education of a committed cadre of trained professionals will be able to secure the traditions of neutrality, impartiality, and independence. In this *Reader* the history and hope of that endeavor seem, to me, to blend and rhyme into a poetic and noble assertion, one of undoubted reality but softened by the romance of universal love. The seeds of experience will, we hope, be allowed to blossom into wisdom. Future generations will have to continue the endless effort to relieve unnecessary suffering and promote universal justice and peace. *History and Hope* should help guide the way forward. That surely is my intent.

PART I

History

History and Hope opens, appropriately, with an essay on the modern history of humanitarian action, and a chapter detailing the ethical and legal foundations of the discipline. Both cite the dangers that recent trends, particularly the "war on terror," pose to hard won, almost universally accepted, positions assuring the independence of international humanitarian assistance.

One of the books in the series, *Technology for Humanitarian Action*, was considered innovative and advanced when published in 2005. But, as already noted, nothing changes faster than the science of modern technology. Each chapter in that book was introduced by a vignette describing the reality faced by a humanitarian fieldworker. Two vignettes introduce a more current contribution by the head of the United Nations Office for the Coordination of Humanitarian Affairs emphasizing the importance of technology as we struggle to provide assistance in complex emergencies.

Humanitarian Action in the Twenty-First Century: The Danger of a Setback

Paul Grossrieder

Humanitarian action as envisaged by Henry Dunant, the founder of the Red Cross Movement, is both simple—it is based on the natural human tendency to respect a fellow human—and original—Dunant wished to apply that common sense principle in systematic fashion, even in war.

A fleeting glance at the past will help us appreciate what was original about humanitarian action as conceived by Dunant, why it goes beyond good intentions or mere charity. Until September 11, 2001, there was no reason to believe that the international community would be tempted by a simplistic view of the world to roll back the concept of humanitarian action that was born with the Red Cross. I do not wish to indulge in facile anachronisms, but will retrace the development of humanitarian idea and action and highlight the challenges as well as the risks of the twenty-first century for humanitarian action.

Ancient Greece (Fifth Century BCE)

War had limits for only some members of humanity. The extent to which the Greeks humanized war can only be understood in the light of their society's division into city-states, competition between which was natural and gave rise to regular conflicts in an attempt to establish which was the best. Fighting between cities of the same culture and the same religion was governed by unwritten rules (*agraphoi nomoi*). The city that lost was always at a disadvantage, but the victor had to respect limits to its conduct with regard to captives. Those rules were not a form of international law, however, as they applied only between Greek city-states, whereas there was no limit to the acts of violence that could be carried out against the enemy in wars between Greeks and barbarians (non-Greeks).

Ancient Greece therefore witnessed the first, very partial endeavor to use rules of law to regulate certain conflicts between Greek city-states. Whether or not those unwritten rules applied depended not on one's condition as a human being, but on one's membership in Greek civilization.

Religion and Respect for Human Beings

On the one hand, all the world's great religions (primitive religions, Judaism, Christianity,[1] Islam, the religions of the Far East) recommend that their followers treat other human beings with respect; on the other hand, each religion is linked to a people, to a culture (or is imposed on others as a culture), and the notion of universality is therefore absent. In addition, violence is often a part of religious behavior, carried out to defend a god or a truth. In any event, it makes sense for every religion to consider itself the best, otherwise why believe? In most past and present conflicts, religious communities have identified with one of the parties to the conflict. The conflicts in the Balkans have provided ample proof of this, but the same thing has happened in the eastern Democratic Republic of the Congo, in Sri Lanka, and in many other countries in conflict. It was therefore not religions that originated and promoted the founding ideas of humanitarian law, neither in the distant past nor in modern times.

Christianity since the Middle Ages: Love, Compassion, Charity

Since the Middle Ages and until the twenty-first century, the notions of love, compassion, and charity, and the activities based on them, evolved principally along two lines:

1. One tradition used love, compassion and charity to fight the established powers. In the face of the self-assigned privileges of the rich and powerful, men such as Francis of Assisi (twelfth century), Joachim de Flore (fourteenth century), and, later, Giordano Bruno (sixteenth century) branded those notions as weapons in defense of the poor and the underprivileged. In some cases, their struggles ended in social and political revolt.
2. In another tradition, represented chiefly by the institutional church, those notions were applied only in respect of the faithful who followed the right path. In that case, nothing took precedence over the established order; charity toward the poor was a means of maintaining that order and a requirement for salvation, but had no intrinsic value. It can even be said that this tradition

substituted charity for justice. Charity was the pretext for not dispensing the justice that could undermine the power of the rich and mighty. This tradition's purpose was to maintain and uphold a political and social order that was unconcerned by equal rights and used charity to contain any hint of rebellion on the part of the lower classes. In that context, the idea of universal humanitarianism had no scope to develop.

The dichotomy between the two traditions prevailed throughout Western Christian culture until the nineteenth century and constituted the political leitmotif of that period.

The Premises of the Modern Humanitarian Idea

A Christian Exception: St. Vincent de Paul

In the seventeenth century, St. Vincent de Paul adopted a systematic approach to poverty in France, with a view to its eradication. To that end, he established two structures, or religious orders: the Daughters of Charity and the Lazarists. St. Vincent de Paul's approach was original in that it tackled poverty as a social phenomenon and established structures to remedy it.

Unfortunately, the system was appropriated by Louis XIV, or more specifically his wife, Maria Teresa of Austria. St. Vincent de Paul's humanitarian endeavor was turned into "internment houses" run by the police, spelling a sad end to a pioneering humanitarian effort and protecting the hierarchical order of the time.

The Concept of "Humanity"

During that period—between the seventeenth and nineteenth centuries—Europe awakened to the revolutionary idea of a human being as an individual (Descartes, Spinoza, Kant, Marx, etc.). Whereas Christian charity as it had evolved in Western societies was compatible with social inequality, the modern concept of "humanity" considered every man and woman as equally "human." Without a doubt, the philosophical development of the concept of humans as individuals fostered the sociological advent of the demand that all men and women be treated equal, and hence the idea that any person, no matter what his social status, was entitled to respect without discrimination.

The First "Humanitarian" Operations (Late Eighteenth to Early Nineteenth Centuries)

1793: relief operation for French aristocrats forced to flee Santo Domingo during a slave uprising;

1812: earthquake in Caracas: the United States organized assistance by boat;

1821: aid for the Greeks (only) during their war against the Turks

Humanitarian action in time of war initially took the form of medical services provided by the armed forces for their troops. Those who pioneered such services were Ambroise Pare (sixteenth century) and Baron Larrey (1766–1842).

The eighteenth century saw the conclusion of the first agreements between combatants for the reciprocal use of hospitals.

1743: Battle of Bethingen—agreement between the Marshall of Noailles (France) and Lord Sain (England)

1759: Seven Years War—agreement between General de Barail and Henry Seymour Conway

Henry Dunant and Solferino

The Battle of Solferino in the Italian War of Unification (1859) marked a decisive moment in the modern concept of humanitarianism, thanks first to Henry Dunant and, subsequently, to the Red Cross in general and the International Committee of the Red Cross (ICRC) in particular. Dunant and the Committee of Five "invented" the principles that underpin humanitarian action to this day. They are based on three fundamental ideas:

The basic idea: A universal space, that of the victim, that respects the neutrality of the victims of war. Henceforth, aid would not be limited to one's own wounded but would be extended to all the victims. As Henry Dunant wrote in *A Memory of Solferino:* "The women of Castiglione, seeing that I made no distinction between nationalities, followed my example, showing the same kindness to all these men whose origins were so different, and all of whom were foreigners to them. '*Tutti fratelli*,' they repeated feelingly" (ICRC, 1986).

The second original idea: Those helping the victims must be part of the same space, the space of humanity. Humanitarian agents help all the victims as members of one humanity. To give effect to this idea, an independent organization, untainted by any military or political commitment, was founded; it was the voice of humanity in the midst of armed conflict. It soon came to be called the Red Cross.

The third original idea: At a time when all man's laws apparently ceased to exist when fighting broke out, Henry Dunant created a space for a contract. Certain laws could be applied universally even in the heat of battle. International humanitarian law was born. In 1865, the States signed the Geneva Convention for the protection of the war wounded, an international treaty that defined a legal space for humanitarian aid.

Thus, Henry Dunant and the Red Cross laid the foundations of contemporary humanitarian action, which seeks to treat enemies hors de combat as equals in humanity.

Contemporary Periods of Humanitarian Action

World War I

Previously a legal and moral authority, the ICRC—and the entire Red Cross—had now to start taking action. The First World War was different from wars of the nineteenth century in that it was total. It involved countries, economies, and populations on an unprecedented scale. The Red Cross was obliged to demonstrate that the principles and rules laid down in the law of war were applicable.

The ICRC went from being a moral and legal authority to an operational organization. Its main fields of action were prisoners of war, repatriations, and tracing activities. Forty-one delegates visited fifty-four prisoner-of-war camps. They repatriated a total of 700,000 prisoners; 1,200 volunteers worked at the International Prisoners-of-War Agency in Basel, restoring ties between prisoners and their families. Two million parcels were sent to prisoners.

In 1917, the ICRC was awarded the Nobel Peace Prize.

The Period between the Two World Wars

The first problem was *practical in nature*: What was to be done with the enormous infrastructure set up during the First World War? The fight against tuberculosis was one of the operations undertaken during this period. A Red Cross poster proclaimed: "Beat the Germans, beat tuberculosis."

There then arose a *political problem*, for after the First World War, pacifism became a force to be reckoned with (President Wilson, Treaty of Versailles, the League of Nations, the Kellogg-Briand Pact). War was to be outlawed.

In order to deal with these two problems, the Red Cross organized itself into two international institutions. At the instigation of the President of the American Red Cross, the League of Red Cross Societies was established; it would be responsible for peacetime activities. The ICRC would specialize in wartime operations, and in humanitarian law and its dissemination.

During the same period, the Save the Children Fund (1919) and the precursor of a High Commission for Refugees (1921) were also established. Both organizations would deal with peacetime issues arising from war.

World War II

For the Red Cross, and in particular the ICRC, this war was marked by the questions and issues posed by totalitarian regimes (Bolshevism, Nazism).

Those regimes manipulated humanitarian aid for their own purposes. In 1921, for example, the USSR had demanded total control of the humanitarian assistance provided to the famine-stricken population of the Ukraine. Under the pressure of public opinion, the Western countries had caved in to its demands.

The Second World War also brought to light shortcomings in international humanitarian law. Specifically, it became apparent during the war in Spain (1936) that humanitarian law did not cover non-international conflicts. Nor did it afford protection to civilians in time of war.

Moreover, the totalitarian regimes, which rejected the international system of the League of Nations, also ignored humanitarian law.

The ICRC, for its part, strengthened by its success during the First World War, approached the humanitarian issues of World War II as though they were a repetition of the first. It focused almost exclusively on prisoners of war. Blinded by its operational approach, concerned to safeguard its activities, the ICRC made the tragic decision not to deal with civilians or the Holocaust. There were several heroic exceptions, the result of initiatives taken by certain delegates in the field. The most spectacular example was Friedrich Born, who saved an estimated 15,000 Jews in Hungary from the death camps.

The Postwar Period

After the Second World War and the horrors committed by the Nazis, the world felt the need to do all in its power to make sure such crimes were never again committed. In that atmosphere of widespread remorse, numerous associations were founded to help the populations of Europe, especially in the United States and among the religions communities (Catholic, Protestant, Jewish): the International Rescue Committee (IRC), Catholic Relief Services (CRS), Church World Services (CWS), the Joint Distribution Committee (JDC), CARE, Oxfam, to name but a few.

It was also during this period that most of the United Nations specialized agencies were founded; that the Geneva Conventions were renegotiated to include common Articles 1 and 3, and that the Fourth Convention, on the protection of civilians, was adopted. These new international instruments explicitly recognized that the ICRC was an "impartial humanitarian organization."

Finally, the Refugee Convention was adopted in 1951.

This was a heady period for humanitarianism, for society and public opinion were eager to correct the serious mistakes of the Second World War.

The Cold War and Humanitarian Action: The Limits Set by Ideology

The universal, independent, neutral, and impartial approach was severely tested by the growing ideological tension and deepening cold war between the East and West blocs. On the one hand, the Soviet Union did not agree to apply humanitarian law and its principles in the countries and regions within its sphere of influence;[2] on the other, the West included the law in its arsenal of weapons against the East bloc. All this took place against a backdrop of public will to do good.

During the same period, the widespread struggle for decolonization brought humanitarian organizations face-to-face with liberation movements and the peoples under their control. Generally speaking, the organizations belonged to one of two schools:

Those influenced by the analyses on inequality and anti-imperialism (F. Fanon, S. Amin),[3]

Those guided by the position of American economist W. Rostow: that poverty fostered the spread of communism.

In the face of these global developments, of the rise and proliferation of liberation movements (the PLO, UNITA, the Sandinistas, RENAMO, etc.), how was the ICRC, the guardian of humanitarian law, to react? How should the law and practice be adapted to encompass these "new conflicts?" How could the basic principles and rules be recognized as applying to the victims of those conflicts? How could the ICRC contact all the parties? Obtain access to all the victims? These questions were the subject of protracted debate, and, in the end, the ICRC decided to adapt the law to the changed situation. That adaptation in no way signified that Henry Dunant's humanitarian principles were to be abandoned, but rather that their field of application was to be enlarged. The ICRC's decision resulted, in 1977, in the adoption of the Protocols additional to the Geneva Conventions.

At the same time, the "borderless" movement was launched as a different approach to the same issues. Doctors seconded to the ICRC by France during the Biafra war, deemed the organization's methods poorly adapted, too rigid and legalistic, to bound up with the authorities, and founded *Médecins Sans Frontières* (MSF, Doctors Without Borders) in 1968.

This new kind of humanitarian organization was set up to counter the ICRC, to circumvent the constraints of humanitarian law, which were seen as an obstacle to humanitarian action. Unfettered by diplomatic and legal considerations, MSF found it easy to be ironical about the timid approach of the Red Cross and the cowardice of the Untied Nations. It has covered interesting ground since then, for today MSF is one of the most fervent defenders of humanitarian law and has published a highly accessible handbook, the most complete manual for humanitarian practitioners in existence.

MSF and the organizations founded on the same model have a number of strengths and limitations. One of MSF's strengths is that it is a private association conducting private operations, which are therefore very independent and free. Its staff tends to go on brief but intense missions, and its operational policy is characterized by enormous flexibility.

In terms of limitations, MSF's political choices, especially during the early years of its existence, prevented it from being impartial (for example, in Afghanistan during the Soviet period, when MSF doctors sided with the mujaheddin). The covert nature of certain activities precluded the development of systematic, large-scale operations.

Things have changed now. MSF's methods are much closer to those of the ICRC, and the ICRC has followed in MSF's footsteps and adopted a more informal style. What remains particularly different is the duty to bear witness, by which MSF staff members are bound, whereas ICRC delegates must follow a policy of discretion, chiefly in order to obtain access to places of detention and prisoner-of-war camps.

The 1980s: The Proliferation of Conflicts on the Periphery: "Le Tout-urgence"

The wars of liberation were followed by what Jean-Christophe Rufin called conflicts on the periphery. These were waged within the context of a return to the Roman *limes* policy, in which "imperial" interests did not extend beyond the limits of a concentric circle outside which war and chaos were allowed to rage. This new form of conflict was contemporaneous with the "dissolution of the bipolar order."[4] The proliferation of bloody and spectacular periphery conflicts, involving little activity on the part of the superpowers (Sri Lanka, Ethiopia, Cambodia) signaled a return to urgency. Humanitarian agents played on the emotions and troubled conscience of people in the West. This period of absolute urgency had its downside, as well. Were we feeding the victims or feeding war? Certain leaders, such as Mengistu in Ethiopia in 1995, considered it judicious, for reasons of internal politics, to foment disaster.

After the Cold War: Humanitarian Action in Spite of Everything

The fall of the Berlin Wall sparked somewhat rash predictions that conflicts on the periphery would end and humanitarians would be out of a job. In fact, the number of regional and local conflicts rose (Afghanistan, Angola, Sierra Leone, Liberia, the Balkans). The anarchic and chaotic nature of those conflicts made them extremely dangerous and rendered humanitarian work hugely complex, as it became more and more difficult to have access to the victims for security reasons. This period was marked by the almost total withdrawal of external political support for local wars. As a result, armed movements replaced their political partners with economic partners and embarked on business activities, at times forming alliances with private commercial firms. They also started to exploit territory or to plunder the population. They became incredibly diverse in nature.

In those circumstances, the plight of the civilian population became increasingly perilous (witness the famines in southern Sudan and Somalia). The ICRC, UNHCR, and the nongovernmental organizations (NGOs) all mobilized to provide emergency aid on an unprecedented scale.

Enter the States: The Politicization of Humanitarian Action

That situation—the proliferation of local conflicts and the growing number of victims who suffered as a result—was compounded in 1990 when the states burst on the humanitarian scene. During the Cold War, direct state intervention had been justified by the fight against "the other side." That justification wore thin after the fall of the Berlin Wall, and when the international community decided, at the behest of the Americans, to intervene in Kuwait, it invoked defense of the law. Those grounds soon proved insufficient. The concept of "peacekeeping," with its humanitarian veneer, was then advanced. Most "peacekeeping" operations had no clear political or military objective and in fact, troops were deployed for no purpose other than to facilitate the arrival of relief supplies for civilians or to bring in those supplies themselves. That is what happened in 1991 in Kurdistan (United Nations General Assembly resolution 688, 1991), and subsequently in Somalia, the former Yugoslavia, and Rwanda.

Those interventions were the tangible expression of the right to intervene. They were generally not well received by those concerned, who saw in them the risk of a new form of legal domination by the north over the south, by the rich over the poor. In practice, those so-called humanitarian interventions were not without political ulterior motives, and were thus selective.

Those interventions also served to heighten the confusion between humanitarian endeavor and military operations. In Somalia, the ambiguous mandate of the allied forces led them to become just another belligerent and resulted in their precipitate withdrawal. In Yugoslavia, international troops undertook humanitarian action while the population was decimated by a siege. In Rwanda, United Nations Assistance Mission in Rwanda (UNA-MIR) was not allowed to bring in more troops and the genocide could not be stopped. Confining the blue helmets to a humanitarian role gave rise to confusion. "How long will our governments persist in their hypocrisy?" Claude Malhuret wrote in *Le Monde* on August 20, 1992. "Incapable of deciding on a course of action, which they know public opinion demands, they instead get involved, to show that they are 'doing something,' in humanitarian assistance that does nothing to remedy the basic problem. How much longer will they try to make us believe that humanitarian action can take the place of political action?"

In reality, there is a wide gap between military humanitarian action and the principles promoted by Henry Dunant. In particular, confusion between what is military and what is humanitarian voids the principle that the victim and the humanitarian agent are neutral, which remains the *sine qua non* condition for the existence of a humanitarian space. The principle of neutrality cannot be implemented by soldiers, only by independent humanitarian organizations.

Post-9/11: The Risk of a Further Drift

The attacks of September 11, 2001, against the twin towers of New York's World Trade Center and the Pentagon in Washington, D.C., naturally represent a paradigm shift in international relations. They open a new phase in humanitarian action and present a major challenge to international humanitarian law.

Following the attacks, the United States decided to launch a "war against terrorism" that, to date, has taken the form of a war against Afghanistan and a pitiless international fight against terrorism and terrorists.

We are therefore faced with two different phenomena, even though they occasionally overlap. On one hand, we have an international war in Afghanistan in which the Geneva Conventions, in particular the Third Convention, apply. On the other hand, another struggle of another kind is being carried out against an international network (Al Qaeda); the American administration calls this a "war against terrorism." It in no way resembles traditional warfare and raises entirely new issues for humanitarian law.

It goes without saying that we must first affirm that humanitarian law is applicable in the international, American-Afghan conflict, and that it must be implemented as closely as possible to the terms of the Geneva Conventions. Strictly speaking, however, humanitarian law is not applicable in the "war against terrorism." We are nevertheless entirely justified in wondering how to classify the situation. In principle, it is a kind of police operation, but President Bush did call it a "war," and the means employed to wage it are indeed reminiscent of war. In addition, the parties represent a break with tradition in that one of them is transnational and transstate. But it is that sufficient reason to remove this new kind of war from the purview of humanitarian law, whose specific aim is to help and protect the victims of war?

In any event, the first step is to demand compliance with the existing provisions of humanitarian law where they are applicable and to do everything possible to ensure that the law does not crumble under political pressure. At the same time, the possibility to act must be ensured. Last, humanitarians must ponder the new challenges and deal with them.

Today, as during the bleakest period of the Cold War, there is a real and present danger that humanitarian law will suffer a setback, its principles subordinated to political interests. We must not allow that to happen, we must hark back to the origins of the law and ensure that the interests of the victims reign supreme.

Conclusion

The definition of humanitarianism and its history reveal an original notion dating from the Enlightenment and Henry Dunant: that humanity takes precedence over war, over politics, race, and religion. The concept of humanitarianism, moreover, has been incorporated into an international corpus of law. The principles must at all costs be preserved so that the victims can continue to be protected and assisted.

The twenty-first century has started with doubts about the law and the Geneva Conventions. Giving in to those doubts would be an unforgivable setback for humanity. Yes, we can become more professional; certainly, the different stages of humanitarian endeavor, from prevention to development, can be more fully integrated with one another. But the first requirement of humanitarianism is and will remain independence and freedom. All else is a matter of method, logistics, and the management of security constraints.

It would be disgraceful indeed if the twenty-first century laid open to question the principles laid down in the nineteenth, notably that humanitarian action aims first and foremost to restore man's lost dignity, with no economic or strategic ulterior motives.

Humanitarian Ethical and Legal Standards

Michel Veuthey

There is a need for the implementation of existing ethical and legal standards,[1] especially regarding the fundamental guarantees of human life and dignity.

International instruments of human rights and of international humanitarian law are not the only sources providing these fundamental guarantees.[2] International law is only one of the many sources of humanitarian standards. Legal mechanisms alone are insufficient to provide for an effective protection of fundamental human values. Many different approaches can contribute to the promotion of respect for fundamental human values in today's conflicts. Historical considerations, including spiritual and ethnic research,[3] could also be among the remedies for today's impasses.

Origins and Development

Spiritual Origin of Humanitarian Standards

Limiting Violence in Order to Ensure the Survival of the Group

Each civilization has formed islands of humanity inside which certain rules limit violence by imposing restraints on the use of force and exist an obligation of solidarity toward victims.

These religion-based rules were of two types, imposing negative and positive obligations:

1. A *taboo* by which it was forbidden to attack women and children, to destroy temples or sacred places, to kill priests or people in religious orders, as well as women, children, and elderly people belonging to the group. In the West, the Peace of God (*Pax Dei*)[4] and the Truce of God (*Treuga Dei*)[5] were such rules.

   Other similar rules can be found in every religion. Some of these rules were more generous in so-called primitive civilizations than in today's international law.

2. The *Golden Rule*, which is found in several civilizations, not only in Judeo-Christian ones, and which can be resumed thus: *So, whatever you wish that men would do to you, do so to them.*[6]

These rules were set to ensure the survival of a group, and forbade behaviors that would have permanently endangered the group.[7] Indigenous people of all continents have aimed to avoid excesses that would turn conflicts into collective suicides. Customs of Melanesians,[8] Inuit,[9] and Nilotic people,[10] as well as of African tribes; religious precepts in Buddhism,[11] Hinduism,[12] Taoism,[13] Confucianism,[14] and Bushido[15] in Asia; Judaism,[16] Christianity,[17] and Islam[18] in the Middle East; and mutual restrictions imposed by chivalry and military honor[19] in Europe, contain examples of rules of "Life-Affirmative Societies," in which the main emphasis of ideals, customs, and institutions is the preservation and growth of life in all its forms.[20]

All these rules were aimed at precluding excesses that would turn clashes into anarchy and hence make peace more difficult to achieve. Thus, in article 6 of his *Project for Perpetual Peace*, Kant wrote: "No State shall, during war, permit such acts of hostility which would make mutual confidence in the subsequent peace impossible."[21]

Recognizing the Human Dignity of Every Human Being   Francisco de Vitoria (1480–1596), a member of the Dominican Order, is often considered the founder of Western international law. He believed in *jus gentium,* a universally valid "law of nations" established on the basis of natural law. Living at the time of the conquest of the Americas, Vitoria developed his teaching partly in the context of his discussions on the appropriate treatment of the native peoples of the New World.

Supported by Vitoria, Bartholomew de Las Casas (1474–1566) devoted himself to the defense of the Amerindians against the ruthless exploitation and ferocious cruelty that they suffered under the Spanish conquerors.[22]

Building Bridges Among Civilizations   St. Francis of Assisi tried to open a dialogue between Christians and Muslims in 1219.[23] All of the world's great religious traditions today emphasize the intrinsic value of each individual human life, and in recent decades, religious communities have recognized their vital role in expressing moral outrage and taking actions to curb the types of inhumanity that people have, time and again, inflicted upon one another over the last century. Religious communities are, without a doubt, the largest and best-organized civil institutions in the world today, claiming the allegiance of billions of believers and bridging the divides of race, class and nationality.[24]

Proliferation and Universality of Standards

International Humanitarian Law (IHL)   International humanitarian law is usually defined as the set of principles and rules restricting the use of violence in armed conflicts, both to spare the persons not (or no longer) directly engaged in hostilities (wounded, sick, shipwrecked members of the armed forces, prisoners of war, and civilians), and to limit the use of methods and means of warfare that causes superfluous injury (or excessive suffering, as in the case of dumdum bullets or with gas warfare[25]), or severe damage to the natural environment, or betrayal of an adversary's confidence in agreed-upon obligations ("perfidy").

The principle of the limitation of armed violence is reflected in contemporary written law, in the Saint Petersburg Declaration of 1868,[26] as well as in Article 22 of the Hague Regulations of 1907[27]: "The right of belligerents to adopt means of injuring the enemy is not unlimited."

The terminology used to refer to international treaties may vary ("humanitarian law,"[28] "international humanitarian law applicable in armed conflicts,"[29] "Laws of war,"[30] "Law of Geneva,"[31] "Red Cross Conventions," "Law of The Hague,"[32] "human rights in armed conflicts,"[33]) but all seek the same objective—namely, to limit the use of violence in war.

Contemporary international humanitarian law is the moving balance between two dynamic forces: the *requirements of humanity* and *military necessity*.[34] It is also the sum of tragic real-life experiences that need not to be repeated: military wounded and shipwrecked—and the humanitarian personnel taking care of them—must be rescued and respected; prisoners of war must be humanely treated and released at the end of active hostilities; and civilians not be killed nor harmed.

Each stage of the codification of international humanitarian law was the result of a postwar shock wave in public opinion and governments, a collective painful process of learning. These codifications occurred as follows:

The Battle of Solferino (1859)[35] between Austrian and French armies was the impetus for the First Convention, in 1864, protecting military wounded on land

The Battle of Tsushima (1905) between the Japanese and Russian fleets prompted adjustments of the Convention on War at Sea, in 1907, extending protection to military shipwrecked

World War II led to the four 1949 Conventions,[36] an extensive regulation of the treatment of civilians in occupied territories and internment

Decolonization and the Vietnam War preceded the two 1977 Additional Protocols,[37] which brought written rules for the protection of civilian persons and objects against hostilities

A worldwide campaign by like-minded governments, United Nations agencies, the Red Cross and Red Crescent Movement, and NGOs in a full partnership that stressed the human suffering and socioeconomic costs caused by anti-personnel mines resulted in the total ban on landmines signed in Ottawa on December 4, 1997

Universality of International Humanitarian Law   The four 1949 Geneva Conventions are universally ratified. The two Additional Protocols are widely ratified, but still lack ratification by the United States and some other countries.

The 1907 Hague Regulations, which establish laws for conducting war on land, are universally considered part of international customary law since the International Military Tribunal of Nuremberg declared on October 1, 1946, binding both signatories and nonsignatories.[38]

Humanitarian law has evolved from a law protecting only certain categories of individuals (from medieval knights to today's prisoners of war) to a set of provisions ensuring fundamental human rights guaranteeing the survival of entire civilian populations in wartime.

The International Criminal Tribunals for the Former Yugoslavia[39] and for Rwanda[40] broke down the distinction between international and non-international armed conflicts regarding the prosecution of war crimes.[41]

Fundamental humanitarian rules and principles are to be respected in all circumstances. This is especially important today, in the case of "collapsed states,"[42] "postmodern wars,"[43] and anarchic conflicts.[44] According to the ICRC's Commentary to the 1949 Conventions: "The words 'in all circumstances' in Common Article 1 of the four 1949 Geneva Conventions refer to all situations in which the Convention has to be applied, and these are defined in Article 2. It is clear, therefore, that the application of the Convention does not depend on whether the conflict is just or unjust. Whether or not it is a war of aggression, prisoners of war belonging to either party are entitled to the protection afforded by the Convention."[45]

The First Geneva Convention of 1864 had only twelve articles. The four 1949 Geneva Conventions and their two Additional Protocols of 1977 count more than four hundred and fifty provisions. One article summarizes international humanitarian law: Common Article 3 of the 1949 Conventions.

The International Court of Justice (ICJ), in the Nicaragua Case (1986), considered Common Article 3 of the 1949 Geneva Conventions as "elementary considerations of humanity" binding all:

> The Court considers that the rules stated in Article 3, which is common to the four Geneva Conventions, applying to armed conflicts of a non-international character, should be applied.
>
> The United States is under an obligation to "respect" the Conventions and even to "ensure respect" for them, and thus not to encourage persons or groups engaged in the conflict in Nicaragua to act in violation of the provisions of Article 3. This obligation derives from the general principles of humanitarian law to which the Conventions merely give specific expression.[46]

Human Rights   The Preamble of the United Nations Charter states the determination of Member States "to reaffirm faith in fundamental human rights, in the dignity and worth of the human person, in the equal rights of men and women, and of nations large and small." Article 1, paragraph 3 defines one of the purposes of the UN as: "To achieve international co-operation in solving internal problems of an economic, social, cultural, or humanitarian character, and in promoting and encouraging respect for human rights and for fundamental freedoms for all without distinction as to race, sex, language, or religion." World War II and regional conflicts prompted the drafting of the United Nations instruments on human rights, disarmament, prohibition of terrorism and mercenaries, protection of the environment,[47] and of the rights of children.[48]

While instruments of international humanitarian law are normally applicable during armed conflicts, human rights treaties are based on a peacetime approach, yet their scope often overlaps, especially in regard to the fundamental guarantees they embody.

The universality of humanitarian standards can also be seen with human rights instruments:[49]

> The 1948 Universal Declaration of Human Rights (see the appendixes for the full text of the 1948 Universal Declaration of Human Rights)
>
> The 1948 Convention on the Prevention and Punishment of the Crime of Genocide
>
> Both 1966 Covenants (International Covenant on Civil and Political Rights and the International Covenant on Economic, Social and Cultural Rights)

The 1984 Convention against Torture and Other Cruel, Inhuman, or Degrading Treatment or Punishment

The 1989 Convention on the Rights of the Child

The universality[50] and indivisibility[51] of human rights was reaffirmed by the UN International Conference in Tehran in 1968[52] and by the World Conference of Human Rights in Vienna in 1993.[53]

The Advisory Opinion on the ICJ on Reservations to the Convention on the Prevention and Punishment of the Crime of Genocide, of May 28, 1951, confirmed that the prohibition of genocide is part of customary international law.[54]

The following regional instruments complement the UN instruments:

The 1950 Convention for Protection of Human Rights and Fundamental Freedoms of the Council of Europe, signed in Rome;

The 1969 Inter-American Convention on Human Rights, San Jose de Costa Rica;

The 1981 African Charter on Human Rights and Peoples' Rights;

The Charter of Fundamental Rights of the European Union signed and proclaimed by the Presidents of the European Parliament, the Council, and the Commission at the European Council meeting in Nice on December 7, 2000.[55]

Two regional instruments prohibit torture:

The 1985 Inter-American Convention to Prevent and Punish Torture;

The 1987 European Commission for the Prevention of Torture and Inhuman or Degrading Treatment or Punishment.

In addition to the first two "human rights generations" (civil and political/economic and social), new human rights—a third generation of "Solidarity Human Rights"[56] are under consideration at the United Nations and at regional fora, among which are:

the right to development,

the right to a healthy environment,[57]

the human right to peace,

the human right to health, and

the right to food.

The "Declaration on the Right to Development" was adopted by the United Nations General Assembly in 1986.[58] The item has been regularly debated at the General Assembly since then.[59]

The "Human Right to Peace" was hailed by Federico Mayor, Director-General of UNESCO, as "a prerequisite for the exercise of all human rights and duties."[60]

The "Human Right to Health" is proclaimed in the World Health Organization's Constitution, as well as in Article 25 of the Universal Declaration of Human Rights, and in the 1988 Protocol of San Salvador.[61]

As for the Right to Food, the Preamble to the FAO Constitution sets "ensuring humanity's freedom from hunger" as one of its basic purposes. The World Food Summit in November 1996 reaffirmed the right of everyone to have access to safe and nutritious food, consistent with the right to adequate food and gave a specific mandate to the High Commissioner for Human Rights to better define the rights related to food and propose ways to implement and realize them.[62]

"Soft Law" Standards Treaty law is not the only source of humanitarian standards. "Soft Law" is also a source of humanitarian standards. One example is the adoption, by the International Conference of the Red Cross in Vienna in 1965, of the Fundamental Principles of the Red Cross/Crescent—humanity, impartiality, neutrality, independence, voluntary service, unity, universality.

Solidarity and compassion have always been widely expressed in both words and deeds in the most diverse cultures.[63] The Fundamental Principles are the result of a century of experience. Proclaimed in 1965, they bind together the National Red Cross and Red Crescent Societies, the International Committee of the Red Cross, and the International Federation of Red Cross and Red Crescent Societies.[64] They were imitated in many ways. The principle of neutrality has even become one of the core principles of organizations such as Médecins Sans Frontières.

The "MSF Charter"[65] also mentions the principles of impartiality, nondiscrimination, independence, and voluntary service.

It stresses the right to humanitarian assistance.

Neutrality should be understood as the capacity of being available to everyone for service, the ability to assist and protect victims without discrimination, enhancing the security of humanitarian workers and the sustainability of their action, more important in its perception by all actors than in actual practice, closely linked also to funding access to victims.

Professional ethics (military,[66] police,[67] medical,[68] and media[69]) also strives for universality.

In 1999, the Secretary-General of the United Nations proposed the "Global Compact" to create a dialogue between business and civil society along nine fundamental principles, drawn from the Universal Declaration of Human Rights, the International Labor Organization's (ILO) Fundamental Principles on Rights at Work, and the Rio Principles on Environment and Development.[70]

Multiplication of Legal Mechanisms

The proliferation of standards is matched by the multiplication of implementation mechanisms for international humanitarian law or for human rights instruments or for both.

International Humanitarian Law Mechanisms The mechanisms provided for in the 1949 Geneva Conventions on the protection of war victims are:

1. The States Party, which undertake to "respect and ensure respect" for the Conventions "in all circumstances."[71] "Respect" clearly refers to the individual obligation to apply it in good faith from the moment it enters into force.[72] "To ensure respect," according to the ICRC Commentary to the 1949 Conventions, "demands in fact that the States which are Parties to it should not be content merely to apply its provisions themselves, but should do everything in their power to ensure that it is respected universally."[73] This collective responsibility to implement international humanitarian rules[74] often takes the form of bilateral or multilateral measures by States Party. Leaving aside the exceptional meeting provided for in Article 7 of Protocol 1 of 1977,[75] States Party to international humanitarian law treaties have used bilateral or multilateral meetings at the United Nations, the Non-Aligned Movement (NAM), regional organizations (OAS, AU, OSCE, the European Parliament, the Council of Europe), as well as the Inter-Parliamentary Union (IPU), to manifest their concern that humanitarian law should be respected.[76] "In all circumstances" means in time of armed conflict as in time of peace, taking preventive steps, in the form of training[77] or evaluation,[78] and prosecution.[79]

2. The Protecting Power,[80] which was widely used in Europe during WW II[81] and much less thereafter.[82] Additional Protocol 1 defines the Protecting Power in international humanitarian law as "a neutral or other State not a Party to the conflict which has been designated by a Party to the conflict and accepted by the adverse Party and has agreed to carry out the functions assigned to a Protecting Power under the Conventions and this Protocol."[83] The role of the Protecting Power is to maintain the liaison between two States at war, to bring relief assistance to the victims, and protection to prisoners of war and civilian internees.

3. The ICRC, which received mandates from the international community in the 1949 Geneva Conventions to:

Visit and interview prisoners of war[84] and civilian internees;[85]

Provide relief to the population of occupied territories;[86]

Search for missing persons and to forward family messages to prisoners of war[87] and civilians;[88]

Offer its good offices to facilitate the institution of hospital zones[89] and safety zones;[90]

Receive applications from protected persons;[91]

Offer its services in other situations[92] and especially in time of non-international armed conflicts.[93]

The First 1977 Additional Protocol adds two mechanisms of implementation:

The United Nations, "in situations of serious violations of the Conventions or of this Protocol" (Article 89 of Protocol 1); and

The optional "International Fact-Finding Commission" (Article 90 of Protocol 1).[94]

The implementation mechanisms of international criminal law[95] was significantly developed as the United Nations Security Council established the ad hoc International Criminal Tribunals for the Former Yugoslavia and for Rwanda,[96] and with the sixtieth ratification of 1998 Rome Statute of the International Criminal Court[97] on April 11, and its entry into force on July 1, 2002.

This is a milestone in the international community's fight to end impunity for war crimes, genocide, and crimes against humanity.

The International Criminal Court will be able to punish war criminals and perpetrators of genocide or crimes against humanity in cases where national criminal justice systems are unable or unwilling to do so. It is vital for the Court's effective functioning that the State Parties rapidly adopt comprehensive implementing legislation in order to be able to cooperate with the Court.[98]

Human Rights Mechanisms   Increasingly, human rights mechanisms, at the international, regional, and national level, deal with human rights as well as with international humanitarian law issues.

The United Nations General Assembly (Third Committee), the Human Rights Council, the Human Rights Committee

For the Americas: the Organization of American States Commission on Human Rights and the Human Rights Court

For Africa: the African Commission on Human and Peoples' Rights, under the aegis of the OAU.

In Europe: the European Commission, the European Court, the European Committee for the Prevention of Torture and Inhuman or Degrading Treatment or Punishment, all under the aegis of the Council of Europe,[99] as well as the relevant organs of OSCE[100] and the European Union.[101]

Informal Mechanisms   In addition to the formal mechanisms of implementation of international humanitarian law and human rights, there is an increasing role for informal mechanisms at the international as on the national level:

good offices,[102]

media (local, regional, and international),[103]

NGOs such as Human Rights Watch[104] or Amnesty International,

engaging nonstate actors[105] to abide by humanitarian rules and principles,[106]

civil society,[107]

ad hoc independent monitors, agreed upon by all parties,[108]

private diplomacy, including private economy (multinational as well as local),

spiritual leaders,[109] including mediators such as the Sant'Egidio Community.[110]

Toward a Renaissance of Fundamental Humanitarian Values

Research Roots

"Renaissance" literally means rebirth, renewal, and return to the source. We need to research the roots of fundamental values in all civilizations in order to move beyond the superficial universality of legal instruments, too often perceived as imposed by Western powers and, in too many cases, poorly implemented.

As the ICRC survey conducted in 1999 for the fiftieth anniversary of the 1949 Geneva Conventions demonstrated, the local spiritual values are often the only efficient, convincing factor, with which motivate the compliance with humanitarian rules in warfare.[111]

Reanchor Awareness in All Civilizations

> The whole idea of compassion is based on a keen awareness of the interdependence of all these living beings, which are all part of one another and all involved in one another.
>
> —Thomas Merton

Without losing the universality attained by the 1949 Geneva Conventions—and in especially Common Article 3—we need to reanchor them in all civilizations in a new awareness of belonging, empowerment and interdependence, a renewed commitment to common humanity (*humanité commune*), and for the respect of common values (*patrimoine commun de l'humanité*) and objects indispensable to the survival of humankind, such as water, food supplies, public health structures, cultural, and spiritual treasures.

Reaffirm Universality of Fundamental Values

We need to underline the common values, to move beyond the twentieth century celebrations of the fiftieth anniversary of the UN Charter, of the Universal Declaration of Human Rights, of the 1949 Geneva Conventions, of the 1951 Convention on Refugees, etc., to reaffirm the universality of fundamental values.

There are divergences of opinion between American and European allies (on the death penalty, for example). There are differences of emphasis between civil and political rights on one hand and social and economic rights on the other. There are also differences of importance of individual and group rights.[112]

We therefore need to reaffirm a common core of human values, in discovering what makes them universal beyond cultural differences:

The right to life

The right to personal security and religious freedom

The right to family life

The right to health care, adequate nutrition and shelter

The principle of nondiscrimination

The prohibition of torture, inhuman or degrading treatment or punishment.[113]

Reinforce Existing Mechanisms

The international community of States Party to the 1949 Geneva Conventions should reaffirm their collective responsibility according to Article 1, common to all four Conventions and to Additional Protocol 1. According to this provision, "The High Contracting Parties undertake to respect and to ensure respect for this Convention an all circumstances." Should measures[114] be limited to diplomacy, adoption of resolutions, or rather the use of sanctions[115] and peace-enforcement operations in order to stop genocide and arrest war criminals? A number of Security Council resolutions, including those on anarchic conflicts, call upon all parties to respect international humanitarian law and reaffirm that those responsible for breaches thereof should be held individually accountable.

According to Article 89 of Protocol 1, "In situations of serious violations of the Conventions or of this Protocol, the High Contracting Parties undertake to act jointly or individually, in cooperation with the United Nations and in conformity with the United Nations Charter." This is a quite important provision, allowing for creativity and flexibility, as needed.

The involvement of the UN in the implementation of IHL took many forms including denunciations of violations of IHL in resolutions by the Security Council or the General Assembly.

Ending the impunity of perpetrators of atrocities is a major challenge.[116]

The most important step taken by the UN in this context is the establishment of international criminal tribunals such as "The International Tribunal for the Prosecution of Persons Responsible for Serious Violations of International Humanitarian Law Committed in the Territory of the Former Yugoslavia;" The Security Council established it in May 1993[117] for serious violations committed there since 1991. The tribunal has competence on the following offenses: grave breaches of the Geneva Conventions,[118] violations of the laws and customs of war,[119] genocide,[120] and crimes against humanity.[121]

The International Tribunal for Rwanda was established by the Security Council in 1994. This is the first time that an international criminal tribunal has been established with respect to an essentially non-international conflict.

Those ad-hoc Tribunals will need adequate resources and political support.[122] Their existence does not do away with the requirement in the 1949 Geneva Conventions for all States Party to see to the punishment of grave breaches wherever they occur, be it by government officials or warlords.[123]

The International Criminal Court needs to be supported. It is only one part of a system that would end impunity to the perpetrators of genocide, crimes against humanity, war crimes, and torture. Such a system could certainly contribute to deter people contemplating such crimes, to allow victims to obtain justice, and to support reconciliation efforts. States Party to the Geneva Conventions have been increasingly aware of their responsibility to respect international humanitarian law not only as individual States but also collectively. The awareness of their collective responsibility is a more recent phenomenon, resulting from the combined pressure of public opinion, the ICRC, and various human rights NGOs,[124] bilaterally or before United Nations bodies. This collective responsibility not only pertains to the enforcement of humanitarian rules, it is contributing to national stability and international security, preventing disorderly movements of populations, uprooting of displaced persons and refugees, and the spreading of uncontrolled violence around the world.[125]

Reinvent Remedies

We need to be more creative in applying remedies[126] to promote the respect of fundamental values in all situations.

Some remedies might include:

1. The reaffirmation of fundamental humanitarian rules, customs, and principles in a simple, easy to understand form, and translation into local languages;
2. Training of arms bearers (military, police, private security groups) in fundamental restraints of violence and essential humanitarian principles;[127]
3. Conducting international, regional, and local public opinion campaigns to promote fundamental humanitarian values[128] and counter-hate campaigns;
4. Mobilization of public role models (such as artists or athletes) in close contact with local traditions who can influence leaders and public opinion at large;[129]
5. Including spiritual leaders in those campaigns, especially when religious and spiritual values have been used to fuel conflicts;[130]
6. Preparing the youth to recognize and defend the distinction between humanity and inhumanity through educational programs.[131] Reintegrate child soldiers into society;[132]
7. Learning from human rights[133] and environmental[134] activists to promote fundamental humanitarian values to allow, in the long run, humanitarian norms to become a part of humanitarian consciousness;
8. Monitoring arms transfers, beginning with light weapons,[135] and promoting innovative disarmament approaches, such as "weapons for food" or "weapons for development";

9. Exerting better targeted bilateral and multilateral diplomatic, economic, and adequate military pressures against violators, in accordance with the UN Charter and international humanitarian law;[136]
10. Fully including the respect of fundamental human values in the framework of the maintenance and reestablishment of international security.[137]

Rebuild Public Conscience

"Public conscience" was introduced in positive international law by the Martens Clause at the Hague Peace Conference in 1899.

It was the result of a compromise reached at the Hague Conference to break a deadlock between great and small powers in Europe over the definition of combatants. In case of doubt, international humanitarian rules should be interpreted in a manner consistent with standards of humanity and the demands of public conscience.[138]

Humanitarian law is, at the same time, rooted in the history of all traditions of humankind, in all parts of the world, and is also very much part of our future, as one essential safeguard for our survival as a species. In the words of Jean Pictet, one of the founding fathers of contemporary humanitarian law, respect for humanitarian law is "necessary to humankind's survival."

In the words of Martin Luther King Jr.: "The chain reaction of evil—hate begetting hate, wars producing more wars—must be broken, or we shall be plunged into the dark abyss of annihilation" and "Either we live together as brothers, or we perish as fools."

As the spiritual dimension was at the origin of universal fundamental human values, we now need to bring back the spirit of humanity into the letter of international humanitarian law.

Humanitarian Vignettes

Nicola Smith and Larry Hollingworth

I

Radio communication is vital in a relief and humanitarian setting; it is relatively cheap to establish—after the initial purchase of hardware—and costs nothing to run. Radio frequencies are normally allocated to various humanitarian actors by the national government; sometimes channels are shared, but more often than not humanitarian actors operate on different frequencies.

Interventions in camp settings become more complicated due to the vast array of humanitarian actors who are involved. Services provided include camp management; health, water, and sanitation; child protection; food distribution; education; shelter, and the list continues. There are many different agencies, both national and international with different capacities and abilities, operating in the same camp. Consistent coordination and communication is essential. Sometimes agencies have shared radio frequencies, but that is not common. In fact, it is extremely rare to have all the agencies in the same camp able to communicate with one another. The importance of communication becomes very apparent during periods of insecurity.

In 2003, I was working in Kandahar in southern Afghanistan. MSF was the health-care provider in a camp for approximately forty thousand internally displaced Afghans. The camp was literally in the middle of the desert and was called Zhare Dasht ("yellow desert" in Pashtun). Space was not a problem, and the camp was well laid out, but there was a problem with a consistent supply of water and security.

The Zhare Dasht camp was the perfect infiltration environment for Taliban and Al Qaeda who were operating against the Coalition in the war on terror. Tragically, in 2003 Osama bin Laden openly declared war against the humanitarian actors in Afghanistan and accused them of working with an illegal government. The assassination of an ICRC delegate was the first in an increasing number of murders of humanitarian aid workers.

By October 2003, security was becoming very difficult. Al Qaeda murdered two humanitarian aid workers who were traveling up the main highway from Kandahar to Herat. Security worsened after an incident occurred in the Zhare Dasht camp. Taliban and Al Qaeda operatives had infiltrated the camp and attacked the demining agents who were working on the periphery removing the mines and unexploded ordinance that litter the country. Thankfully, the execution of the aid workers was thwarted, and the operatives fled the scene. That day a security incident was averted, but more ominously only two humanitarian agencies out of seven operating in the camp could communicate with one another to share information. If technology could help provide a fast, user-friendly way of allowing improved communication among different agencies, it could literally mean the difference between life and death.

—Nicola "Nicky" Smith

II

Every message needs a messenger. The speed at which the message is delivered, the number of people it reaches, and the effect it has can change lives.

In natural disasters the earliest hours are the most critical. Few die after the opening hours. The knowledge of where to go, what and where to avoid, and what to send and where to send it saves lives.

In manmade crises sometimes it is better to stay than to move. If you move, you need to know to where and how and what dangers you will encounter. When you return you need to know what awaits you—mines or booby traps, friends or foe.

In interethnic violence the media has proved to be both a force of evil and of power. Radio stations have spewed forth venom and bias, TV images have fueled insurrection, and the written word has published false gospels. Governments and factions have manipulated the news to their own ends. Even the most independent media stations have struggled to remain impartial in their output.

In the Balkans and in Central Africa, TV and radio stations are attempting to reunite communities by using soap operas that emphasize the common bonds and older values that existed before the violence. The difficulties of return and reintegration, forgiveness and reconciliation are played out in tightly scripted daily episodes.

The obscene aftermath of indiscriminate mine-laying, the loss of limbs, the loss of livelihoods, and the loss of self-respect can be mitigated by an awareness of the danger. Mine-awareness programs can save more lives than mine-clearance activities. Posters and banners in schools and community buildings, advertisements in newspapers, warnings on radio and television can prevent children from playing and farmers from planting and tilling in suspect areas.

In crises, people need to know more than ever what is happening and who is winning, who is causing the pain and who is curing it. Rumor spreads faster than fact. It is more difficult to correct misinformation and disinformation than it is to disseminate truth. If desperate people believe that transport is waiting to take them away to safety, if starving people believe that food is to be distributed and both of these are untrue, the blame will be placed upon the shoulders of the agency, not on the authors of the untruth. The reaction and response may range from distrust to destruction and rioting.

The major media companies are eager to cover "breaking news" crises, their pictures and their comments are accepted as the facts, and when general public interest wanes or the news becomes routine, they move on, leaving an information vacuum in the very place where news coverage is needed most. Switching off the camera lights falsely implies that the crisis is over, whereas for the local population the long journey to recovery has hardly begun.

—Larry Hollingworth

Humanitarian Response in the Era of Global Mobile Information Technology

Valerie Amos

Technology is among the most difficult topics to tackle in a chapter designed to be relevant for more than a few months. The digital revolution has brought, and is still bringing, many positive changes to the world. In the humanitarian sector, technology has revitalized worldwide volunteerism through crowdsourcing, driving closer cooperation between the humanitarian and the for-profit sectors. It has empowered people who receive humanitarian aid and improved the way we manage information.

These changes have challenged old assumptions and reshaped existing systems in deep and unexpected ways. In this chapter, I will set out what new technology offers us across the humanitarian sector; highlight the mutual benefits of the sector's newly formed relationship with the technology sector; and suggest how we can improve the partnerships we are building to tap the full potential of information technology in our work.

Building Resilience

The first step in crisis response starts well before disaster hits. Developing resilient early warning systems helps communities withstand even major hazards. Mobile technologies offer improved ways of doing this.

Social and economic data, including maps, are essential to building resilient communities. Most conversations about public safety and assistance take place around a map. Mobile technology enables us to compile, share, and update maps more quickly and accurately than ever before, so that we can put our resources where they will be most effective, at both local and national levels.

The Grassroots Mapping Project (www.grassrootsmapping.org) uses inexpensive techniques, like balloons and kites, to compile maps that are aimed at changing how people see the world in environmental, social, and political terms. The organization worked in the New Orleans area in 2010 to map the BP oil spill, and is now broadening its scope to explore inexpensive and community-led means to measure and explore environmental and social issues.

Interactive mobile technology can also enhance the ways maps are used, making them a valuable tool for advocacy and development—crucial elements of building resilience. In Somalia, the Danish Refugee Council (DRC) is running an online map of its development projects in rural areas. The map shows every village with a project funded by the DRC. Clicking on a village reveals details about the project, its aims, and its progress. Somalis in the diaspora have started to use the map to decide on the best villages for their donations. These diaspora communities are even topping up the original funding offered by the DRC—an unexpected side effect of the project.

Interactive mapping has been taken up at the international level by the World Bank, which launched the Mapping for Results platform in October 2010. This initiative visualizes the location of World Bank projects and enables citizens and other stakeholders to provide direct feedback, enhancing the transparency and social accountability of these projects.

For select countries, the platform provides not only geographic information about World Bank–financed programs, but also allows users to overlay disaggregated poverty, population density, and human development data (i.e., infant mortality rates, malnutrition, etc.). Population density is available for 107 countries; data on mortality, maternal health, and malnutrition data are available for forty-three countries; and poverty data for thirty-one countries. Such moves toward transparency will undoubtedly have implications for funding and development in the future.

Mobile cash transfer programs, which deliver vouchers or cash directly to recipients, can also play a crucial part in building resilient communities, help people to withstand slow-onset crises, and build sustainable livelihoods. Programs can be integrated with national social security systems to maximize impact. As in so many areas, humanitarians are only beginning to investigate the possibilities that this technology offers.

Local Action

In all disasters, local communities form the front line of the crisis response. If local people have access to cutting-edge technology during an emergency, they can be extremely effective in communicating the needs of affected communities to each other and to local, regional, and international aid organizations.

The formation of local social networks to spread news, including tips and warnings about impending weather events or volcanic activity, is another important way in which mobile technology has contributed to disaster prevention and recovery. These tools are increasingly being used in disaster-prone areas. For example, civil authorities in Mexico City have recently rolled out a free mobile application that will warn people when an earthquake is imminent. The application triggers an alarm on the phone once an earthquake of magnitude 6.5 or higher has been detected. During the 2010 eruption of Mount Merapi outside Jogjakarta in Indonesia, a local communications group called Jalin Merapi used Twitter, Facebook, SMS, and local radio to keep the community informed in real time and to understand and communicate emerging needs.

Local filmmakers in Thailand also used digital technology to spread the word during a flood emergency in 2011. They posted a series of ten videos on YouTube aimed at bringing home to people the seriousness of the situation. In one, they represented the billions of cubic meters of water bearing down on Bangkok as an equivalent volume of blue whales. The main video in the series has been viewed more than a million times.

Looking to the future, it is clear that local mobile networks also have much to offer in disseminating information during a crisis. The response to a tornado that hit the town of Joplin, Missouri, in May 2011 was partly coordinated through a Facebook page. The page, Joplin Tornado Information, was set up within two hours of the tornado striking and began connecting needs, resources, transportation, and storage requirements. It soon had nearly 50,000 fans. Relief organizations, churches, and news sources started to post information on the page, including the news that water trucks had arrived in the town.

Similarly, social media was a primary source of communication after an earthquake and tsunami struck northern Japan in March 2011. Within an hour of the earthquake, an estimated 1,200 tweets per minute including references to the disaster were being posted on Twitter. Many Japanese people used Facebook, Twitter, and the Japan-specific site Mixi to share information and keep in touch. These examples from highly connected countries with robust infrastructure show what will be possible in an increasing number of countries in future.

Many of the most useful new mobile platforms are also accessible to locally based groups and even those affected by crises. For example, Crowdmap (www .crowdmap.com) allows anyone to set up a mapping project on the Ushahidi platform (www.ushahidi.com), a tool to crowd-source information using multiple channels. This technology has recently been used by people in Syria to track unrest there in real time.

Early Warning

Information saves lives, and the UN is heavily investing in global systems to alert early responders in the event of a major sudden-onset crisis like an earthquake or typhoon. The UN Office for the Coordination of Humanitarian Affairs (OCHA) runs a web-based real-time information channel for affected countries and bilateral responders used immediately after major disasters. This channel, known as the Virtual On-Site Operations Coordination Centre (OSOCC) is used by most Member States and regional organizations. Since 2004, the Virtual OSOCC has been part of the Global Disaster Alert and Coordination System (GDACS), which is an international network of disaster information systems aimed at facilitating information exchange and coordination in the first hours after a natural disaster. GDACS includes an automatic disaster alert and notification system, as well as automatic feeds of related disaster maps and satellite images. GDACS alerts are submitted to subscribers by e-mail and SMS text message minutes after disaster events to inform about the possible humanitarian impact of disasters.

A major initiative in this area is the UN Global Pulse, which was created by UN Secretary-General Ban Ki-moon in 2009 to explore opportunities to use real-time data to gain a more accurate understanding of well-being, and assess levels of stress, particularly on vulnerable people. Global Pulse tracks the human impacts of crises as they happen, and enables the UN to access feedback in real time on how well its responses are working.

The strategy has three interdependent areas of activity: "Data Research" to assess community well-being; a "Technology Toolkit" of free and open source software tools so development experts can mine data, share ideas, and make evidence-based decisions; and the "Pulse Lab Network," an integrated network of country-level innovation centers, bringing together government experts, UN agencies, academia, and the private sector to apply new applications of data to development challenges. Global mobile communications technology plays a crucial role in all these areas.

Global Pulse stresses the importance of creating actionable information, that is, policy recommendations, from raw data. The project detects what it calls "digital smoke signals" that indicate changing conditions and behavior. For example, if people start to reduce unnecessary expenses and sell off property and livestock, this is an early predictor of food insecurity and malnutrition. The initiative's main technology tool is a social network called Hunchworks, which helps experts share hypotheses, collect evidence, and make decisions.

In addition to this major international push, national and regional disaster management agencies also recognize the importance of using mobile technology in early warning systems. Social media was used widely during the January 2012 floods in the Philippines, which has the fifth-largest number of Facebook users in the world. Some 130,000 people made use of the government's Weather Watch website to receive updates on conditions for travel by road and sea. The site issued warnings on collapsed roads and dangerous sea conditions for fishermen. Many Filipinos who lack access to computers used their smart phones to receive this information.

Saving Lives in Crisis: An Evolving Picture

The scope for technology to help emergency responders was first explored after the magnitude 7.0 earthquake that hit Port-au-Prince, Haiti, in January 2010. With hundreds of thousands of people dead and more than a million homeless, governments pledged hundreds of millions of dollars, but ordinary citizens also contributed enormous amounts of money. Much of this was raised through mobile phone text messages, marking the dawn of a new era of instant electronic donation.

Amid the chaos, one utility was up and running within days: the mobile phone network. Over the previous five years, Haiti had undergone a transformation. Two mobile phone networks run by Digicel and Voila covered almost the entire country. These networks had become the country's leading industry. Haiti in 2010 was the poorest country in the Americas, but its people could communicate with each other, and with the world, even after the earthquake. This meant that they could share information via local and international radio and online networks and participate in online mapping projects.

Volunteers gathered online to look for ways to communicate with Haitians and map the crisis, using a raft of innovative tools from SMS messages to collaborative mapping platforms and systems to mine data from social media sites like Twitter. Within hours of the earthquake, the collaborative mapping platform Ushahidi set up a site to collate and map data from text messages, social media, official situation reports, and other sources of information.

An SMS short code, 4636, was established with Digicel for local people to send and receive emergency-related messages. (Short codes work like the emergency numbers 911 or 999 as easily memorized shorthand for longer "traditional" numbers.)

OpenStreetMap,[1] a collaborative system to mark names and key points on a publicly available online map, started charting the transformed city of Port-au-Prince; this became a vital resource for aid responders. A Haitian OpenStreetMap team formed a close relationship with the International Organization for Migration and their work informed the entire aid effort.

All these steps produced an incremental change in attitudes toward the use of mobile technology in a disaster zone and this had a significant impact during the Libya crisis of early 2011. Part of the challenge in Libya was that the UN did not have physical access to much of the country and was struggling to get a clear picture of what was happening. Although there was data available online, there was no way to verify and process this information. The Standby Task Force (SBTF)—a self-organized group of volunteers born from the Haiti experience—responded by creating the Libya Crisis Map.[2] The map worked by collating data from dedicated collaborators and the general public to plot incidents or trends, such as refugee flows, on a map in real time. A UN specialist reviewed the data, looked for patterns, and found ways to use this information.

Another significant step forward came during the largest humanitarian crisis of 2011: a massive regional drought in eastern Africa. The United Nations High Commissioner for Refugees (UNHCR) approached the SBTF, which activated a network of volunteers to analyze thousands of images and chart settlements, tagging over a quarter of a million features.[3] This helped to identify newly built urban areas and to get a better picture of the numbers there who needed help.

Mobile Phones Change the Game: Two-Way Communication and Electronic Cash

The spread of cheap communications technology also promises to change the entire aid model fundamentally by changing the relationship between humanitarian workers and those affected by emergencies and disasters. A 2011 study by the U.S. government-funded Internews Media Support NGO examined the experience of Somalis in the world's largest refugee camp in Dadaab, Kenya, and found that establishing two-way communication with affected communities was not a high priority for aid workers:

> Serious communications gaps between the humanitarian sector and refugees . . . are increasing refugee suffering and putting lives at risk . . .
>
> > Large numbers of refugees don't have the information they need to access basic aid; more than 70 percent of newly-arrived refugees say they lack information on how to register for aid, and similar numbers say they need information on how to locate missing family members.[4]

Some aid organizations have begun to contact affected communities using communications technology. The International Federation of Red Cross and Red Crescent Societies (IFRC) is aiming to set up formal agreements with mobile phone providers in fifty disaster-prone countries. They will be able to see how many people are connected to each telephone aerial, and send out mass text messages. These could be carefully targeted in the case of localized flooding, or used for early warning of hurricanes or other adverse weather events. The connection could also be used to seek feedback on crisis conditions in an area, or even to locate people trapped under rubble.

Another development that will have a significant impact on the relationship between donors, humanitarians, and affected communities is the rise of mobile electronic cash. This has the potential to transform the humanitarian sector through direct transfers to large numbers of people affected by emergencies and through targeted transfers to individuals to conduct specific tasks, including monitoring, assessments, purchasing medicines for a clinic, and so on.

In crisis after crisis, markets have been shown to provide supplies extremely quickly. The problem is that the most vulnerable people cannot afford to buy anything. Instead of meeting this shortfall with huge, expensive international logistics chains that undercut the market, the advocates of mobile cash transfers argue that it is cheaper and more effective to provide vulnerable people with money or vouchers to buy what they need.

This proposition is fraught with controversy. Transferring cash creates many logistical challenges, and will not always provide what is most badly needed. The World Food Programme (WFP) says it chooses which kind of aid will be most appropriate depending on various factors, including cost-effectiveness and availability of food. "When appropriate," it states, "cash and vouchers can meet more closely the needs of targeted vulnerable people."[5]

Several programs are already using electronic money and vouchers. In 2009, the WFP launched a mobile delivery and tracking system based on electronic vouchers in Zambia, redeemable through mobile phones thanks to a technology platform provided by Mobile Transactions Zambia. Recipients registered by uploading a national registration card into the system. They then received a scratch card that they could redeem at specific vendors.

A program in Niger in West Africa shows that this technology has potential even where mobile phone ownership is low. In 2010, the international NGO Concern joined forces with the mobile network operator Airtel to facilitate mobile money transfer to four thousand households affected by drought-related food insecurity, in an attempt to reduce operating costs and increase benefits to recipients. Other households received cash in envelopes. Concern partnered with Tufts University to investigate the impact of the mobile money transfer. They found that receiving mobile money saved time for recipients, who did not have to walk to a distribution point or wait for a delivery. The mobile money recipients also bought a greater variety of food types and nonfood items and grew a wider variety of crops; the reasons for this were not clear. Even illiterate households had no problem accessing the money; they sought help from relatives and neighbors.

Private Sector Involvement

Another element of this changing landscape is the growing interaction between the aid sector and the private sector. This interaction has brought the energy and financial power of the private sector to benefit humanitarian causes. It has also benefited the private sector, with a growing acknowledgment from companies that encouraging healthy societies provides many tangible and intangible benefits.

After the Haiti earthquake, one of the country's mobile phone providers, Digicel, provided its 2 million customers with $5 of free credit, which enabled them to get in touch with each other and the outside world, and build a better picture of the situation at the height of the crisis. Digicel also donated generators, phones, and credit to fifteen radio stations in Port-au-Prince to help them reach their listeners. This provided an essential conduit for humanitarian aid responders to get their message out to the general public.

Partnership with mobile phone providers also provided information on a grander scale in Haiti. A study by researchers from Sweden's Karolinska Institute and Columbia University[6] showed that it was possible to track the movement of displaced people by following their mobile phones. The study indicated that some 600,000 people had left the Haitian capital in the nineteen days after the earthquake, with clear implications for the provision of humanitarian aid. This tracking technology was also used after the Japanese earthquake and tsunami of 2011, and offers great possibilities for future emergencies, displacements, and epidemics, provided due attention is paid to privacy issues.

Partnerships between the UN and the private sector were initially philanthropic; the UN and partners would raise money from the private sector to fund projects that were often not related to the core business of the company in question. Today, these are genuine collaborations. An innovative partnership between the Vodafone Foundation and the UN Foundation known as the Technology Partnership has brokered relationships between UN agencies and some of the biggest companies in the world. WFP is working with partners including PepsiCo, Caterpillar, and Unilever. The IFRC has a long-running partnership agreement with Nestlé.

These partnerships reached a turning point when the technology sector began to make products cheap and robust enough to be relevant to the developing world. In December 2011, OCHA and Ericsson celebrated the eleventh anniversary of their global partnership for the provision of GSM (Global System for Mobile Communications) and related services and expertise in support of humanitarian relief operations. Ericsson Response is the company's volunteer program that works to help OCHA in emergency situations by setting up mobile networks for voice and data communication. The team has been deployed fifteen times since

2001, most recently in Haiti in 2010, when its mobile network provided an average of five thousand free calls per day to humanitarians for six months.

UNHCR, in partnership with Microsoft, is using communications technology to improve UNHCR operations and develop programs to help refugees rebuild their lives, store their data, and access new opportunities through education and connectivity. Microsoft supports UNHCR by providing technological expertise, while UNHCR contributes its fifty years of know-how in addressing challenging refugee issues. Google is working on several projects, including the improvement of financial tracking of donor contributions and is providing Google Earth services to some aid operations.

Private organizations contribute resources such as employee mobilization or secondment, funds, in-kind donations and expert services, cause-related marketing, and expertise to support humanitarian actors in relief and rehabilitation efforts. The private sector also brings leadership, assets, access to global networks, and a unique perspective that can greatly benefit our work.

For their part, companies are eager to partner when they add value. Working in the humanitarian sector provides a narrative that shows that they are making a sustained difference and builds a business case for their work, creating value for the company.

Ericsson says that their volunteer program empowers employees to make a difference in society and adds another dimension to employees' jobs, making them feel more motivated. In addition, the experience and knowledge gained through working in emergency situations enables them to develop resilient and sustainable technical solutions that will be relevant to their business in the longer term.

Both the humanitarian community and the private sector still have a lot to learn from each other. Companies have far more to offer than the aid sector is currently equipped to ask for. We know there are potential private sector partners who are struggling to understand the humanitarian system and how to play a part in it.

Overcoming Challenges: The Future

I see three main challenges to maximizing the value of new technology for aid work: defining and working with the physical limitations of the technology; transforming our institutional frameworks to take account of the changing environment; and dealing with cultural and even psychological barriers to the adoption of new working practices.

First, we need more experience and research to clarify concrete areas in which mobile technology offers significant benefits. One simple example is that in some cultures, mobile devices and computing power may be under the control of male heads of household, which could present problems in delivering messaging, information, or cash transfers to women or the elderly. Building trust in new financial instruments like cash transfers will be crucial to ensuring that they are taken up and used effectively.

There are also valid concerns about the "consumerization" of disaster communications, ranging from fears over what happens to user data in politically insecure environments to the proliferation of "white noise"—the paradox of being utterly overwhelmed with information but still unable to find the information needed for decision making.

These efforts must take into account the need to mitigate the risks associated with ad hoc messaging in a disaster or a war zone, including managing expectations and avoiding any perception of political bias or putting in danger those that are highly vulnerable or at risk of political persecution. The technology must be used wisely if it is to be as effective as possible.

At an institutional level, the international community has built large and complex systems over the years to collate, analyze, distribute, and act upon information. These tend to be driven by experts, and organized hierarchically. Some of these structures are necessary and important to deal with issues of privacy, quality control, economies of scale, security, and political sensitivity. But working with new technology and new partners—including the new volunteer and technical communities, and those from the commercial sector—has demonstrated that these may be a barrier to full collaboration.

At a cultural and behavioral level, research has shown[7] that aid agencies typically perceive new technology as being expensive or difficult to use, requiring specialist knowledge and support. Senior managers can often be the most reluctant to embrace change as they may hold on to a traditional view of how programming should work. It will require vision and leadership to overcome this reluctance and move from the "pilot" phase to the wide-scale adoption of new technologies. Financial controllers must also be supportive in order for change to happen, and must be made aware that initial investments will yield efficiencies or cost savings over time.

A short chapter on such a rapidly evolving subject will inevitably leave out more than it contains and many of the specifics may quickly become out of date. However, it is possible to draw one conclusion that will stand the test of time. The uptake of new technologies is more than a technical phenomenon: It is essential to ensuring that aid work is as effective and relevant as it needs to be.

PART II

Principles/Values

In this section, some of the humanitarian communities most distinguished practitioners reflect on fundamental principles and values. The former Directors of Doctors Without Borders and Amnesty International provide cautionary advice—how one can sacrifice gains to the cause of expediency. There are three chapters describing serious fault lines in so-called civilized societies that must be recognized and exposed, or we risk becoming partners in gender exploitation, terrorism (or unbridled counterterrorism) and torture.

Neutrality or Impartiality

Alain Destexhe, M.D.

The construction of a new world order and the evolution of the United Nations after World War II have been guided by the principle: Never again! The Nazis' unprecedented crimes became a benchmark for an international community founded on certain basic values: opposition to genocide, the search for world peace, and respect for human rights. However, over the years, that determination has been replaced by pragmatism. The United Nations, rendered powerless as a result of superpower hostility, found its role restricted to the provision of development aid. The end of the Cold War raised again the idea of an international community based on shared values, administered by international institutions, and defended by democratic countries. In the face of an increasing number of crises, the UN is now called upon regularly to encourage negotiation, to interpose itself, and to assist people at risk. However, the window of opportunity that seemed to be opening with the end of the Cold War is rapidly closing, and the idea that the UN could be the guarantor of world peace is far from being realized. The honeymoon period and the dreams of a "new world order" seem to be over. The major powers have made it clear that they will neither sanction the UN to be the world's police force nor take on the role themselves, not even the United States.

Fifty years after the creation of the UN and five years after the end of the Cold War, the international community showed its true colors: in Rwanda, it failed to react to the first indisputable genocide since that perpetrated against the Jews; in former Yugoslavia, it failed to react to the return of war and "ethnic cleansing" at the heart of Europe. Under the pretense of neutrality, its only response was humanitarian aid.

The Shortcomings of the "New Humanitarianism"

There has been an unprecedented enthusiasm for humanitarian work throughout the world during recent years, yet it is far from certain that this is always in the victims' best interests. The end of the Cold War ushered in a "new humanitarianism," or "emergency ethic," that has become increasingly prevalent. There was an end to the practice of judging individual victims from an ideological perspective, seen as "good" or "bad," depending on which sphere of influence they were from (communist or noncommunist). Now, they became simply fellow human beings deserving of compassion. However, we were too quick to forget that Cold War values were also combined with realpolitik and that it was moral outrage converted into action that, above all, helped to counter totalitarian thinking. From Afghanistan to Angola, from Nicaragua to Cambodia, no one major Western power used humanitarian aid as its sole weapon against the Soviets, the Cubans, or the Vietnamese: political or military interventions were key components in a strategy of containment in which humanitarian aid played only a minor role.

However, the examples of Bosnia and Rwanda demonstrated that this "new humanitarianism" can rebound on those it is intended to help. These fellow human beings, fighting to defend values we share, have become "victims" to be assessed in terms of their immediate suffering; hungry mouths to feed, if they survive. Protesting that it was essential to remain neutral, Europe, and later the UN, provided humanitarian aid as their only real response to Serb aggression in Bosnia; the same response, based on the same claim to neutrality, was proffered in Rwanda—when the genocide was over and it was too late to influence the situation. Here the massive deployment of aid to the huge number of refugees became the focus of the world's attention, disguising the culpable failure of the international community to come to the assistance of the Tutsi people. In Bosnia humanitarian aid, elevated to the status of official policy, encouraged and fostered aggression while convincing public opinion to accept both the *fait accompli* by the stronger party and an "ethnic" reading of the conflict.

A Brief History of Neutrality

From a humanitarian point of view, the principle of neutrality cannot be separated form the history of the Red Cross. The movement was founded by Henry Dunant in 1863, in reaction to his horror at the slaughter he witnessed at the Battle of Solferino.[1] This led him to define the principle enshrined in the first Geneva Convention for the protection of wounded soldiers and to set up the neutral Red Cross agency to care for them. Subsequent Conventions extended this neutrality to other noncombatants: civilians and prisoners of war. The almost universally acknowledged Geneva Conventions remain the cornerstone of the Red Cross, a movement that has seen an enormous expansion in membership over the years. The

Geneva Conventions represent a fundamental stage in the history of humanitarian action, first, because they enshrine the principle of neutrality applied to noncombatants, and second, because of the importance of the International Committee of the Red Cross, universally recognized for its total respect for the principles of neutrality and impartiality.

Dunant did not invent the concept of neutrality. Indeed, since the earliest times there have been many examples of neutral behavior during conflicts and of bilateral agreements aimed at respecting the wounded, civilians, and prisoners. But it was Dunant who had the genius to see that the principle enshrined in a convention would be universally respected. His wish has been realized; the four Conventions now in force, signed in 1949, have now been ratified by almost every country in existence today. Thanks to Dunant, the Red Cross is an agency backed by international law, to which it can refer when calling on warring parties to respect a certain number of basic rules in regard to the treatment of the wounded, both prisoners and civil populations.

However, despite this undeniable progress, the Red Cross principle of neutrality was soon brought into question and the difficulties that it presents have not been resolved. First, the principle of neutrality certainly could be applied to pitched battles between the armies of European countries that shared much of the same ideology. But it was rendered null and void when, in the name of civilization, the white man attacked "barbarians." Then humanitarian law ceased to apply. The British, for example, after the battle of Omdurman, in the Sudan, did nothing to assist fifteen thousand wounded enemy soldiers. Yet this was 1898, thirty years after Britain had signed the first Geneva Convention.[2] The principle of neutrality was conceived with a civil war in mind, or a war of two opposing comparable forces. What relevance did it have in a war of aggression or in a case of systematic genocide such as that perpetrated by the Young Turks against the Armenians? Chateaubriand, the French writer, gives the answer: "Such a neutrality is derisory for it works against the weaker party and plays into the hands of the stronger party. It would be better to join forces with the oppressors against the oppressed for at least that would avoid adding hypocrisy to injustice."

Second, although the Red Cross is a private institution, it has always depended on national governments to enforce respect for humanitarian law. In order to avoid embarrassing Convention signatories, it has constrained itself to the discrete silence that is an essential part of the Red Cross image. In fact, over several decades the International Committee for the Red Cross (ICRC) has limited itself to transmitting protests from one party to another during a conflict without ever commenting on their validity. Meanwhile, many national Red Cross organizations, far from being apolitical or neutral, seem to have taken on the role of faithful government helpers.

The Red Cross grew up at the end of the nineteenth century, in a period of liberal ideas. Lenin and, to a greater extent, Hitler confronted it with regimes that were fundamentally opposed to the values on which it is founded. Forced to decide between respect for humanitarian principles and the universality of the movement, the Red Cross has always chosen the second alternative, persuaded—and not without reason—that only thus could it continue to play the role of a neutral intermediary in conflicts. The Red Cross has never broken off relations with a country's government—not with Mussolini, not with Lenin, and not with Nazi Germany, not even when Jews were expelled from the German Red Cross.

Although this was not clearly understood at the time, it was when faced with the "Final Solution" that the limits of humanitarian action really showed themselves. The Red Cross, as well as the Allies and the Vatican, knew about the terrible reality of the Nazi extermination camps. And today it is still reproached for never denouncing them and keeping silent about the largest-scale genocide in the twentieth century. Worse still, despite everything, the Red Cross tried to assist those held in the death camps by handing over aid packages for them, without any control whatsoever, to the German authorities. No matter the reasons the Red Cross presents as justification for its silence, the stance it took represents a black page in the history of the movement.[3] One result has been that the role played by the ICRC in other domains (prisoners of war, tracking down and reuniting family members, and so on) has received less attention than it deserves. Neutrality might have been an issue in regard to the German and Allied armies, but how could it be evoked in the face of the Nazi extermination camps? Organizations that aim to be "*sans frontières*" ("without borders") were founded on lessons learned from that experience. The inhuman must not be humanized; it must be denounced and it must be fought against. Such organizations consider that they have a dual role to play: they provide aid to victims in the field, but they also speak out as witnesses to intolerable events.

The Biafra crisis was another important stage in the evolution of the humanitarian movement. On one hand, it again underlined the limits of the Red Cross's "neutral" approach. It was unable to achieve an agreement between the two parties in order to allow food to get through to the Biafran enclave. It was a group of churches that finally decided to disregard the objections of the Nigerian government and the Red Cross and launched an air bridge to the encircled Biafran secessionists.[4] The churches thus invented the modern concept of humanitarian intervention, while making a significant breach in the principle of sovereignty that has so often been used as an excuse for nonintervention, and that is still invoked today.

The stance taken by the Western powers during the Biafran crisis foreshadowed the treatment of the Bosnian crisis, when all the major powers played the humanitarian card without ever looking for a political solution. France, for example, openly encouraged Biafra to secede, but it neither recognized the secessionist government nor provided arms to allow it to stand against Lagos. Unfortunately, Biafra's leaders soon learned that pictures of their starving children were the best weapons for ensuring an international response and famine became inseparable from the conflict itself.[5] When the time came to sum up, it was clear that the amount of humanitarian aid provided was always ridiculously small in comparison with the scale of the tragedy, although sufficient to allow the great powers to maintain the illusion of an international commitment. The world was convinced that it had flown to the rescue of Biafra: television images were proving more convincing than reality.

The guerilla-style conflicts of the 1980s are an even clearer illustration of the limits to neutrality. The Red Cross and UN agencies, refused access to guerilla zones, had to chose between maintaining a presence that provided support exclusively to the government side or withdrawing completely. "*Sans frontières*" organizations were much better suited to provide assistance in that period of guerilla wars. They could intervene clandestinely in most of these conflicts via neighboring countries, in defiance of international law and the niceties of national sovereignty. Unlike the Red Cross, this type of organization does not rely on humanitarian law but on the backing of public opinion aroused by witness accounts of massacres and aggression. Most of the larger-scale conflicts of the 1980s were indirect consequences of the growing influence of the USSR and her allies in developing countries, which became the battlefields where the Cold War was fought by proxy. As a result, consciously or unconsciously, humanitarian aid became a powerful instrument in the anti-Soviet struggle throughout the world as more than 90 percent of refugees during this period were fleeing from "progressive" regimes allied to the USSR. Humanitarian assistance was provided both to populations that could only be reached by the clandestine intervention of "*sans frontières*" organizations, and to those in refugee camps set up on the borders of neighboring countries, which also served as sanctuaries for the guerillas. It was at this time that the UN High Commission on Refugees (UNHCR), working in such refugee camps, developed into one of the most important agencies in the aid system.

If it was during the 1980s that the serious flaws in the concept of humanitarian neutrality became very apparent, it was in former Yugoslavia and in Rwanda that they came to be seen at their most perverse.

Bosnia: The Placebo Effect

The war that was fought in Bosnia for over three years claimed two hundred thousand victims, most of them civilian, and turned four million people into refugees and displaced persons. This conflict, the first on European soil since 1945, began in April 1992, the day the Republic of Bosnia-Herzegovina was recognized by the European Community (EC) and the United States. When Bosnian Serb forces, with the support of the Yugoslav federal army, quickly seized almost 70 percent of the new republic's territory, the Western powers appeared to acquiesce in this *fait accompli*, confining their response to reopening Sarajevo airport and deploying Blue Helmets in an attempt to help those most in need.

Although newspaper editorials had forecast war in Bosnia month before it finally broke out, there were no attempts to try to prevent it. The populations of Bosnia's towns and villages forced to leave their homes were not only the principle victims of the combat, but also the target of the whole pitiless conflict. Europe, reduced to the role of a charitable though powerless witness, raised no obstacle to ethnic cleansing in Bosnia, which was at times carried out under "humanitarian protection."

In fact, in a war being waged with the ultimate aim of excluding and expelling a large part of the population, humanitarian workers faced an impossible dilemma. There were two choices. Either they assisted people to evacuate so that they could be protected, which inevitably helped to achieve the objectives of ethnic cleansing, or they refused to ally themselves with such inhumane acts and left people to endure even more terrible suffering. The major preoccupation was no longer to provide material assistance but to protect the people, which has never been in the mandate of humanitarian organizations, but should have been included in that of the Blue Helmets. Thus, humanitarian action was reduced to feeding the mass of refugees. UNHCR representatives, delegated by the UN and EC to coordinate aid in the former Yugoslavia, had to decide countless times during the conflict which as the lesser of two such evils. Trying to protect refugees without having the power to prevent them from becoming refugees in the first place not only undermines humanitarian principles but actually aggravates the problem.

Paradoxically, humanitarianism, while siding with the victims, also became an arm of the aggressors. The Serbian army quickly realized the advantages to be gained from opening up "corridors of ethnic cleansing" for those they were expelling and bringing them to the "humanitarian front line." Indeed, on several occasions, the UN Protection Force (UNPROFOR) directly contributed to the enforcement of ethnic cleansing by "helping" in the exchange of population. In some ways, the humanitarian effort unintentionally served to help achieve Serbian military objectives because the ethnic cleansers were only too happy to hand over responsibility for the victims of their crimes to the international community.

The distribution of aid was subject to the acquiescence of the Serbs who opened and closed the tap to the aid pipeline as and when it suited them, but never without deducting a substantial levy. For more than a year, the encircled towns and villages of eastern Bosnia received no aid at all as UNPROFOR convoys never used force to get through.

Humanitarian arguments are used to explain the failure of governments to make clear strategic decisions. But the real question is whether humanitarian work should have been entrusted to UN troops in the first place. When peacekeepers are sent into the middle of a way, they may be expected to use their weapons. If relief work is impeded by violence, then the obvious role of armed UN troops is to protect relief convoys and oppose the people who are obstructing them. Unlike Somalia, in Bosnia the humanitarian problems were not the result of a general breakdown of order but of Serbian aggression. If force had any role to play in relieving human suffering in Bosnia, it should have been used to protect the population against the armed thugs who were massacring, raping, looting, and driving away people from their homes. But that was never the intention.

Many NGOs wish governments would leave humanitarian work alone and concentrate on the roles proper to them, which are political and military. In Bosnia humanitarian problems had political causes that governments failed to acknowledge and deal with. UNPROFOR was used in a humanitarian role as the alibi for the international community's disastrous cop-out, making it appear something was being done while failing miserably to react in the politico-military sphere, the only arena for resolving the root causes.

From Total War to Total Humanitarianism

World War II taught Western democracies that no spoon is long enough for supping with the devil. "Never again!" cried Europe in unison, and a whole generation grew up under the influence of this, rejecting all ideas of racial purity and territorial ambition. But this belief system was shattered the first time that Europe was again confronted from within by a racist policy based on religion and ethnic group. From that moment, history was forgotten and all the certainties and idealism flew out of the window; the countries of Europe started to behave as if they had learned nothing. Admittedly, there seemed only a small risk of the conflict spreading and becoming more generalized. Admittedly, Milosevic, or Karadzic, is not Hitler. Nevertheless, the Bosnian disaster flouted all the ideals on which the European democracies were founded in the aftermath of World War II, and no real attempt was made to defend them.

It was Winston Churchill who developed the concept of a "total warfare against Nazism, enforcing land, sea, and air blockades that even prevented food getting through to Occupied Europe. The deterioration in health that inevitable resulted was seen as a weapon in this form of total war where politics forced humanitarian-ism off the stage. Although this concept posed a dilemma from a humanitarian point of view, the Allies were convinced that it was justifiable. In Bosnia, we passed from one extreme to the other, from the concept of "total war" to that of "total humanitarianism"; people were provided with food but not protection, and no real political pressure was put on the aggressor. The logic of humanitarianism pre-vailed over the logic of a politics that did not dare exercise its prerogatives for fear of endangering humanitarian efforts in the field. The question of what would have been the best course of action from the victims' point of view was made totally sub-ordinate to that of how the international community could avoid involving itself in military intervention. Certainly food got through to Sarajevo most of the time and the impressive humanitarian effort saved the life of tens of thousands of people throughout the area. Certainly the presence of the Blue Helmets on the group had a moderating effect. But what about Vukovar, Gorazde, and Srebrenica? Should we really be congratulating ourselves that fifty years after the creation of the UN we were unable to stop that kind of slaughter?

Despite the sop it offered to European public opinion, in the short term, humanitarianism achieved little. In the longer term, it served as an alibi for politi-cal impotence. Finally, in September 1995, under strong pressure from an American government that finally decided to involve itself more actively, air strikes were directed at Serb military targets and the Dayton Agreement led to the establishment of a NATO-led international task. But it was all too late to avoid the inevitable: the separation of Bosnia into separate, ethnically based ministates that may yet divide even further. When they were confronted once again with Milosevic's intransi-gence, this time in Kosovo, Europe and the United States utilized the hard lessons learned from Bosnia.

Rwanda: From Indifference to Compassion

What took place in Rwanda between April and July 1994 was a genocide: and excep-tional event in twentieth-century history. The term was first coined in 1944 by

Raphael Lemkin[6] and is the basis of the UN General Assembly's convention committing member countries to punish and prevent genocide.[7] This convention, passed in 1949, defines genocide very specifically as those "acts committed with intent to destroy a national, ethnic, racial, or religious group." By applying it too generally, this specific meaning has been so watered down, taken out of context, and misused by those seeking to draw attention to other horrors that the real intention behind this particular crime has been lost and the word genocide has become synonymous with any act of mass murder. In fact, only three instances of mass slaughter the twentieth century can correctly be called genocide: the massacres of Armenians under the Ottoman Empire in 1915 and 1916, the extermination of the Jews and Gypsies under the Nazis, and the 1994 slaughter of almost 1 million Tutsis by Hutu militias in Rwanda.[8]

When the massacres first began in Kigali, the world turned its back and the UN decided to pull out its main body of Blue Helmets. Yet the death toll was increasing daily, and within four weeks it was estimated that almost a million people had been killed. But the genocide could have been stopped early on if two moves had been made. The UN could have used its troops to protect the churches, hospitals, schools, and other places where Tutsis were desperately seeking refuge, and the UN could have clearly recognized the Rwandan Patriotic Front (RPF) as the legitimate government of Rwanda and broken off relations with the government that initiated the genocide. Such measures would have changes the course of Rwanda's history, but they were not implemented. Again, the Security Council of the United Nations decided to remain neutral and not to take sides with the RPF.

By the end of June 1994 the crises in Rwanda was seen exclusively as a humanitarian catastrophe affecting hundreds of thousands of (Hutu) refugees, arousing international compassion, and completely distracting attentions from the genocide that had more or less run its course because there were no more (Tutsi) victims available for slaughter. As the RPF troops advances, the architects and instigators of the genocide organized a mass exodus of the Hutu population into rapidly erected refugee camps in Goma (Zaire) and Tanzania, or into the French-controlled security zone within Rwanda. The former government planned this deliberately so they could claim that the RPF might have won the land, but not its people.

Humanitarian aid poured into the camps, fueled by the generosity of a public moved by television pictures of cholera victims in Goma. However, although such aid may well be intended and based on sound principles, as had already been pointed out, it can never be totally neutral. In this case, as so often elsewhere, it represented almost the only source of food, equipment, and jobs in the camps and thus became a major stake in the power struggle for control over the refugees.

Humanitarian workers were continually confronted with the same problem: how to aid the victims without getting caught up in the power game being played by their oppressors, or in this case militias who were acting as the strong arm of the politicians in the camps.

The problem was (is) that the refugees settled commune by commune in the camps under the direction of the local leaders who had accompanied them. But this situation posed a major ethical problem inasmuch as these leaders, who were also implicated in the genocide, retained their authority over the refugees and passed on instructions to them from the former government-in-exile. It is with such people that the aid agency had to collaborate.

It is useful to draw a parallel here with the way in which the Khmer Rouge were able to gain power over Cambodian refugees by manipulating humanitarian aid. At the beginning of 1979 the Khmer Rouge, who were responsible for the massacre of a million of their fellow Cambodians, fled before the advancing Vietnamese army. Using force and propaganda, they took with them hundreds of thousands of civilians into refugee camps in the frontier area with Thailand, where they experienced dreadful famine. The international community mobilized, although more slowly than would happen today, and thousands of lives were saved. But the humanitarian effort also fed the Khmer Rouge and inadvertently helped them to establish their control over the refugee population, enabling them to continue the conflict for a further decade.

It is clear that the international relief effort in Rwanda created a similar vicious circle, fed by aid that could at worst grow into a future conflict and at best ensures that the Hutu refugees remain in the camps. This is the result of treating the Rwandan crisis as a purely humanitarian matter when it was first and foremost a political issue. Other measures could have been taken, for example, early deployment of human rights observers in Rwanda, increasing the amount of aid distributed directly though Kigali, reestablishing the justice system as quickly as possible, and organizing a Nuremberg-style trial for the main instigators of the genocide. If the right conditions had been provided, many humanitarian organizations were convinced that most of the refugees would have returned home. Instead, it is very likely that the world will have to assist two million refugees for a period that could stretch into years, war may well break out again, and further aid will be required for future victims. Political inaction thus risks a much stronger negative effect on the situation than the positive effects of the outpouring of solidarity that swept the world in 1994.

Humanitarian action provided a way of responding to the crisis while continuing conveniently to overlook the fact that a genocide had taken place, until the situation had evolved to the point where it could be ignored completely. In a world where humanitarian aid seems almost the only international response to a crisis, aid that neither can nor will make a distinction between different categories of victim, all catastrophes are treated alike and reduced to their lowest common denominator—compassion on the part of the onlooker. Certainly all victims merit our care and consideration, whether they be Tutsis suffering as a result of genocide or their murderers forced to become refugees and struck by cholera. Humanitarian action is at the service of all victims: it seeks to care for and feed them and does not take sides. But goodwill on its own is not enough and humanitarian aid is useless if it is not accompanied by political action and efforts to achieve justice.

Humanitarian action transforms any dramatic event—crime, epidemics, natural disasters—into catastrophes for which it seems that nobody is every given the blame. Humanitarianism also masks the obligation and the necessity to intervene in other ways and acts as a defense against any possible future accusation of nonassistance to persons in danger. There are only a handful of individuals who might risk speaking out in the middle of a catastrophe, when donations are rolling in, to point out that giving food and drink to people who have lost everything in the wake of horrendous massacres is only the least that can be done. Unfortunately, any kind of debate along these lines is usually pursued when it is too late to be anything other than theoretical. It only can be usefully carried on while a crisis is occurring and some practical resolutions can be reached. Leave it too long and those who should be accused of mass murder have succeeded in rehabilitating themselves politically and become parties to the debate.

In short, confronted with the first unquestionable genocide since the Nazi Holocaust, the world reacted with indifference. It was the sight of hundreds of thousands of refugees pouring out of Rwanda and the subsequent cholera epidemic that aroused compassion and led to a purely humanitarian intervention. This was a convenient cover-up for nonintervention at the political or military level and allowed Western governments to look good because they appeared to be doing something. The refusal of the UN and the principle countries that should have been involved to take a firm stand against the former criminal regime in Rwanda allowed them to remain neutral in the face of the planned extermination of a population. But the concept of neutrality has no sense when genocide is being carried out.

The Limits of Humanitarian Action

Humanitarian action has acquired a monopoly on morality and international action in ongoing wars of a local nature. But if it is not coupled with political action and justice, it is doomed to failure: it can work as a palliative, not as a panacea. Even worse, when held up to the limelight by the media for its work during a major crisis, it becomes little more than a plaything of international politics, a conscience-saving gimmick. There is an enormous disparity today between the principles and values proclaimed by our democratic societies on the one hand, and the measures taken to defend them on the other. In summary, although we may take great satisfaction in commemorating past victories over tyranny, the historical lesson was not sufficiently well absorbed to move us into action against the first indisputable genocide since World War II in Rwanda or the return of ethnic cleansing to the heart of Europe.

For the international community to claim neutrality is a shaky defense of inaction. To be neutral is defined in the dictionary as "not assisting either party in the case of war between other states."[9] The Red Cross is more specific: "In order to maintain the confidence of all parties, the Red Cross withholds from taking sides in hostilities and never takes sides in political, racial, religious or philosophical controversies." This is a radical interpretation of neutrality that suits the very specific mandate of the Red Cross (especially in regard to prisoners of war). However, if applied generally by the international community, NGOs, the UN, and individual states, there may be disastrous consequences for populations in danger.

A claim of neutrality makes no sense at all in the case of genocide, where neutrality is reduced to the weakest possible definition of "indifference" and succeeds only in removing every distinction between the victims and those who victimize them. A number of humanitarian organizations have founded a very comfortable refuge in neutrality on the intellectual level, which provides them with an excuse not to question the sense or the consequences of humanitarian action. Indeed, neutrality can become a refuge large enough to accept inhuman policies.

Whether working at the heart of conflicts, the course of which they influence, or whether faced with governments and totalitarian parties that are void of any scruple, humanitarian organizations are always faced with two recurring and related questions in the long term: first, to use the expression of William Shawcross, "how to feed the victims without also providing aid to their tormentors,"[10] and second, how to avoid humanitarian aid involuntarily having a negative effect on the victims instead of improving their situation. These questions often take on sharper meaning in extreme crisis situations. It is self-evident that humanitarian action saves human lives. But it also risks a series of induced and secondary consequences that are extremely important. In Somalia, food and other resources provided by the humanitarian organizations help keep the conflict alive because gangs of armed bandits also benefit from it. Such aid often helps to prolong and modify the course of a conflict in other ways, because humanitarian organizations require authorization from the warring parties in order to have access to victims and this renders them vulnerable to blackmail, manipulation, and all sorts of other pressures.

Alternative Reactions

Diagnosis

A doctor's duty toward a sick patient is first to establish a diagnosis before under-taking a treatment, and this principle should be applied just as systematically by the international community when faced with a crisis situation. We have too often seen a cure attempted before any serious analysis of the situation has been carried out. This results in a rash and unreflective prescribing of the type that largely explains the failures in international responses to Rwanda and the former Yugoslavia. Intervention should be a question of timely reaction motivated by political rather than humanitarian intentions. When the UN has to deal with a deadly conflict, it should analyze what is at stake for the parties involved, particularly the civilian population, and then base its response on a clear distinction between two kinds of conflict.

On the one hand, there may be a clear-cut, unilateral aggression by a very much stronger party against another. In such cases, the UN cannot remain neutral. It must stand with the victims and the "weaker side" against the aggressor, and mili-tary intervention should at least be seriously considered. However, given that this might entail a risk of involvement over a long period, urgent consideration should also be given to other possible actions, including the use of diplomatic or economic sanctions. What is important is that the international community show a clear signal that it will no longer stand by helplessly in the face of massacres and the slaughter of civilians.

In Bosnia, during the spring and summer of 1992, a choice had to be made between allowing Serbia's Milosevic and Karadzic to seize territory and practice ethnic cleansing and supporting the multinational government led by Bosnia's President Izetbegovic. The second alternative was the only one worthy of honest consideration. In Rwanda, as soon as it became obvious that Habyarimana's regime and his armed forces were conducting a genocide, the only morally responsible choice was to support the forces of the RPF, who could have halted the genocide. In cases such as these, it should be clear which is the right choice to make.

On the other hand, the conflict may take the form of a general breakdown in civil order with no clear-cut issues, no central authority in command, and an increasing number of warring factions and militias out of control. This would describe the situations in Somalia. The UN must recognize that very little can be done to prevent or stop this kind of conflict without force, and that its role is to avoid the ultimate collapse of the state and the prolonged suffering of civilians. Every diplomatic measure must be considered, and the earlier the better; the art of preventive diplomacy should be practiced far more often. Humanitarian assistance must, of course, be maintained impartially throughout the course of this type of conflict.

Most crises are a complex mixture of both models and there are some conflicts that do not fit neatly into either description; therefore, diagnosis is even more essential. Other political considerations complicate the situation even more. It is clear that it is not possible to react in the same way to Russia's intervention in Chechnya as to, for example, an attack on Belize by Guatemala. The principal point that must be recognized is that the international community and the UN failed in Rwanda and Bosnia because of a refusal to define and categorize the crises before responding to them.

Impartiality

"Neutrality" is a highly problematic concept. By the official Red Cross definition, "it means not taking sides—military or ideological—in hostilities or engaging at any time in controversies of a political, racial, religious or ideological nature." This is a radical definition. This definition presumes that no distinction is made between, for example, a racist authoritarian regime and democratic forces, between victims and their executioners. It also presumes that the crimes committed cannot be qualified because the parties to a conflict will never agree on the meaning of terms such as genocide or crimes against humanity. This definition of neutrality seems dangerous as it takes no account of the necessary distinction between criminal and other politically motivated actions, or the level of gravity of the acts committed.

There is an alternative to neutrality that does not pose these kinds of problems and that is impartiality. Whereas neutrality focuses on the warring parties, impartiality focuses on the victims as individuals. In this sense, impartiality means making no distinction between the victims with regard to race, ethnic origin, political, philosophical, religious, or other beliefs. In humanitarian terms, it primarily means to stress equality of all those who are in distress, with only priority given based on the acuteness of the need for help. It does not mean reserving judgment of a political nature, but rather recognizing the validity and rights of an individual in distress. Were this concept to be emphasized by the international community and its official bodies (the UN and so on) in situations of deadly conflict, the rights of the victims would pass before that of any such ambiguous concept or excuse of neutrality of sovereignty. There would then be greater freedom to react in a variety of ways, and countries could no longer refuse to do more than provide an exclusively humanitarian response.

Justice

It is essential that those responsible for formulating, instigating, and carrying out genocide, crimes against humanity, or ethnic cleaning be brought to trial. Justice is not only a moral imperative but also a political necessity: Ensuring that justice is seen to be done will discourage others from carrying out further mass crimes. Justice is necessary not only for the victims, but also for international order. There is an enormous potential in the world today for crises with an ethnic dimension. The greatest threat to society internationally is the rebirth of racist ideologies, with their racial hierarchies that reject and exclude all others. Only the threat of punishment for mass murder will make leaders think twice before playing the ethnic card to tighten their slacking grip on power. Justice must play a more important role in international relations and could become a powerful instrument of preventive diplomacy.

Conclusion

Humanitarian action sometimes shows humanity at its most noble, providing assistance to victims, fellow human beings trying to regain control over their own destiny. When the international community, supposedly still acting in the name of humanity, reduces human beings to the status of mere biological organisms by providing food in the place of the military and political support they so desperately need and ask for,[11] then it must stand accused of complicity in a massive crime against humanity: nonassistance to people in danger. It must be states one more time that passing food through the window when nothing is being done to get the assassin out of the house is not a humanitarian act. When hostages are taken, the first priority is to overcome the hostage takers, not to feed the hostages while they are eliminated one by one.

To sum up, humanitarian problems are always the result of some more profound problem and cannot be solved by humanitarian means alone. In cases of aggression, crimes against humanity, and genocide, the international community can no longer invoke neutrality and be satisfied with an exclusively humanitarian approach, rendering it an accomplice to the most criminal regimes. If humanitarian assistance is to be worthy of its name, it must work in parallel with efforts to meet the demands of justice and respect for human rights.

Torture

Timothy W. Harding, M.D.

Torture has been and remains a constant in human society; its history is closely linked to the evolution of state powers and the exercise of authority.[1] In all circumstances, the notion of torture has two essential elements: the purposeful infliction of pain, usually described as excruciating, and an ulterior motive in the interests of the authority responsible for the torture.[2] The pain can be either physical or psychological in nature, and most authorities would accept that provoking intense fear through mock executions or threats to family members can be considered a form of acute psychological pain. Furthermore, the notion of humiliation is considered by many authorities as central to the process of torture, being antinomic to the principle of human dignity at the origin of modern concepts of human rights.

The most frequently cited motive for torture is the extraction of a confession or the obtainment of information during interrogation. The Japanese word for torture, *gōmon*, is made up of two *kanji*, the first, rather rarely used in Japanese language, meaning "to flog" or "to beat," and the second a commonly used *kanji* meaning "to question." However, torture is also used as a form of punishment, intimidation, and coercion outside the interrogation process. The use of torture on a large segment of the population, including rape and mutilations, is recognized as a means of intimidation against populations or minorities.[3]

The word for torture in most European languages is derived from the Latin "to twist" or "to distort," reflecting techniques of torture involving forcible extension of the body or twisting of limbs, provoking intense musculoskeletal pain. The word can also be taken to reflect the fundamental distortion in the human relationship between the torturer and the tortured person. It should be recognized that, as well as the tortured person's losing his or her fundamental human dignity and suffering long-term consequences, both psychological and physical, the torturer is also debased and humiliated by his activity. A key question, therefore, is why individuals are prepared to torture. At one time, it was thought that only particularly sadistic individuals were capable of committing torture. However, psychological experiments show clearly that most normal individuals are capable of inflicting even apparently intense pain under experimental conditions.[4] It is the perception of the victim and his or her difference and inferiority, as well as dangerousness, that allows individuals with a normal psychological makeup to commit acts of torture. A striking example is the systematic rape of civilian women by soldiers during armed conflict, for example when the Japanese Imperial Army entered Nanking in 1937,[5] or, by Serb forces during the war in Bosnia. In both instances, there was an open permissiveness and even encouragement by senior military officers, as well as a perception of Chinese or Muslim women as racially inferior.

Brief Historical Review

Paradoxically, it is easiest to provide a well-documented account of torture in early civilizations in ancient Greece and Rome, as well as in the Middle Ages in Europe up until the eighteenth century, than in the modern world.[6] This is because torture was openly practiced and was part of judicial procedure, both during investigation and as part of punishment. In both ancient Greece and Rome, slaves were systematically tortured if they were involved in a judicial procedure, whether as accused or simple witnesses, in order that their testimony could be heard in court. The earliest debates about torture come from Roman times, when both Seneca and Cicero criticized the torture of free men as being likely to lead to false confessions: "Even the innocent may lie when tortured." This is a utilitarian and legalistic argument against torture, rather than a moralistic or humanitarian opposition. Saint Augustine is often cited as the first to oppose torture on the grounds of its moral perversity. However, even his opposition is centered on the risk of punishing a person for a crime falsely confessed under torture. He did not take a clear position against the humiliation and infliction of pain during criminal procedures or as part of punishment.

The late Middle Ages and the period of the Reformation and Counter-Reformation saw an institutionalization and reutilization of torture; many woodcuts of this period give explicit details of torture instruments and methods. The use of torture was common during the times of religious divide. The use of torture during the period of the Inquisition in Spain has probably been exaggerated and its main victims were not religious dissenters but the Jewish and Moorish minorities.

In the eighteenth century, during the period of the Enlightenment, the first clearly enunciated oppositions to torture on moral and humanitarian grounds were published by Voltaire, Rousseau, and Hobbes. Their philosophical position was linked to the new concept of the relationship between the individual and the state enshrined in the American Constitution and the Declaration of Rights of the Citizen following the French Revolution.

Torture was first abolished in Sweden in 1734, and almost all European countries had abolished torture from the provisions of criminal procedure by the early nineteenth century.

There is surprisingly little written about the effects of this prohibition on interrogation procedures, and only fragmentary accounts of torture exist after its abolition in nineteenth-century Europe. Many political activists claimed to have been beaten or subject to prolonged solitary confinement, particularly in czarist Russia. In North America and Europe, the term "third degree" method came into use for police questioning of difficult suspects, and certainly involved methods that today would be considered as torture. It was the unprecedented and systematic abuses committed by the Third Reich and the Japanese Imperial Forces in the form of genocide, other forms of mass murder, human experimentation, and abuse of prisoners that led to the Universal Declaration of Human Rights and the outright prohibition of torture in any form.

It is only a little over sixty years ago that torture was prohibited in a series of interlocking provisions of international law; nevertheless, all objective assessments about the prevalence of torture in the world today lead to the conclusion that systematic torture occurs in one form or another in the majority of states despite the fact that they have confirmed their adherence to the Universal Declaration of Human Rights and have ratified the United Nations' International Covenant on Civil and Political Rights. Article 7 of this covenant reads: "No one shall be subjected to torture or to cruel, inhuman, or degrading treatment or punishment."[7] Torture is also prohibited in times of armed conflicts by the Common Article 3 to the Geneva Conventions. It is outlawed by the 1994 United Nations' Convention Against Torture. In the statute of the International Criminal Court, torture is recognized as a crime against humanity when it is committed as part of a widespread or systematic attack directed against a civilian population.

Torture is, therefore, one of the few issues in which international human rights and humanitarian law is unambiguous and for which no exceptions are provided. For example, under the European Convention of Human Rights, any high contracting party may take measures derogating from its obligation under the Convention in time of war or other public emergency threatening the life of the nation. However, no derogation is permitted for Article 3, prohibiting torture.[8]

The provisions of international law prohibiting torture did not give clear definitions of what would constitute torture. In most texts, the concept is linked to that of inhuman and degrading treatment, while the International Covenant on Civil and Political Rights (1966) indicated that being subjected to medical or scientific experimentation without free consent is a particular form of torture or cruel, inhuman, or degrading treatment.

The definitions were to come from several sources; first, through the work of the European Court of Human Rights (and later the complementary European Convention for the Prevention of Torture and Inhuman or Degrading Treatment or Punishment of 1989). In the decision concerning the case of Ireland versus the United Kingdom over techniques of "interrogation in depth" carried out by the British Army in Northern Ireland, the court ruling included a detailed account of wall standing, hooding, subjection to noise, deprivation of sleep, and deprivation of food and drink, which were considered as a violation of Article 3 of the European Convention. The reports emanating by the Committee for the Prevention of Torture and Inhuman or Degrading Treatment or Punishment (CPT), set up by the 1989 Convention also give some detailed consideration as to what constitutes torture.

Second, the reports of the special reporter of the UN Commission of Human Rights investigating torture on a global scale also provide descriptions of the wide variety of abuse and treatment that should be considered as torture.

In 1975, the United Nations General Assembly adopted a declaration on Protection from Torture, in which torture is defined as "an aggravated and deliberate form of cruel, inhuman, or degrading treatment or punishment." The essential elements in the definition are the intentional infliction of severe pain or suffering, whether physical or mental, at the instigation of a public official. Torture is thus defined as an intentional act under the authority of the state with the purpose of obtaining information or a confession, but also as a punishment or to intimidate. The 1984 United Nations Convention Against Torture has a closely similar definition, although the role of a "public official or other person acting in an official capacity" is widened to include not only direct infliction but also instigation, consent, or acquiescence. Both definitions from the United Nations exclude "pain or suffering arising only from, inherent in, or incidental to lawful sanctions."

Torture is most commonly associated with attempts by security forces to deal with dissent, insurrection, terrorism or other perceived threats to the authority of the state. One example is the widespread and indiscriminate torture by security forces in Syria[9]. Those in Britain, France and the United States who condemn the abuses in Syria should not forget the systematic use of torture by the British during the Mau Mau uprising, 1952–1960, and by the French during the Algerian War, 1952–1960.[10] In both cases the use of torture by the colonial power provoked "retaliatory" torture by the other side. Military occupation is a potent trigger of torture, as in the territories occupied by Israel or in the aftermath of the Iraq war of 2003. Although public attention was seized by photographic records of the abuse of detainees in Abu Ghraib prison, the violations were part of a much wider pattern of ill treatment of persons detained by Coalition Forces revealed in a report of the International Committee of the Red Cross (ICRC) to the United States government in 2004.[11] The ICRC refers to "prisoners of war and other protected persons under the Geneva Conventions." This was in fact a contentious issue, since the US attorney general at the time, Alberto Gonzales, considered that such detainees should be considered as unlawful combatants and therefore not under the protection of the Geneva Conventions. He also considered detainees held at the Guantanamo Bay detention center as "unlawful combatants," thus authorizing an array of techniques used during interrogation which amount clearly to torture.[12] Some of the methods were reminiscent of those used by the British security forces in Northern Ireland during the 1970s and condemned by the European Court of Human Rights in 1978 but in addition "waterboarding," a refinement of simulated drowning ("submarine") used by security forces in Latin America with the knowledge and tacit approval of US security services in the 1970s. However spurious Alberto Gonzales' argument may be in international law, it clearly illustrates the tendency of executive authorities to legitimize torture as a response to terrorism. The Turkish authorities had the same reflex in their handling of detainees during the uprising by the Kurdish minority and also of members of left wing revolutionary movements.

However, torture can readily become a pervasive practice by the police in dealing with "ordinary criminals" as was the case in Turkey until recently and is still frequent in many post–Soviet bloc countries. For this reason, a case study, "the Angelova affair," is recounted to underline that torture occurs in apparently banal circumstances.

Case Study: The Angelova Affair

A seventeen-year-old boy was seen by the police hanging around parked cars in a small town in Bulgaria.[13] He was chased and apprehended by a policeman and was then seen by members of the public handcuffed to a tree while the police carried out a search of the area. He was taken to the local police station. No written detention order was issued and the register did not have an entry for him. The following morning, the boy was taken by the police to a local hospital, where he was pronounced dead shortly afterward. An autopsy established that the cause of death was internal bleeding in the brain as a result of a fractured skull around the left eyebrow. The autopsy report established that the trauma had occurred between four and six hours prior to his death. There were also marks of recent trauma on several other parts of the body. The medical legal conclusions were therefore clear: the boy had died as a result of a blow received while in police custody, furthermore, there had been a delay of several hours before the boy was brought to hospital; when he arrived, it was too late to provide any care.

Since the police were involved, the criminal investigation into the boy's death was taken over by a military investigator, who appointed five medical experts from the police and military to reexamine the conclusions. Without providing any fresh evidence or arguments, the experts concluded that the trauma could have been received more than ten hours before the death, and, therefore, prior to his arrest. On this basis, the investigation was terminated. No administrative or discipline reaction of any kind was taken.

So ends a typical case of death in custody, giving rise to serious suspicions of ill treatment and possible torture by the police, investigated by another state authority, which concluded clearly that no abuse had occurred. If we add that the victim belonged to the Roma ethnic group, a minority subject to discrimination and social exclusion in many Eastern European countries, we can understand easily why such a boy could be subject to abuse by the police and why the government's investigation was so half-hearted and inconclusive.

The story would normally end there, had Bulgaria not ratified the European Convention of Human Rights in 1992. With the support of an NGO and a human rights activist lawyer, the boy's mother made an application to the European Court of Human Rights on the basis of Article 2 of the European Convention, which guarantees the right to life. The mother complained simply of an unexplained death in police custody, the failure to provide adequate medical care, and the ineffectiveness of the subsequent investigation. The proceedings before the court established that the police had manipulated the detention records and that the government's explanation of the death was implausible. The police had delayed provision of medical assistance and this contributed in a decisive manner to the fatal outcome. Therefore, there had been a violation of the state's obligation to protect the life of persons in custody. Furthermore, the court considered that the investigation carried out by the military authority lacked the "requisite objectivity and thoroughness." In particular, the police officers were never asked to explain why detention records had been forged and why they had given false information on the boy's arrival at the hospital.

The court went further in its condemnation of the Bulgarian government by concluding that the injuries shown at the autopsy were clear signs of inhuman treatment. It was therefore concluded that a violation of Article 3, which prohibits torture and inhuman or degrading treatment, had also occurred.

Finally, the court considered the mother's complaint that the police's abusive treatment was based on their discriminatory perception of him as a gypsy was grounded on "serious arguments," but proof beyond the reason brought out had not been provided.

The mother received €19,000 in nonpecuniary damages.

This case is recounted in some detail in order to demonstrate how easy it is for inhuman treatment amounting to torture and death to occur while in custody, particularly when the victim is from a minority group; and how difficult it is to investigate and bring to account the perpetrators.

Allegations, Denial, and Impunity

The clarity of the legal prohibition of torture is limited by the difficulties of investigation, which in turn leads to the widespread problem of impunity and denial. On each occasion, when reputable human rights organizations such as Amnesty International or Human Rights Watch provide well-documented reports of torture in a particular country, there is a ritual exchange of documented allegations followed by official denials.

One example of such an exchange: on Monday, February 12, 2001, the BBC World Service reports as a main news item:

> The human rights group Amnesty International says torture and ill treatment of prisoners and detainees in China has become "widespread and systematic;" the victims are members of the banned Falun Gong spiritual movement, Muslim separatists in Xinjiang, prisoners in Tibet, many of whom who were reported to have died in custody. Amnesty suggested that the Chinese government's commitment to curb torture was often undermined by its directives to use "every means" in anticorruption campaigns and political crackdowns. Furthermore, the torture and inhuman treatment were often carried out almost publicly in order to "instill fear and discipline."

The message is therefore clear: commitments to end torture do not survive government drives against political opponents or what are perceived as dangers to the fabric of society, such as corruption or separatist or religious movements.

The following day, Tuesday, February 13, 2001, the BBC World Service News carried the rejection by China's Foreign Ministry of the report by Amnesty

International. "The allegations are totally groundless," the Foreign Ministry's spokesman was quoted as saying. Later in the same week, the BBC News carried a further item in which a senior Chinese government official denied the allegations of torture and inhuman treatment of members of the Falun Gong spiritual movement. This spokesman accused the Falun Gong of being politically motivated and "maiming and killing people." He gave the example of the recent immolation of five Falun Gong members in Tiananmen Square as a testimony to the group's inhumanity and deadliness. Furthermore, the official protested about the interference from the outside in China's internal affairs, in particular the protests by the European Parliament at that time concerning violation of human rights in Tibet, the destruction of mosques, and the arrests of teachers of the Koran.

We can see therefore that the problem of torture is not limited to individual occurrences of ill treatment in police custody, prisons, or other state detention centers, however common they may be. Torture is intimately linked to the powers of the state, the belief by those in authority of the need to defend, at all costs, the state's authority and policies, and the perception of individuals and groups as dangerous to the state. The denial of torture by governments is always accompanied by reminders of threats against the state and the dangerousness of certain minorities. The unspoken message is, of course: if torture does occur, it is because it is necessary to defend the state.

The ritual waltz between human rights organizations and governments, with its well-defined, prearranged steps of allegation and denial, occurs dozens of times every year. China, Egypt, Burma, Israel, Russia, Guantanamo, Turkey—the list goes on and on, and the dance always remains the same. And, to be honest, our own perception of these allegations is invariably related to our feelings about the regime concerned. The ritual exchange quoted here took place early in 2001. Since then, of course, the ritual has evolved further: every government response to allegations of torture mentions the threat of terrorism.

Is the Prohibition of Torture in International Law Credible?

The issue of torture today therefore exposes not only the deep-seated fault line about the relationship between the state and vulnerable individuals or groups, but also the very credibility of International Human Rights Law. We have to ask the question whether we are not living an illusion. The unequivocal outlawing of torture in human rights instruments has become a cruel farce in relation to what actually happens in police commissariats, interrogation centers, and prisons in most countries of the world. By participating as lawyers, medical experts, international civil servants, or academics in the ongoing debates and processes at the international level, while ignoring what really happens in the shadows of states' power and structures, we are actively participating in this farce. Would it not be more honest to face up to the ineffectiveness, the impotence, of International Human Rights Law in the face of the power and prerogatives of individual states?

Such a position might seem heretical to most observers of the human rights scene and participants in international organizations and NGO militants. It would be seen as an acknowledgement of defeat, a surrender, or, in more subtle terms, an appeasement. However, such a position would be more in line with historical reality. Torture has existed under all civilizations. (We should perhaps pause a moment to note the paradoxical nature of this simple statement: Can torture really be part of a civilization? Or does civilization necessarily imply some form of state authority that, in turn, opens the way to torture and inhuman treatment?) Well, according to historical perceptions of civilization, torture has almost always been an integral part of it; the question is whether it always will be. As indicated above, for most of recorded history, torture has been a formal part of juridical procedure, used for obtaining information, forcing confessions, and also for punishment and execution. In China and Japan, torture practices are reflected in specific language and terminology, which was found also in the detailed, almost obsessional, inventory of torture techniques and instruments developed in Europe in the late Middle Ages and during the Inquisition.

The persistence of torture in the so-called modern era of human rights since 1948 leads us to two kinds of analysis. First, whether torture is the inevitable response of the state under threat, for example in time of war, when faced with acts of terrorism or deep-seated social ills, and second, how it is that the complex and wide-ranging provisions of international law are so consensual in public discourse and so ineffectual in reality. Law can only be understood in a historical context, and International Human Rights Law is no exception. The preamble of the Universal Declaration describes the context clearly: "Whereas disregard and contempt for human rights have resulted in barbarous acts which have outraged the conscience of mankind . . ." It is therefore a reaction to the horrors of the Third Reich and the Japanese Imperial occupying armies in the middle of the last century. The preamble also places the inherent dignity of all members of the human family as the foundation of freedom, justice, and peace in the world.

This was a period when the concept of the state was undergoing a fundamental change. Keynesian economics and the foundation of the welfare state were changing the relationship between the individual citizen and the authorities. It was clearly seen that genocide, torture, mass rape, and abusive human experimentation undermined the dignity not only of victims, but also of perpetrators and the state itself.

Eleanor Roosevelt described the "basic character" of the Universal Declaration in these terms: "It is not a treaty; it is not an international agreement; it is not . . . a statement of law or of legal obligation; it is a declaration of human rights and freedoms . . . to serve as a common standard of achievement for all peoples of all nations." It was time, therefore, that the people and the nation could be placed on the same footing with an appeal to the dignity of both. The powers of the state should be limited and could not be used to undermine or threaten human dignity. The aim was clearly to eradicate the kind of relationship that had existed between the Nazi regime and Jews, gypsies, and the mentally ill, or the Japanese military forces and the civilian population in Nanking or Manchuria.

The failure of International Human Rights Law to reduce substantially the practice of torture is part of wider failure of international public law. The proliferation of conventions covering women, children, minority groups, indigenous peoples, the disabled, the mentally ill, and many others, are all flawed by the absence or the inadequacy of enforcement procedures. The special reporters of the United Nations Commission of Human Rights are often hampered in their work by governments, and there is more and more resistance to the idea of international investigative powers and jurisdiction. The idea that International Human Rights Law would progressively influence national law has had some success, and many countries have enacted laws criminalizing torture. However, there has been little success in fields such as the investigation, exposure, and sanctions against torture. Many government leaders express satisfaction about the growing body of Human Rights Law but are resistant to its direct application for vulnerable people. A substantial part of International Human Rights Law law is therefore essentially cosmetic.

The European Exception

The most fertile ground for the realization of the human rights approach has provided, without any doubt, to be Europe. The political and economic context, the recent traumatizing experiences of the Second World War, lent themselves to a proactive approach to human rights, going further than the hortatory tone of the United Nations' texts. Thus, the Convention for the Protection of Human Rights and Fundamental Freedoms signed in Rome in 1950 opens with the statement that the "Western European" governments were resolved "to take the first steps for the collective enforcement of certain of the rights stated in the Universal Declaration." However presumptuous this might seem to the rest of the world, it is undoubtedly true that investigation and enforcement are excessively weak, if not entirely absent, from almost all International Human Rights Law. It is, therefore, hardly surprising that the investigation and punishment of torture is so ineffective and weak at the national level. However, the European Convention did put into place procedures that allowed for the first time an independent supranational body to investigate allegations of human rights violations committed by state parties themselves. Furthermore, the complaints could be launched not only by other state parties, but also by individuals. Thus, in 1978, the court condemned the United Kingdom for systematic violations of Article 3 during the interrogation of Irish Republican Army (IRA) suspects arrested and interrogated by military investigators in Northern Ireland. The court has rendered a number of other decisions on the Article 3 of the Convention in recent years, for example the interrogation of detainees in Chechnya (also the subject of two public statements made by the CPT).

It was rapidly recognized that the impact of the court was limited by its lack of investigative power, especially in situations of detention and interrogation. The revelations at the end of the 1980s and in the early 1990s of abusive interrogation techniques and falsification of evidence in cases against suspected terrorists in Britain, which had led to prolonged imprisonment of many innocent individuals, shocked many people.

It was at this time that the Council of Europe introduced a new convention with extraordinary powers of access to places of detention and with the explicit objective of preventing torture and inhuman or degrading treatment: the CPT. In the early years of the CPT's work, visits and investigations were carried out, which allowed, for the first time, a rather detailed picture of the anatomy, physiology, and pathology of systematic torture to be described. It is not surprising that the early reports of the CPT on visits to Turkey remained unpublished for many years (the reports from the early 1990s detailing widespread and systematic torture were only made public in 1998). Although the sinister interrogation rooms that were a constant feature of Turkish police commissariats have been replaced over the last few years by less intimidating premises and allegations of torture are less frequent, elsewhere allegations of police violence are on the increase. Clearly, both the European Court and the CPT have much work to do, especially as their remit now extends from Lisbon to Vladivostok. The commitment of the forty-odd members of the Council of Europe to collectively prevent and banish torture has therefore achieved some impressive results. Furthermore, the CPT has widened the scope of its work progressively to cover not only police stations and prisons but also psychiatric hospitals, detention centers for immigrants, and juvenile detention centers. However, the existence of the European Court and the CPT did not prevent the extrajudicial detention of terrorist suspects subject to rendition in at least two European states.

From the earliest years of the Council's existence, there was, however, a deeply hypocritical vein to this commitment. France and Great Britain, the self-declared defenders of human rights and democratic values, were becoming embroiled in long and drawn out colonial wars. We now have convincing evidence of the systematic and extensive use of torture and illegal killings as the violent struggle for independence evolved in Africa and Southeast Asia. It is now clear that the most senior military commanders and government ministers were fully aware of these abuses over the period of 1952–1960 and, indeed, provided additional resources and expertise. Thus, in both Malaya and Kenya, the British set up so-called reeducation camps for terrorists, involving prolonged sensory deprivation, humiliation, mock executions, and unrelenting physical abuse. France is trying to come to terms with the admissions by most senior military officers of widespread torture and illegal killings during the Algerian war, 1954–1962. The revelations and apologies or, in a least one case, unrepenting justification are at the same time moving and disturbing.

All these instances of documented and confessed torture help us to understand better the nature of torture and the fundamental distortion of human relationships that are implied. The Bulgarian policeman's perception of a Roma adolescent is of the same order as the Japanese soldier's perception of a young woman in Nanking when the Imperial Army entered in 1937, the same as British interrogation officers' toward Catholic terrorist suspects in Northern Ireland, or of the British and French army faced with military uprisings by people who, until then, had been colonial subjects.

The Medical Profession and Torture

It is widely believed that doctors can and should play an important role in the fight against torture.[14] First, they have the competence and expertise to detect and document torture. When they examine prisoners or ex-prisoners, they may observe physical lesions or the psychological consequences of abuse. Doctors who work regularly in prisons or visit police stations can use epidemiological models to follow the incidence of certain kinds of injuries and draw conclusions about the overall prevalence of physical abuse. They are also able to observe certain patterns of injury and correlate them with type of torture. The forensic pathologist has a special role for cases of death in custody, providing objective and irrefutable evidence of traumatic lesions, their pattern, and timing.

However, this role is limited by the fact that some doctors working for the state are not free to speak out and may be fearful of authoritarian regimes. Indeed, there are many well-documented cases of doctors who have spoken out about cases of torture who have been arrested, mistreated, and even tortured themselves. Doctors, who occupy a privileged position in all societies, should be able to criticize the authorities more freely than ordinary citizens, especially if they have the support of professional organizations. However, this is not always the case, despite the fact that most national medical associations are affiliated with the World Medical Association, which has codified the responsibilities of doctors in relation to torture in the 1975 Declaration of Tokyo. Another limitation is the fact that many doctors are not trained to carry out forensic examinations; few doctors can accurately detect the signs of asphyxia and interpret different kinds of bruising or abrasions. The British Medical Association has been particularly active in leading the campaign of "doctors against torture." The association published a substantial report on torture in 1986,[15] followed by a remarkable publication, *Medicine Betrayed: The Participation of Doctors in Human Rights Abuses*, published in 1992,[16] in which the active role of doctors in a process of torture and human rights abuses is extensively documented. The conclusions about doctors' motives for participating in torture are probably applicable to other professional groups working for the state, particularly police officers, army interrogation experts, and prison guards. The seminal study in this field is Lifton's account of the Nazi doctors, which puts emphasis on the way in which societal pressures progressively distorted medical ethical values.[17] This view has been elaborated by Staub, who also emphasizes the role of military training and obedience, the tendency to "blame the victim," and, above all, the discrimination against and labeling or devaluing of a victim group.[18] Nazi doctors were thus living in a society where fundamental human values had been denied; they, therefore, yielded to the psychological process of fear and threat of loss of their professional identity by adopting the credo of assigning a subhuman status to Jews, gypsies, and the mentally ill.

An important stimulus to medical involvement in the fight against torture has been the role of medical journals. Until 1985, there were very few articles or editorials in the field of prison medicine, human rights, or torture published in medical journals. Since then, the lead has been taken by certain editors, in particular in the *Lancet, British Medical Journal*, and *New England Journal of Medicine*, to open their columns to accounts of torture by doctors working for humanitarian organizations, as well as to more scholarly accounts of torture victims. Overall, the number of papers on the subject of torture (to be found in citation lists) has grown from between ten and twenty in 1985 to well over a hundred articles published each year since 2000.

Ambivalence

Torture and inhuman treatment are a fault line that runs deep and long in almost every human society. Its history is as long as the history of state power and its geographical distribution is planetary. Since the prohibition of torture in international human rights law, we can best describe the attitude of the state authorities toward torture as ambivalent. The risk factors, to employ a public health model, are clear: detention for interrogation, deep-seated perception of inferiority of the victim, and the conviction that the state is under threat (the so-called war on terrorism syndrome) certainly increase the risk of torture of those arrested as terrorist suspects.

Methods of Torture

1. Beating: Kicks, fists, truncheons, canes (*lathi*), whips (*sjambok*), electric cables, plastic bags, *falanga* (beating of soles of feet), *telefono* (beating of both ears with palms)
2. Postural: Prolonged standing, suspension (Palestinian hanging), extension, binding/fixed position, confined space
3. Burning: Cigarettes, acid, hot metallic objects, hot water
4. Electric Shocks: Electrodes (with hand-driven generation), shock baton (battery driven), metallic bed (attached to main electricity)
5. Piercing: Genitals, tongue, hands, fingernails
6. Asphyxia: Plastic bag, gas mask (*elephant*) submersion (*submarine, la banera*), waterboarding, strangulation
7. Psychological: Pressure, threats, mock execution, anticipation (in earshot of torture), humiliation, ridicule
8. Extrajudicial killings: Faked suicide, "attempted escape"

Principles of Treatment of Torture Victims

1. Listening
2. Documentation
3. Avoid encounters reviving torture experience
4. Psychomotor approaches: relaxation/massage/exercises
5. Psychotherapy—cognitive, supportive
6. Psychopharmacology
7. Psychosocial rehabilitation

Today, just as there are international networks of crime, money laundering, corruption, and terrorism, there is also an international network of repression and torture. There is no doubt that security forces, antiterrorist agencies, and secret police maintain contact and share information, not only about investigations and suspects, but also about techniques of interrogation and torture. There is no doubt that the police officers and military investigators concerned believe sincerely that their corporation and the resort to interrogation amounting to torture is justified, whether in Chechnya, Israel, China, or Turkey. In every case, this belief, this justification, is underpinned by a distortion in the perception of the human relationship concerned.

The pessimistic but realistic conclusion of this analysis is that existing human rights law and procedures are powerful enough to counteract this network. Despite this, it is fundamentally important to face up to the historical realities of torture, whatever political, religious, or national affinities may be. Thus, the case brought against General Pinochet and the details of torture carried out under his regime informed public opinion both about the reality of torture and also its underlying purpose as an instrument of state terror. Another case, which has had the same effect of forcing a reluctant public's attention, is that of Teniet El-Hdd, who was born to a sixteen-year-old Algerian girl who had been tortured and repeatedly and brutally raped by more than thirty French officers in an Algerian internment camp. In 2001, a French court awarded damages to the son, thus breaking the preexisting taboo about official recognition of torture and rape by the French army in Algeria.

The final example, of belated recognition of torture and illegal killing is drawn from Geneva, Switzerland, home of many international and human rights organizations. Many visitors include in their itinerary the impressive and monumental Wall of the Reformers, at the foot of the old town of Geneva, commemorating Jean Calvin and his fellow Protestants. The visitor can have little doubt of the pride that underlies such a memorial. Few visit another memorial, just next to Geneva's medical school, which is in memory of Michel Servet de Villeneuve d'Aragon, who was tortured and burned at the stake in 1553, one of the many Catholic victims of the theocratic regime of Jean Calvin. The inscription reveals the deep-seated ambivalence that exists when condemning torture: "Respectful and grateful sons of Calvin our great reformer but condemning an error which was that of his century and strongly attached to liberty of conscience according to the true principles of the Reformation and the Evangile we have erected this expiatory monument." It is a clear illustration of the ambivalence toward the perpetrators of torture and the failure to recognize the fundamental flaw in the relationship between the state and the individual, which underlies such abuses.

Issues of Power and Gender in Complex Emergencies

Judy A. Benjamin

Two key issues dramatically affect the lives of women and children caught in the chaos of complex humanitarian emergencies: protection and equal access to relief goods and services. Equal access means that women and girls have the same access and rights to relief items, shelter, health services, access to clean water, sanitation facilities, training, employment, and education opportunities. Protection's role includes safeguarding displaced people—women and girls, in particular—from rape, abduction, forced sexual slavery, genital mutilation, forced marriages, exploitation, torture, and murder.

The Fundamental Right to Basic Human Needs

Conflict is the main reason people become refugees or internally displaced. Women and children comprise an estimated 80 percent of displaced populations. In situations of complex humanitarian emergencies, women assume primary responsibility for the survival of their families. Women keep the social fabric intact by maintaining cultural practices and traditions even during conflict and displacement.

The basic human needs embody the fundamental rights of all people. Basic needs include food, water, shelter, nonfood items (blankets, clothes, cooking pots, etc.), health care sanitation, education, and opportunities for self-support, as well as freedom from persecution.

Power, Gender-Based Violence, and Access to Food

The entry point for preventing abuse and violence against women is the food distribution line. It is there that gender-power relationships are manifested in harmful ways. Food ranks as the most valuable commodity in a refugee camp. Food can be readily sold, traded, or bartered for cash and other items. Power rests with those who control access to food. Women do not enjoy equal access to food in nearly all of the hundreds of refugee and IDP camps I have visited during the past ten years. Sex exploitation scandals[1] in the camps in Guinea, Sierra Leone, and Liberia point to food as the main resource exchanged for sex. Food and other humanitarian relief items provided by the international community fall under the control of men. Poor monitoring by relief agencies permits the sexual exploitation of women and girls. Other men, including international peacekeepers, military forces, and UN and relief agency employees exploit the severe poverty conditions suffered by the refugees by offering to women and young girls small sums of money or "gifts" in exchange for sex. The majority of the victims of exploitation are females under the age of eighteen—the most vulnerable recipients of humanitarian assistance.

Equal participation in relief programs and services will not guarantee that women will not be pressured into providing sexual services or that they will not be cheated on their rations as they pass through the distribution lines, but the chances of blatant abuse will be lessened with women in decision-making roles and actively engaged.

Refugees versus Internally Displaced Persons

Most conflicts today occur inside the boundaries of the affected country; therefore, the global number of IDPs exceeds that of refugees. In the writer's experience, refugee and IDP camps are much the same. In general, IDPs receive less international assistance than refugees do for several reasons. IDPs fall under the jurisdiction and responsibility of their own government, although in many situations the government may be the cause of the displacement, or may not have the means to offer support to its displaced citizens. The UNHCR's mandate does not normally include responsibility for IDPs, although in some cases they take on the task when requested to do so by the UN Secretary-General. International relief agencies may not be operational in IDP camps unless the conflict has high visibility or has gained international attention.

Applying a Gender Analysis in Humanitarian Assistance

What are the major issues of concern to refugee and displaced women and girls? What steps can the assistance community take to address and ensure the rights of women in emergency situations? How can the gap between policy and practices be closed? What can individual humanitarian workers do to ensure the protection of the rights of vulnerable refugees and displaced persons?

Gender analysis requires a basic understanding of the premise upon which gender theory rests. Gender refers to the female and male roles within a given culture. These roles and the expected behaviors of men and women are based on cultural practices formed over time. We cannot study gender by focusing on females or males to the exclusion of the other sex because gender involves dynamic interactions between women and men; to understand gender-power relationships, we must examine those interactions.

As a concept gender often raises more questions that answers. In many cultures the word gender does not translate into local languages and dialects. Although an understanding of gender and the idea of gender equality has evolved in recent decades, and has become part of the global development and relief vocabulary, in situations of forced mobility, whether caused by conflict or natural disaster, people tend to behave according to the gender norms in their society. Extraordinary events, however, may result in behavior that deviates substantially from social norms or personal standards.

Gender as a Social Construct

How gender is constructed explains the position of women in society. Women in developing countries negotiate their lives within a gender framework set by their particular cultural groups. As Caroline Moser has rightly noted, when lives drastically change, as in the case of forced migration and conflict, women often lose their negotiated positions of strength and revert to less equitable social statuses.[2] If gender is about a socially constructed concept that describes how men and women interact within a particular society and how they define their roles in that culture, then gender constructs are brought with refugees in exile along with other remnants of their culture.

The Gender Dimensions of Refugee Life

A review of refugee literature points to a gap in classifying refugees in gendered roles. Development anthropologist Elizabeth Colson called the gap "biased toward undifferentiated people without gender, age, or other defining characteristics." References to refugees in international agency and media reports often omit reference to gender, age, or other defining characteristics except ethnicity. Media accounts merge refugees into one mass of starving, malnourished people wearing the same bitter, hungry expressions. Such ethnocentric attitudes add to the problems women and children face in the camps. The representation of women refugees[3] has been that of passive, dependent homogeneous victims treated as nameless faces in masses of humanity—individuality and personal identity missing. Harrell-Bond (1996) rejected the idea that women refugees are helpless and dependent. Rather she saw their vulnerability stemming from their lack of participation in humanitarian aid upon which their lives so much depended. The categorization of women as helpless victims marginalized them in the sense that they are not afforded respect and, therefore, not afforded the opportunity to become leaders and decision makers in the camps.

The term "victim" evokes images of helplessness and weakness. Images of resourcefulness, stamina, and fortitude must replace the negative depictions of women to support their becoming important members of their societies.

Tools for Gender Analysis

UNHCR uses a planning tool that they promote in field locations for staff training called the People-Oriented Planning (POP) method. POP examines, among other things, who does what, who owns what, and who controls what within a community. In other words, to better understand how the division of labor, economics, and control over resources are broken down by gender.

The POP method uses a simple framework to analyze gender. The three components are (1) Refugee Population Profile and Context Analysis, (2) Activities Analysis, and (3) Use and Control of Resources Analysis. These analytical components can be charted to facilitate useful checklists for field use.

Gender Violence Associated with Conflict and Forced Displacement

Conflict-imperiled women have been subjected to gender-specific abuses, including rape, sexual slavery, and forced marriages to members of various fighting forces. Systematic and widespread rape and other sexual violence have been a hallmark of many internal and external conflicts around the globe. Sexual violence has been directed against women of all ages, including very young girls. Thousands of reported cases include individual and gang rape, sexual assault with objects, and sexual slavery among other violent acts. All parties to armed conflict have committed human rights abuses, however, the international community has paid little attention to gender-specific violations to date.

Gender violence in conflict situations violates the fundamental human right to mental and physical integrity as protected under the Universal Declaration of

Human Rights,[4] the Convention on the Elimination of All Forms of Discrimination against Women (CEDAW),[5] and the Convention Against Torture and Other Cruel, Inhuman or Degrading Treatment or Punishment.[6] Sexual violence is the chief source of fear for displaced women and girls.

Conflict situations greatly increase the violence inflicted upon women and girls—at no other time are they more vulnerable. Frequently during conflicts women not only lack the protection of their families and spouses, but also are under threat by armed soldiers, who may regard them as spoils of war. Even when abuses are not aimed at them personally, women suffer violations of their human rights disproportionately when the normal codes of social conduct are ignored because of conflict. Teenage rebels have ignored custom and social mores by raping women old enough to be their grandmothers.

When Short-Term Coping Equals Long-Term Risks

Both unequal access to food and gender-based violence lead to coping strategies that may endanger women including increasing their exposure to harmful diseases such as HIV/AIDS and other sexually transmitted infections. These two concerns are among the most critical problems women and girls face when uprooted by circumstances that force them from the relative safety of their homes and villages into temporary living situations fraught with danger and high risk.

What Is Gender-Based Violence?

Gender-based violence refers to violence targeted to people because of their gender, or because of their special roles or responsibilities in their society. In many cases women have sole responsibility for their households. Certain responsibilities of women's gender roles put them at greater risk of injury. Crossing landmine fields or walking near military encampments in the course of their gender-defined task of searching for water and firewood subjects women to maiming, crossfire injuries, and sexual attacks. Gender-based violence may be manifested in several ways: domestic violence, rape, and forced prostitution and marriages. Although rape and other sexual abuses are recognized as serious crimes in humanitarian laws, only recently has the international community addressed these forms of violence as serious infringements of fundamental women's rights.

Rape is a deliberate tactic used in war to dehumanize and dishonor not only women but also husbands, families, communities, or ethnic groups. The humiliation and degradation of rape are only compounded by the impunity of the perpetrators. The incidence of rape against refugee and internally displaced women is higher than what is actually reported. Women IDPs are often reluctant to report rape for fear of retribution from the perpetrators. Other forms of sexual coercion are rife in refugee and IDP settings where young girls may be abducted and forced into marriage or prostitution. Awareness of the problem and special programs are needed to reduce the likelihood of such occurrences.

What Constitutes Vulnerability?

In general, the greater the mobility of displaced women and girls, the greater their vulnerability. Program interventions in emergency situations need to pay special attention when women become highly mobile. War-affected women often find themselves without male household members who under normal circumstances would provide protection to them and their children. When people are forced to flee their homes and seek refuge they often escape with only the clothes they are wearing. Women are usually the ones who must secure the household's necessities, including food, water, and cooking fuel.

In situations of forced migration women without husbands or fathers in their households are more vulnerable to abuse than women with make adults present in the home. Since most emergency situations today are the results of conflict, in many refugee settings women outnumber men. In war zones many men die in conflict, become prisoners, or actively engage in ongoing fighting. Vulnerability also increases during periods of food shortages and scarcity.

Who Is Responsible for Protection?

In the case of refugees, the host state is responsible for the protection of refugees (under the 1951 Refugee Convention obligation). However, the responsibility for protection is also an international one that calls on assistance from UN agencies and NGOs as well as host communities. UNHCR is the primary UN agency with a mandate to provide for the protecting of refugees. Other UN agencies who have taken on protection issues for both refugees and internally displaced people are UNICEF, WFP, WHO, UNDP, and OCHA.

Why Is Response to Sexual and Gender-Based Violence So Inadequate?

Implementing agencies often lack clear and coherent policies regarding gender issues. Even when international organizations' headquarters endorse strong gender policies, the field offices often do not implement programs. This can be due in part to the high rate of staff turnover that makes it difficult to provide sufficient training on critical issues. The tendency to compartmentalize sector activities in the field leads to vertical programming that does not integrate well into other sectors. Gender issues crosscut through all sectors.

Inexperienced Western fieldworkers are sometimes intimidated by unfamiliar cultural practices. Their ignorance creates fear to the extent that they may not respond to events they would not tolerate in their Western environments. Domestic violence is a huge problem in camps. Women are seriously injured and even murdered, but relief workers are reluctant to interfere in household conflict. They may not recognize cases of child abuse or exploitation of child labor. Large poor families sometimes send their older children out to fend for themselves in order to reduce the number of mouths to feed. Some of those children become virtual slaves for their employers.

Cultural Relativism

"It's cultural, there is nothing we can do," is a response often heard from aid workers to excuse themselves from responding to cases of human rights abuse. Humanitarian organizations that work with refugees or IDPs in various cultural settings must be prepared to address misconceptions regarding cultural practices. Assistance agencies must take action to educate their local and international staff about human rights, refugee laws, UN conventions and resolutions, agency policies, and operating practices in order to combat harmful practices that violate international standards. Agencies must clearly state their policies, and staff must be held accountable for carrying out their agencies' policies and intended practices. One of the founding principles of human rights law is that it is not culturally relative—basic human rights are universally applicable as a matter of law.

Most NGOs working in refugee or IDP camps to not consider protection to be their responsibility. Women and girls are insecure and at risk of sexual abuse and exploitation from the time they leave their homes, during the exodus, and ongoing during their refuge in camps. Border guards, police, and military factions demand sexual favors of women in transit. Once inside refugee camps women may fear venturing out of their shelters because of harassment or sexual assaults. In a large IDP camp outside of Herat, Afghanistan, women were afraid to visit feeding centers or health posts because of the number of sexual assaults that took place in those locations.

What Steps Can Be Taken to Increase Protection?

Structural

Changes in camp layout and structures will increase protection and reduce the risk of violence against women and girls living in camps. Such measures include providing lighting, especially around water collection points and latrines; locating latrines safe distances from shelters or setting up smaller latrines to be shared by four to five families; changes in camp layout of latrines and water pumps to less secluded locations; employing women as guards; establishing women's "safe haven houses;" and setting up community night watches.

Protection overlaps into all sectors within camp settings—health, education, income generation, shelter, water, and sanitation. Because of severe water shortages in camps, women often must stand in line for hours both before dawn and after dark for water. Many are attacked or forced to provide sex in exchange for water.

Awareness-Raising

Humanitarian agencies can support women and help build their capacity to survive with dignity. Agencies can help prevent gender violence by raising awareness about gender-based violence within the affected community by providing rights-based programming and by working to prevent physical and psychological abuses associated with forced displacement. The UNHCR *Guidelines on the Protection of Refugee Women* and *Sexual Violence against Refugees: Guidelines on Prevention and Response* are excellent resources. These guidelines should be more widely implemented by international and local agencies.

Basic everyday chores become risky when women have to venture outside camps in search of firewood or water. Some refugee and IDP sites provide truckloads of firewood within the camps. Another approach engages the labor of refugee men to cut wood to supply roadside wood depots. These solutions can be expensive and require donor funding but they provide some protection.

Loss of Social and Cultural Ties

Displaced women generally lack community support. The disintegration of community unity increases the vulnerability of women and children and weakens their coping mechanisms. Women and adolescent girls become easy targets for abuse when they are separated from normal support systems, husbands, and other male family members.

Skills Training and Income-Generation Activities

After basic needs are met and protection ensured, people need assistance to get them on the road to self-sufficiency. Women especially need opportunities to learn how to support themselves so they do not have to resort to harmful and degrading practices. The desperate need of refugee women heads of households to secure food for their children can push women into prostitution. Humanitarian agencies should be aware of the coping strategies of women without male household contributors and help women make healthy choices. The most important help organizations can provide to women is to ensure equal access to all resources offered in the camp. Skills training and income generation are vitally important to improving conditions and in helping to empower women and decease vulnerability.

Protection Under the Law

International and local organizations cannot protect the rights of people under their care without understanding the basics of international human rights and refugee laws. The Geneva Conventions, put into effect in 1950, are the core of international humanitarian law. Humanitarian law is also referred to as the law of armed conflict and covers the wounded and sick in the armed forces, treatment of prisoners of war, and the protection of civilians in time of war—Article 3 of the Geneva Conventions.

The Convention on the Elimination of All Forms of Discrimination against Women (CEDAW) was adopted by the U.N. General Assembly in 1979 and took effect in 1981.

Discrimination against women violates the principles of equality of rights and respect for human dignity, is an obstacle to the participation of women on equal terms with men in the political, social, economic, and cultural life of their countries ... and makes more difficult the full development of the potentialities of women in the service of their countries and humanity.

The Convention on the Rights of the Child (CRC) went into effect in 1990. The CRC definition of a child is "Every human being under the age of eighteen."

Both CEDAW and CRC merge civil and political rights with economic, social, and cultural rights, including the rights to life, nationality, expression, association, assembly and thought, conscience, and religion.

International Response to Gender Violence

The UN Special Rapporteur on Violence Against Women's post was created in 1994 in the wake of crimes committed against women in Bosnia and Herzegovina. The post involves fact-finding missions around the world and reporting findings to the UN High Commissioner on Human Rights, but the post has no enforcement power. The UN can only expose and use diplomatic measures against such practices.

Repatriation and Reintegration

Women from the affected communities should be involved in determining the postconflict needs of women and girls, and they must be fully taken into account in the formulation of repatriation and resettlement plans, as well as during the demobilization and disarmament process.

Rehabilitation and reintegration programs must take into account the wide extent of sexual assault and rape and formulate programs to address the specific needs of survivors. Special initiatives must be developed to ensure that the security and subsistence concerns of war widows and other female heads of household are addressed.

NGOs and UN agencies can provide valuable assistance by sharing their program reports, lessons learned, and experiences of working with refugee and IDP populations with agencies dealing with repatriation and reintegration of the same population. To date such collaboration and cooperation have not occurred effectively.

Governments in IDP countries and all parties should abide by and ensure enforcement of the Guiding Principles on Internal Displacement introduced by the United Nations in 1998. Governments must adopt effective measures to guarantee that the particular security concerns of women and children displaced by the conflict are met, including measures against rape and other gender-based violence. Governments and the international community should take immediate action to ensure that IDPs have access to basic services, particularly in regard to food, shelter, health, education, and protection.

Gender-Based Violence Management in Refugee and IDP Camps

The physical structure and design of camps should be done in consultation with the displaced with the input and guidance from women. Full participation of refugee women in planning and providing services is essential. Female community leaders should play significant roles in camp management, especially regarding protection, the allocation and layout of shelter, and in setting up safe havens for at-risk women and girls. Women beneficiaries should be involved in setting up mechanisms to meet the needs of unaccompanied adolescents, the elderly, and the disabled.

Women should be properly registered and should carry their own documentation. Female-headed households should be regularly spot-checked to assess food security and shelter. Latrines, water sources, clothes washing, and bathing facilities should be central, secured with locks, and well lighted. Female security guards should be stationed at locations frequented by women and children.

Ensuring Compliance by Local NGOs and Refugee Camp Officials

International NGOs and UN agencies should not assume that local NGO partners understand gender equity or international human rights and humanitarian laws. Therefore, their services should be monitored and their activities spot-checked to ensure that women have equal access to entitlements and that gender-based violence or exploitation of vulnerable people does not occur. Monitoring, supervision, and training must be done at the point nearest to service delivery because that is where violations occur. Visual, unannounced, spot-checking by experience staff is the best deterrent to abuses during distributions of food and nonfood items, at wood and fuel distribution points, and at water collection sites. Large illustrative posters strategically placed at distributions points are also very helpful in reminding women and other beneficiaries of their rights but also in reminding male staff to respect the rights of women and the rules and policies of the organization they work for.

International NGOs and UN agencies can promote gender equality by requiring local NGO implementing partners to hire gender-balanced staff. International organizations should insist that women are represented on refugee management teams in appropriate percentages based on the population of the camps. Unless women participate in camp management their voices and concerns will not be heard. Neither literacy nor the ability to speak English should be requirements for active participation in camp management. Those skills would not be required for women to participate in civil society in their home villages and towns.

Suggestions for Field-Based Relief Workers

All fieldworkers need training in gender awareness, human rights laws, and the convention on the rights of the child. Field staff—international and national— must be able to recognize exploitation and abuse of women and children and know what correct actions to take.

Fieldworkers are well positioned to make tremendous differences in the lives of women and children in emergency situations. Once fieldworkers understand the issues and know how to recognize the signs of gender-based violence and child abuse, they can be the best advocates for change.

Conclusion

The source of much of the suffering of women and children in emergency situations stems from their lack of access to food and other entitled resources and services provided for refugees and IDPs. When refugee women heads-of-households receive the basic items to which they are entitled—food rations, plastics sheeting, pots and pans, blankets, equal job and training opportunities—they are much less likely to enter into sexual bartering or to accept exploitative and abusive living arrangements with inappropriate partners. Not only are such coping measures harmful to women but also they represent violations to the rights of women. The denial of equal access to food and other entitlements goes against the policies of the United Nations, international NGOs, and donors who provide with assistance to refugees and IDPs.

Women refugees' voices are too rarely heard. They have little say in camp management, design, or operations, and yet women and children make up approximately 80 percent of the population in most camps. Women in refugee and IDP camps are less likely to be selected as camp managers, leaders, or community educators and trainers than men because fewer women speak English, and hiring English speakers is a convenience to international workers—not a requirement for efficiency.

A gender perspective must pervade all activities in humanitarian assistance. International and local organizations' staff need to be trained in gender principles so they may be sensitive to and understand the different roles, rights, and obligations men, women, and children hold in the cultural groups with which they work. The "gender-blindness" of refugee aid must end.

Terrorism: Theory and Reality

Larry Hollingworth

The semantics of studies on terrorism seem to strive more for political correctness than for presenting an accurate picture of the soil in which these terrible acts are usually born, gestate, and explode. Definitions divorced from reality offer, at best, a two dimensional view of a multifaceted problem. To focus solely on acts of desperate individuals and to not equally consider official or state terrorism is not only a simplistic approach but also one that fails to make the obvious linkage of violence to violence.

I have served as a humanitarian worker for refugees and displaced persons, and as a negotiator, in areas of armed conflict in many parts of the world. I have personally witnessed the perverse impact of occupying governmental forces on innocent civilians in Srebrenica, Chechnya, Aceh, East Timor, Rwanda, and Palestine.

Where there is an overt government policy to terrorize civilian populations into a dependent, even supplicant, state, the silence of the oppressed can be very deceptive. Hatred breeds when homes, fields, schools, hospitals, water and electricity supplies, and vital records are wantonly destroyed; when well-equipped armies use overwhelming force against entire townships, killing and maiming women and children; when targeted assassinations and torture instead of the rule of law are used by sovereign states.

In this chapter, I shall offer the reflections of a fieldworker on some commonly used definitions in the "war on terrorism," and then provide a view of terrorism as perceived and experienced on the ground by civilians under army occupation.

Definition

Look up "terrorism" on the web search engine "Google"; there are more than fifty pages of entries, many clamoring to define what it is. In the excellent book *Political Terrorism*, the authors Alex Schmid and Albert Longman offer twenty-six choices.[1]

Noam Chomsky, in one of his numerous papers on the subject, offers two approaches to the study of terrorism: the literal and the propagandistic.

> Pursuing the literal approach, we begin by determining what constitutes terror-
> ism. We then seek instances of the phenomenon—concentrating on the major
> examples . . . and try to determine causes and remedies. The propagandistic
> approach dictates a different course. We begin with the thesis that terrorism is
> the responsibility of some officially designated enemy. We then designate ter-
> rorist acts as "terrorist" just in the cases where they can be attributed (plausibly
> or not) to the required source; otherwise they are to be ignored, suppressed, or
> termed "retaliation" or "self defense." It comes as no surprise that the propagan-
> distic approach is adopted by governments generally, and by their instruments
> in totalitarian states.[2]

The U.S. Department of State definition is, "Terrorism is premeditated, politically motivated violence perpetrated against noncombatant groups by sub-national groups or clandestine agents usually intended to influence an audience. International terrorism is terrorism involving citizens of the territories of more than one country."[3]

The U.S. Army *Operational Concept for Terrorism Counteraction* pamphlet 525-37 of 1984 defines terrorism with a commendable economy of words as "the calcu-lated use of violence or threat of violence to attain goals that are political, religious, or ideological in nature. This is done through intimidation, coercion, or instilling fear."

Igor Primoratz, a philosopher at Melbourne University, defines terrorism, "for the purpose of philosophical discussion . . . as the deliberate use of violence, or threat of its use, against innocent people, with the aim of intimidating some other people into a course of action they otherwise would not take." Thus, he states, "terrorism has two targets. One person or group is attacked directly, in order to get at another person or group to intimidate them into doing something they would not do. In terms of importance, the indirect target is primary and the direct target secondary. The secondary, but directly attacked target is innocent people."[4]

Rakesh Gupta presents a simpler "philosophical" offering. "In any discussion on terrorism—whether it is criminal or political—denial of the right of life would be the basic philosophical category of analysis." This statement seems to suggest that political terrorist acts may be legal. But Gupta continues and clears up the doubt: "Since a terrorist action today is a small group action against innocents and is against either national or international law, it is criminal."[5]

Back to Igor Primoratz to define who the victims of terrorism are:

The innocents . . . persons not guilty of any action or (omission) the terrorist could plausibly bring up as a justification of what he does to them. They are not attacking him; therefore he cannot justify his action in terms of self-defence. They are not waging war on him, nor on those on whose behalf he presumes to act; therefore he cannot say that he is merely waging war. They are not responsible, on any plausible understanding of responsibility, for the (real or alleged) injustice, suffering, or deprivation that is being inflicted on him or on those whose case he has adopted, and which is so grave that a violent response to it can be properly considered.[6]

Primoratz importantly further defines the "innocents": "In the context of war, according to the mainstream version of just war theory, this includes all except members of the armed forces and security services, those who supply them with arms and ammunition, and political officials directly involved in the conflict. In the context of a political conflict that falls short of war, the category of the innocent has similarly wide scope: it includes all except government officials, police and members of security services."

This seems to imply that, at least "philosophically," soldiers, politicians, and police are "legitimate" victims of acts of terrorism.

Violence

The key word in most definitions of terrorism is "violence," an action that has been around since Cain slew Abel. Is there good and bad violence, a violence that liberates and a violence that enslaves? St. Thomas Aquinas maintained that, "violence is good or bad depending on the use or purpose to which it is put." In his book *Violence*, Jacques Ellul stresses the importance of who is responsible for an act of violence and introduces the concept of "force" by quoting the well-known example used by the theologian Suarez: "a man cannot lawfully kill his neighbor, nor can two men together, nor ten thousand, but a judge can lawfully pronounce a sentence of death. His indisputable legitimate power derives from the state. There is all the difference between violence and force."[7]

Does this "force" absolve a state from a crime of violence? Not all states and state decisions are necessarily just or right. The power that condemns to death may be tyrannical or oppressive or simply make a mistake. How legitimate is the state? Did the state or the ruler of the state achieve power justly or unjustly? Does the state's use of force conform to law—national and international? Jacques Ellul again: "Force used by a state is just when its use conforms to the laws; when it does not conform to the laws, it is still force—not violence—but unjust force." Scant comfort for the victim but encouragement for retribution.

Ellul has five rules, which he cautions all who contemplate violence to remember:

1. Once begun there is continuity to violence
2. There is reciprocity: violence begets violence
3. Violence begets violence . . . and nothing else (I am not happy with this one)
4. There is sameness to violence—there are proportions and shades but essentially violence is violence
5. The perpetrators of violence always try to justify the violence and themselves

The Cycle of Violence, the Tandem of Responsibility

"Who started it?" Is there a parent or teacher who has not asked this question?

How often do we hear spokespersons, especially in parts of the Middle East, say, "In response to . . . we have carried out . . ."? In any major crisis over the past decade, it would be very difficult to define when the crisis began and by whom: Sudan, Somalia, former Yugoslavia, Rwanda, Chechnya, Aceh, and Palestine, and I only choose some of those where I have served. But each and every side can point to the last incident as the one that they must revenge, and so the cycle continues. Once the violence begins it is difficult to effect reconciliation. A leader at any level who is prepared to attend talks with the other side risks the accusation of weakness or collaboration. But unless both sides can at least glimpse the view from the other side, there is no hope.

The French Franciscan Father Maillard, when Director of Frères du Monde, published in their magazine this observation: "It is always the violence of the oppressor that unleashes the violence of the oppressed. The time comes when violence is the only possible way for the oppressed to state their case." Again, speaking only from personal experience, I cannot fault this.[8]

The black power leader Pastor Albert Cleage Jr. said after the race riots in Detroit: "Now we are no longer afraid; now it is the white man who is afraid." The violence of the oppressed transfers fear to the oppressor previously secure in his dominance. This is particularly so today in Israel where the Palestinian retaliation includes a weapon that truly frightens the Israeli population: the suicide bomb. Rattle the bars of a caged lion and you must expect to be scratched or bitten.

The Perpetrator

Who is a terrorist? It depends on who applies the label. One man's terrorist is another man's freedom fighter. Or, to quote Noam Chomsky: "actions undertaken against oppressive regimes and occupying armies (are) considered resistance by their perpetrators and terrorism by the rulers, even when they are non-violent."[9]

Terrorists espouse a cause. The focus of the cause can be any shade of the rainbow. They may represent the have-nots—no land, no access to education, no money, no status, no resources; the religiously oppressed; the racially oppressed; the politically oppressed; or the culturally oppressed. More often they are to the left of the political spectrum but some of the most virulent are from the right wing. They can be from minority groups, fascists, racists. They come from all walks of life and all strata of society.

Jihad and Martyrs

A number of terrorist groups operate in and out of states where Islam is the major faith. Their campaigns are labeled "jihad" and their dead are honored as "martyrs."

"Jihad" is the verbal noun of the verb meaning "to strive," "to struggle," "to exert." While a number of other nouns can be linked to jihad to give it different connotations, it is now best known in its meaning "armed struggle" and, more specifically, "armed struggle against unbelievers." In effect, it has the same meaning as "crusade"! Jihad is often mentioned in the Koran as *is qitaal*, which means "fighting." The most relevant references are: K22:39, "Leave is given to those who fight because they were wronged"; K3:157–158, which encourages participation in the fighting; and K169–172, which promised rewards in heaven to those martyrs (*shuhaada*) who die in battle. K2:190–194 has a chilling relevance in the Middle East today: "And fight in the way of God with those who fight you, but aggress not: God loves not the aggressors. And slay them wherever you come upon them, and expel them from where they expelled you."[10]

As scholars pore over holy books and interpret them in different ways, the Koran is no exception. There are at least two distinct schools, the Modernists and the Fundamentalists, and two different ways of approaching the interpretations; one is to take each verse in traditional order and to examine its content in depth, the other is to gather together all the verses on one topic and to examine their relationship. The latter produces the more moderate interpretation.

Rebels

Gupta is keen to point out the difference between a terrorist and a rebel. He labels Bal Gangadhar Tilak, "who has no fetish for nonviolence," as "a mass leader and not an alchemist of revolution," and similarly labels Mahatma Gandhi "a rebel with his entire pacifist menace." I am happy so far but have reservations with his next statement that: "[a rebel's] commitment is to the cause of his people and not to himself or his group, which is the commitment of a terrorist." This may be true in the Indian examples he gives; I am not certain it is when applied more generally. I suspect that many, if not most, terrorists believe that they represent the true voice of the people. They may be deluded but their zeal is genuine.

Edward Herman and David Peterson, in *Z Magazine*, introduce the concept of "retail" versus "wholesale" terror. "Bin Laden and his network . . . is a 'retail' terrorist network, like the IRA or Cuban refugee terrorist network: it has no helicopter gun ships, no offensive missiles, no 'daisy cutters,' no nuclear weapons. Really large scale killing and torture—'wholesale' terrorism—is implemented by states, not by non-state terrorists."[11]

State Terrorism

State terrorism is a taboo term. Politicians never utter it. Newspapers rarely describe it. Academic "experts" suppress it. It is by far the most menacing form of terrorism.

—John Pilger

We must recognize that by convention—it must be emphasized only by convention—great power use, and the threat of the use, of force is normally described as coercive diplomacy, and not as a form of terrorism.

—Michael Stohl

There are states that support terrorism domestically, states that support terrorism externally overtly, states that support terrorism externally covertly, and states that do all three.

William Blum is the recorder par excellence of the activities of the United States as a purveyor of state terrorism. In his highly readable books he chronicles the participation of the U.S. interventions around the globe. In *Killing Hope*, there is a chapter for each intervention. And there are fifty-five chapters![12] The second book is entitled *Rogue State*. It has three sections: "Ours and Theirs: Washington's Love/

Hate Relationship with Terrorists and Human Rights Violators"; "United States and the Use of Weapons of Mass Destruction"; and "A Rogue State versus the World."[13]

Mavis Cheek, who chose the book as one of the books of the year in the UK Sunday newspaper *The Observer*, wrote, "William Blum, once of the U.S. Department, gives a chilling reminder that while there may be no justification for September 11, there may be reasons."

William Blum is not the only U.S. citizen to criticize U.S. policy. "The guiding principle, it appears, is that the U.S. is a lawless terrorist state and this is right and just, whatever the world may think, whatever international institutions may declare" (Noam Chomsky).

John Pilger, who is much more catholic in his range of targets, writes in a post-Bali bombing report: "Today, largely unreported, the Indonesian military, with the tact approval of the United States, Britain, and Australia, is terrorizing the populations of Aceh and West Papua. Most of the 'human rights violations' in these provinces—the euphemism for state terrorism—have been part and parcel of 'protecting' the American Exxon oil holdings in Aceh as well as the vast Freeport copper and gold mines and BP holdings in West Papua."[14] He refers to research by Edward Herman and Gerry O'Sullivan: "Covering the period since 1965, which points to the killing of several thousand people by nonstate terrorists such as al Qaeda, compared with 2.5 million civilians killed by state-sponsored terrorism. These include the violence of South African apartheid regime, the Suharto regime in Indonesia, the "Contras" in Nicaragua, and other American-backed terrorist states."

The U.S. State Department, which, if Mr. Blum is right, should know a thing or two about the subject, itself maintains an annual list of State Sponsors of Terrorism. It includes Cuba, Iran, Iraq, Libya, North Korea, Sudan, and Syria.

Is a state that pursues terrorism a terrorist state? Primoratz: "I suggest we reserve this label for states that do not merely resort to terrorism on certain occasions, but employ it in a lasting and systematic way and, indeed, are defined in part by the sustained use of terrorism against their own population. These are totalitarian states."[15]

It is, however, important to note that a few nontotalitarian states have used terrorism against their own population.

Is there ever a need for external interference? Irving Kristol believes so: "Insignificant nations, like insignificant people, can quickly experience delusions of significance. . . . In truth, the days of 'gunboat diplomacy' are never over. . . . Gunboats are as necessary for international order as police cars are for domestic order."[16]

A Case Study: Palestine

I choose Palestine for the simple reason that I was United Nations Relief and Works Agency for Palestine Refugees (UNRWA) Emergency Coordinator in Jenin Camp on loan from the Center for International Health and Cooperation. I left there six weeks before writing this chapter. I begin with a caveat: it is difficult to serve in an occupied Palestinian community and be true to the tenets of our humanitarian faith—neutrality, impartiality, and independence.

"What is the difference between state terrorism and individual terrorist acts?" asks Lev Grinberg of the Humphrey Institute for Social Research at Ben Gurion University in an oft-quoted article from the May–June 2002 *Tikkun* magazine. "If we understand the difference," he continues, "we'll also understand the evilness of U.S. policies in the Middle East." He then answers the question he posed. "Israel's state terrorism is defined by the U.S. officials as 'self-defense,' while individual suicide bombers are called 'terrorists.'"[17]

Grinberg is not soft on Palestinian terrorists: "Suicide bombs killing innocent citizens must be unequivocally condemned; they are immoral acts, and their perpetrators should be sent to jail . . . However, they cannot be compared to state terrorism carried out by the Israeli government. The former are acts of despair of a people that sees no future, vastly ignored by an unfair and distorted international public opinion. The latter are cold and 'rational' decisions of a state and a military apparatus of occupation, well equipped, financed, and backed by the only superpower in the world."

"Palestinian violence receives worldwide condemnation" (Chomsky),[18] with the silent rider booming in our ears that Israeli violence rarely does.

It is bitterly ironic that the modern state of Israel, conceived by a biblical promise, born out of a terrorist/freedom fighter struggle, growing up with a population of victims of generations of oppression and constantly led by leaders whose roots lie in the Holocaust, is not able to understand the aspirations and desires of their neighbors with whom they share the land. "Do unto others what you would have them do unto you" is replaced with, "Do unto others what was done unto you."

It is sad that in the international arena "Palestinian" is associated closely with "terrorist," in some circles to the point of being synonymous. This image was beginning to change in the early days of the Second Intifada with frequent television coverage of the new "Davids" slinging stones at the new "Goliath" in his armored vehicle. Unfortunately, a faction of militant Palestinians—how easy it is to label all actions as Palestinian—returned to the suicide bomb as its most successful weapon. More unfortunate was the choice of target. If the suicide bombers had blown themselves up at checkpoints, in Israeli barracks, and in Israeli Defense

Force headquarters, and all their victims were military, I am sure they would have maintained the tide of sympathy and may even have earned admiration for their desperate courage. Better still would have been protest suicides outside embassies or other high-profile buildings where the suicide was the sole victim. Sadly, they chose civilian targets and killed and maimed innocent women and children. They have frightened the Israelis beyond expectation, but have brought upon themselves a ruthless military retaliation and return of the dreadful epithet "terrorist."

I was in Jenin in late April 2002 after the Israeli incursion. The talk was of a massacre. A UN mission headed by Mary Robinson, UN High Commissioner on Human Rights, was refused entry into Israel. The United Nations assembled in Geneva a team of the most respected of international senior persons: Mr. Martti Ahtisaari, former Prime Minister of Finland; Madame Sadako Ogata from Japan, former UN High Commissioner for Refugees; and M. Cornelio Sommaruga, former President of the International Committee of the Red Cross from Switzerland, to go to Jenin to investigate what had happened. This fact-finding mission was agreed to between the UN Secretary General and the Israeli Foreign Minister and had the full support of the UN Security Council. The mission was refused entry into Israel! As well as an insult, this was a grave strategic error. Human Rights Watch (HRW), with a speed and accuracy that should be a model for all agencies, produced in early May a comprehensive investigation report that stated that there was no massacre but many severe human rights violations. I will dwell no more on this incursion but recommend the reader to view the HRW report, which is available on the Internet and whose findings I fully support.[19]

I further recommend the more comprehensive and measured report *Israel and the Occupied Territories, Shielded from Scrutiny: IDF Violations in Jenin and Nablus*, issued by Amnesty International on November 4, 2002. This covers the period of April–June 2002.

I left Jenin in early June and returned in mid-August to a Jenin under curfew. What did this mean? I soon discovered. The Israeli Defense Forces occupied the West Bank. It was not possible to get in and out without passing IDF checkpoints, which was time-consuming for internationals and almost impossible for the majority of Palestinians. The curfew was an added inconvenience. It was imposed either with warning or without. If with warning, the start time was given but rarely the end time.

If it was without warning, tanks and armored cars swept into the town, at least one with a loudspeaker. The population was told, "It is forbidden to move around. Go home and close your doors." From then on anyone who moved risked being shot.

The population of Jenin camp is 13,900. Together the town and camp number 41,000.

Forty-one thousand citizens were expected to clear the streets and get home rapidly. Not too easy; very difficult when you take into consideration that more than a third of the work force of Jenin live in outlying villages. Clear the streets, clear a checkpoint with no warning. Clear the schools, clear the hospital clinics. It would be easy with a considerate occupying force. It would be safe with an occupying force with tight rules of engagement: having clear rules of when they can shoot, at whom they can shoot, and with what warning. With aggressive and often nervous troops who were told that their own safety was a paramount importance, bursts of machine gun fire were common. Fatalities and injuries were frequent events. The terrorizing of the population, constant. It is hard to imagine the fear a tank generates as it growls along narrow streets sinisterly swiveling its main barrel from object to object. And if the barrel stops on you, there is a heart-stopping moment while you silently pray the tank commander has recognized that you present no threat. More than a dozen innocent civilians were shot dead during my time in Jenin. They included women and children. Some youths were shot dead throwing stones at tanks. In every exchange of weapon fire between Palestinian and Israeli, the Palestinian was the underdog, the odd-on favorite to lose. The Israeli response was so unequal, so disproportionate. There was no weapon in any hands in Jenin that was capable of penetrating tank armor. If there had been, they surely would have used it. The IDF could have fired pain ball or smoke or tear gas or rubber bullets and dispersed the Palestinians at no risk to themselves.

After weeks of on and off violence, more on than off, the IDF lifted the curfew and replaced it with a lesser imposition: closure. This was a reward for a lull in the attacks on Israelis.

Closure meant that the town and camp were completely blockaded. There were heavy armored checkpoints at every entrance and exit. Sounds easy. Stay within the camp and town and no problem. But what about the third of the work force who live outside the closed area? This included doctors, dentists, nurses, teachers, tradesmen, humanitarian agency staff, the mayor of the town, the governor. And what about the staff of the schools and the clinics and the university who live within the closed area but whose workplace is in outlying villages? What about farm produce, grocery stocks, medicines, baby milk powder that comes into the town from outside?

Did everything stop? No. So what happened? Everyone from the mayor to the vegetable dealer used taxis to come into or out of the town using fields, tracks, culverts, whatever cover was available. Did the IDF turn a blind eye? It knew that this must happen, had to happen. No, taxi drivers and passengers were killed and wounded. Why?

Unfortunately, there were further suicide bombs, so closure was revoked and military operation mounted. This was curfew and closure with a vengeance. Nothing moved. Houses with good views were commandeered, snipers were placed at vantage points, and armored vehicles were positioned at numerous static checkpoints or roamed the town at will. Anyone on the streets was shot at. It did not take many days before there was little food in the town, no baby milk, and, more importantly, no water. Because of two or three suicide bombers whose mission was not known by any more than a handful of controllers, 40,000 citizens suffered severe deprivation. After a while, some pipelines for essential personnel were opened. Passing through these checkpoints was time-consuming and humiliating. Hundreds were arrested; some interrogated and released, others disappeared into Israeli detention centers. Few were charged. Fewer released. Houses of known terrorists were demolished, their bewildered families left homeless.

When the town was on its knees and morale at its lowest, the operation ended, and, thanking the Lord for small mercies, we gratefully accepted the comparative liberty of closure.

I handed the office over to my successor, another international. Seven days later, he was shot dead by Israeli gunfire in the UN compound during an unannounced military operation. The IDF delayed the arrival of an ambulance, not that it would have been of any help.

It is hard to know where to begin categorizing the breaches of human rights. It will be fairest if I end this chapter with an extract from the list of recommendations of the Amnesty International report. Although written to cover April to June 2002 in Jenin, every observation is valid today.

It is not difficult to conclude that the population of Jenin is terrorized by the IDF.

It is also indisputable that suicide bombers came from Jenin. It is indisputable that there are terrorist cells operating within Jenin. It is indisputable that there have been bomb-making factories in Jenin. It is indisputable that there are armed men shooting at Israeli troops in Jenin. Perhaps they number fifty or sixty. Because of them, 39,950 are collectively punished. IDF soldiers killed more Palestinians than suicide bombers killed Israelis. No one placed curfews or closure in their towns. They are, however, now fencing themselves in, creating prisons for themselves mentally and physically.

Their tactics are increasing the numbers of hardliners in the camps and towns.

They fail to see that they escalate the cycle of violence. Suicide bombs are a reaction to violence, not an initiator of violence. Both sides have told me that there is no alternative to their tactics.

Sadly, the answer lied with the United States. As I write, an Israeli team consisting of the Defense Ministry director general, the Prime Minister's bureau chief, and the Finance Ministry director are in Washington to present a request for $4 billion for special defense aid and $8 billion in loan guarantees. Few doubt that they will get it.

"It is absurd that we are still witnessing, in the twenty-first century, a case of occupation where the dominant side is seen as the victim" (Lev Grinberg).[20]

Summary of Amnesty International Recommendations

Amnesty International calls on the government of Israel to:

Ensure the IDF operations are conducted in full respect of international human rights and humanitarian law

Initiate a full, thorough, transparent, and impartial investigation into all allegations of violations of international human rights and humanitarian law, including those documented in this report, and to make the results public

Cooperate with United Nations investigations

Bring to justice those alleged to have committed serious violations of international human rights or humanitarian law in proceedings that meet international standards for fair trial

Ensure prompt and adequate reparation for victims of serious human rights or humanitarian law violations

Respect and protect the human rights of all persons living in the Occupied Territories without discrimination

Include the practices of Israeli authorities in the Occupied Territories in all reporting to UN human rights treaty bodies

Take immediate action to prevent the IDF from compelling Palestinians to take part in military operations or to act as "human shields" and to take measures against any soldier or military commander who undertakes or sanctions such practices

Fulfill its international legal obligations by ensuring that medical staff and ambulances are allowed to carry out duties without undue delays, and with safe passage

Ensure safe access for humanitarian and medical supplies

Immediately stop the use of lethal force to enforce curfews

End collective punishments, including house destruction, closures and curfews, and cutting off water and electricity

End torture or other ill treatment of those in custody

End administrative detention and release all administrative detainees unless
they are to be brought to trial for a recognizably criminal offence in a trial
which is in accordance with UN fair trial standards

Accept an international monitoring presence in Israel's Occupied Territories
with a strong human rights component

Amnesty International calls on the Palestine Authority to:

Take all action to prevent anyone under its jurisdiction from attacking or otherwise endangering the safety of civilians

Amnesty International calls on the Palestinian armed groups to:

Respect fundamental principles of international law that prohibit the killing
of civilians

End any use of children in armed operations[21]

Addendum

Since I wrote the preceding, there has been a lot more reality and no less terrorism.
Osama bin Laden is dead and buried at sea; Al Qaida has not gone away but has
opened branches elsewhere. There seems to be no shortage of volunteers for suicide
missions. The planting of improvised explosive devices has taken a heavy toll of
lives notably in Afghanistan. Kidnapping, especially of aid workers has dramatically
increased, gangsters colluding with terrorists raise the ransom demands and complicate negotiations. The continuing lawlessness in Somalia has caused one refugee
camp in Kenya to swell by one thousand new arrivals per day. Dadaab is now the
largest refugee camp in the world, with upward of 500,000 displaced, making it the
third largest city in Kenya. In the same region piracy abounds.

I concentrated in the chapter on field examples where I had played a role. I
touched on state terrorism and chose a Middle East example. Sadly I intend to do
the same in this addendum.

I worked in Lebanon during the 2006 war. This was a confrontation between
a State and a nonstate actor, a war between Israel and Hezbollah. It is hard to
choose a start point in the lead up to the war but very easy to pinpoint when it

began. On the evening of the 11th of July 2006 Lebanese went to bed after a normal day of work or school or leisure with no warning of what the following day would bring. On July 12, 2006, a stunned Beirut awoke to the sounds and sights of totally unexpected Israeli military action, damaging Beirut airport, destroying roads and bridges, blockading the ports, and invading south Lebanon. 730,000 Lebanese were displaced within Lebanon and a further 230,000 fled to neighboring countries. It was an unequal confrontation, which immediately posed the following questions:

What are the implications of a conflict between a State and a nonstate actor in a neighboring country?

What is the impact on the principle of State sovereignty?

Does a State have a responsibility to deal with its internal 'troublemakers?'

What is an acceptable trigger for the right to self-defense?

How do we measure proportionality?

What is the impact of a conflict on international humanitarian law? And what are the consequences if it is breached?

The humanitarian response began as ever with the assessment and fulfillment of needs to the degree possible. It took a little while before it was realized that the protection of the population was the real need, which could have been achieved with the halting of the Israeli invasion. It took thirty-four days before the international community effected a cease-fire, despite humanitarian and human rights agencies pleading for pressure to be placed on the invading force to stop the fighting, halt the shelling, lift the blockade and permit the safe passage of aid.

The toll of the 34-day war was:

1,183 Lebanese killed and 4,054 injured

At the height of the conflict, 1 million people were displaced

151 Israelis killed (119 soldiers) and 418 injured

5 UN peacekeepers and 1 Red Cross worker killed, 16 UN peacekeepers wounded

Tons of heavy oil polluted 87 miles of the Lebanese coast

6,800 private homes or apartments, 630 roads, 70 bridges and 30 installations (airports, ports, water treatment plants and power stations) damaged or destroyed

778 sites in south Lebanon contaminated by cluster bombs

A reconstruction bill exceeding $7 billion

All of this left us humanitarian responders asking a simple question: "Is a humanitarian response purely the manifestation of the politically possible or just the politically convenient?"

Back to today and to the future. My thoughts concern the harvest from the Arab Spring and the uncertain seasons following it which bring into sharp focus the quandary of a clear definition of who is a terrorist and who is a freedom fighter. History is full of good guys becoming bad guys and bad guys becoming good guys. My grandfather once said to me "Tell me who your friends are and I will tell you who you are" It is becoming increasingly difficult to recognize our friends, "our guys."

A Human Rights Agenda for Global Security

Irene Khan

> Where . . . do universal human rights begin? In small places, close to home—so close and so small that they cannot be seen on any maps of the world. Such are the places where every man, woman and child seeks equal justice, equal opportunity, equal dignity without discrimination. Unless these rights have meaning there, they have little meaning anywhere.
>
> —Eleanor Roosevelt

Human rights are often used by governments as a cloak to put on or cast off according to political expediency, and the UN is often powerless to render states accountable for their adherence to international law and human rights performance. In the words of Michael Ignatieff: "Human rights treaties, agencies, and instruments multiply and yet the volume and scale of human rights abuses keep pace. In part, this is a problem of success—abuses are now more visible—but it is also a sign of failure. No era has ever been so conscious of the gap between what it practices and what it preaches."

That gap was accentuated in the aftermath of the September 11, 2001, attacks as governments geared up to fight "the war against terrorism." It deepened with the military attacks on Iraq. The drive for global security appeared to be trumping human rights with impunity.

This chapter identifies the key challenges posed to human rights by the global security agenda. Recognizing that a narrowly focused security agenda has failed to make the world either safe or free, it argues for a paradigm shift in the concept of security. At the center are not the concerns of states but the human rights of people in the quest for a safer, more just world.

Security for Whom?

In September 2002, when I was Secretary General of Amnesty International, I led a delegation to Burundi just days after a massacre in which some 174 civilians had been killed by the army in a remote village. There were only four survivors. My colleagues and I went to the local hospital to meet them. One of them was a girl of six named Claudine. She could not remember her family name, but she recalled in vivid detail the way in which her grandfather, father, stepmother, and two sisters were killed and her baby brother was bayoneted to death by soldiers. She had somehow managed to crawl between the legs of the soldiers and escape in the commotion without being noticed. A neighbor found her wounded, naked, and unconscious in the forest and had brought her to the hospital, but neither the neighbor nor the hospital had the means to buy her any clothes. That is why Claudine, the youngest of the four survivors of a bloody massacre, was still wrapped in a blanket ten days later when we saw her.

The next morning in my meeting with President Buyoya, I asked him what action he would take to protect civilians in the conflict. He replied, "Madam, you do not understand—we are fighting a war to protect our national security."

There was an unfortunate familiar ring to his response. How often have those words—"national security"—been used by governments to justify the killing of civilians, the torture of dissidents, the persecution of minorities, or the attack on political opponents?

Backlash Against Human Rights

The erosion of human rights by governments in the name of security is not new. What is new is the zeal with which governments have launched a frontal attack on the very framework of human rights in recent times.

In the days, weeks, and months that followed the attacks of September 11, almost every country in the world—from Australia to Zimbabwe—expanded its powers, lawfully or unlawfully, to investigate, arrest, detain, and to restrict people's rights of assembly, free speech, and fair trials.

Between 2000 and 2011 the United Kingdom adopted a range of counterterrorism laws that expanded the definition of terrorism, increased the period of pre-charge detention, introduced and modified the control order regime and increased the use of closed tribunal proceedings and stop and search powers and curtailed the right to protest.

The United Kingdom had adopted a tough antiterrorist law in 2000 that had already led to the banning of twenty organizations, including al Qaeda. Yet, within weeks of September 11, the British Parliament rushed through another piece of legislation permitting the government to detain, on the basis of secret evidence and without charge or trial, foreigners suspected of involvement in terrorism but who could not be deported. The United Kingdom was the only country in Europe to seek derogation from the European Convention on Human Rights to allow introduction of such a measure. Seventeen men were imprisoned under the Act in high security institutions. Following a ruling by the Law Lords, the highest Court in the UK, the men detained under the Act were released in 2005, but immediately put under "Control Orders," tough measures akin to administrative detention in their own homes, imposed by the Home Secretary. Control Orders were abolished in 2011 with the Terrorism Prevention and Investigation Measures Act (TPIM) and replaced with a TPIM notice by the Home Secretary, which has greater judicial oversight and a two-year limit but is basically a control order in almost all but name. Until a 2005 ruling to the contrary by the House of Lords, the Special Immigration Appeals Commission, which hears the detention hearings, took the position that evidence extracted from a third party through torture could be relied on by the Commission to rule on the detentions.

Many repressive regimes have used the so-called war against terrorism as a license to clamp down on political dissidents or minority groups. Others have escaped international scrutiny and censure of their appalling human rights records by professing to join "the global coalition against terrorism."

The enthusiasm of governments to fight "terrorism" has not been dampened by the absence of a common international definition of the term. On the contrary, governments have chosen to define it as broadly or as narrowly as their national, strategic, or political interests call for, making it a shifting concept that is tied to political and ideological interests and, therefore, open to abuse and misinterpretation.

At the international level, for many governments, terrorism signifies an act of violence for what they do not consider to be a good cause. At the domestic level, antiterrorist laws often cover acts that are already criminalized, and so the focus is not on the act or its impact but on the motive. The propensity for abuse is aggravated by the fact that antiterrorist laws are notoriously vague.

In September 2001 the UN Security Council adopted resolution 1373 which imposed binding obligations on all UN member states to take counter-terrorism measures in a broad range of areas, including border control, information exchange, asylum and refugee policies, and extradition, but failed to remind States of their obligation to do so without undermining human rights obligations. It took another two years for a Security Council resolution relating to terrorism to make any mention of human rights. Even the UN has deferred to security over human rights.

Leading the Pack

It is interesting to note the use of the term "war on terror" by the George W. Bush administration. By speaking of "war," it sought to deny the applicability of human rights. By speaking of "terror," it tried to avoid the application of international humanitarian law. By combining the two into a war without geographic or temporal limits, it tried to create a zone of action that is a legal black hole. By taking it one step further to the doctrine of preemptive attack, it made the world a potentially more dangerous place.

Under the Bush administration, the United States arbitrarily detained hundreds of its Arab and Muslim residents. It designated two of its own citizens as enemy combatants, depriving them of legal counsel and *habeas corpus*. It did both without even resorting to the draconian provisions of the Patriot Act, which was rushed through Congress in the wake of the September 11 attacks in 2001.

Doublespeak brings disrepute to human rights but is a common phenomenon among governments. While professing to promote justice, the Bush administration actively tried to undermine international justice and the International Criminal Court through bilateral agreements granting impunity to its own nationals. The message that there is one set of laws for the powerful and another for the rest of the world not only promotes impunity for abuse but also undermines the universality of human rights.

While professing to make the world more secure, the Bush administration undermined the collective security that international law and international institutions offer. It detained hundreds of prisoners (including minors) at Guantanamo Bay, in defiance of the provisions of the Geneva Conventions (a policy the Obama administration continued despite promises to the contrary). Detainees were threatened by the Bush administration with military trials that would violate U.S. as well as international standards of justice, leading one commentator to describe the violations as "the Pentagon's Kafkaesque justice system." In Britain, Lord Justice Steyn, a judicial member of the House of Lords, described the U.S. military commissions as kangaroo courts, a concept derived, as he put it, "from the jumps of the kangaroo . . . the idea of pre-ordained arbitrary rush to judgment by an irregular tribunal which makes a mockery of justice." The U.S. government has ignored allegations of torture and ill treatment by its officials at Bagram in Afghanistan. It has refused to investigate mass murder by its allies in Afghanistan or ill treatment of civilians by its soldiers in Iraq. Some of its actions in Iraq were reminiscent of the violations of international humanitarian law by the Israeli army in the Occupied

Territories: house demolitions, humiliating restrictions on movement of civilians, and failure to investigate civilian killings.

Some governments have seen the actions of the Bush administration as an encouragement to jettison human rights in times of crisis. Others have used it to vindicate their own practices. For instance, the Israeli government has quoted the missile attack by the United States on al Qaeda suspects in Yemen as justifying its own targeted executions of Palestinians in the Occupied Territories.

Collateral Damage

In a climate of fear where even the most powerful and protected feel vulnerable, people are easily persuaded that the price for safety is the erosion of liberty. Yet there is no empirical evidence to show that restraining freedom strengthens security on a sustainable, durable basis. On the contrary, the drive for security at the cost of human rights, far from making the world a safer place, has made it more dangerous by encouraging secrecy, shielding governments from scrutiny, promoting double standards, undermining international institutions and the rule of international law. To those consequences of the backlash against human rights must be added others. The "war on terror" and the war in Iraq have created a deep sense of injustice and alienation that has permeated and deeply divided societies and communities in a way not seen since the end of the Cold War. There is also a growing cynicism about the universal value of human rights. Discriminatory antiterrorist laws in some countries targeted only foreigners or foreign-born citizens or encouraged racial profiling. This kind of stigmatizing is a source of danger, encouraging a climate in which xenophobia and racism flourishes. Muslims, Arabs, and Asians are easy targets of Islamophobia. On the other side, anti-Semitism has also reemerged with the resurgence of Islamic and other political extremism. Political rhetoric about "good and evil,"—"you are with us or against us," "the forces of evil," "them and us"—has widened this gulf.

New seeds of social discord and insecurity are sprouting between citizens and noncitizens. Racism and xenophobia are latent in all societies, but in some European countries they feature blatantly as some politicians exploit people's fears and prejudices for short-term electoral gains. Some aspects of the media have played into this strategy, dehumanizing and demonizing foreigners, foreign-born citizens, refugees, and asylum seekers. They are pointed out as a source of danger and become an easy target for hate speech and violence. Those who need their rights protected the most have become the ones most at risk of attacks.

The increasing polarization between communities has strengthened the hands of those who have always feared the powerful appeal of human rights and who, in turn, are using arguments based on cultural and religious norms to undermine human rights in the Islamic world and in Islamic communities in the Western world. Cultural relativism is being used as a ground to delegitimate the universality of human rights, not only by some fundamentalist and extremist groups but also by some governments in non-Western countries.

Whether at the hands of Christian, Islamic, or Hindu fundamentalists, a common casualty of the "war on terror" has been women's human rights. Western countries manipulated the global security agenda in the name of women's human rights but did little to protect women in Afghanistan or Iraq. The backlash against human rights and the growth of fundamentalism have combined to tighten restrictions on women in Iraq, for instance, and have reinforced the excuses for violence against women in the name of religion, custom, culture and tradition.

Heightened security concerns have also increased pressure on human rights defenders. In many countries, governments have clamped down on activism as a security threat in itself. Activists and particularly small local groups have found that their space for action has shrunk, and that they are viewed with suspicion and even hostility.

In some countries, it has become more difficult to garner public support for human rights work. Human rights advocates work through the pressure of public opinion. The basic premise of their work is that human rights violations anywhere are the concern of people everywhere. It is difficult to mobilize public opinion in affluent societies in favor of human rights when people fear that their own safety might be at stake. It is difficult to promote international solidarity for human rights among ethnic minorities, among the poor and the vulnerable, when they see themselves as the targets, rather than the beneficiaries, of the international security agenda.

Human rights groups have been accused of double standards: of failing to condemn armed groups and "terrorists," while criticizing governments who respond to them. The truth is that most armed groups are not as susceptible to the tactics that human rights advocates apply. "Naming and shaming" is hardly likely to have any impact on al Qaeda! Undoubtedly, human rights groups need to do more to find the levers of pressure on armed groups—for instance, through pressure on allies and supporters, or through exposing the "sources" that provide arms and funds to these groups. But there is no doubt that attacks on civilians by armed groups are a clear violation of international human rights and humanitarian law and can sometimes amount to crimes against humanity and war crimes. Those who commit such crimes must be brought to trial in accordance with international standards. Those who support them, whether governmental or private actors, should be exposed as being complicit in the crime and therefore also liable under international law.

An Agenda for Change

Restrictions on liberty have not paid dividends in greater security. The backlash against human rights indicates that the world today is less free. But the insurgency in Iraq, the anarchy in Afghanistan, and the spate of suicide bombs and attacks in crowded cities from Mumbai to Moscow also show that the world today is less safe.

Building a safer world requires a paradigm shift in the approach to security. Real security comes through respect of human rights and the rule of law. Insecurity and violence are best tackled by effective, accountable states that uphold, not violate, human rights. A trade-off between human rights and security is both unprincipled and shortsighted.

Security and human rights are not incompatible. Governments have the right, indeed the duty, to protect people from attacks by armed groups or individuals but they are obliged to do so within the rule of law and the framework of international human rights. It is possible to carry out both obligations within the human rights system. Human rights treaties are drafted by governments that are acutely aware of security concerns that range from internal subversion to international armed conflict. The treaties therefore grant governments the power to protect legitimate security interests without unduly restricting fundamental freedoms.

Governments are not entitled to respond to terror with terror. Just as criminal violence is best addressed through better—not brutal—policing, so too insecurity and violence are best tackled by effective, accountable states that ensure the security of their people by upholding, not violating, their rights.

There is now—slowly but surely—a better understanding of the balance between security and liberty, at least among some parts of the judiciary. The U.S. Supreme Court decided to examine the legality of detention of some of the people held at Guantanamo and ruled several times against the Bush administration. A U.S. Circuit Court of Appeals panel issued a ruling barring the President from declaring a U.S. citizen an "enemy combatant" without Congressional authorization. A German court upheld the right to a fair trial of a man suspected of terrorist activities and dismissed the charges against him. Legislatures in the United Kingdom and the United States have been less ready to expand antiterrorist powers of the executive. European governments have refused to extradite to the United

States any suspected terrorists without a guarantee against the application of the death penalty. A number of countries, including Brazil, have refused to sign bilateral impunity agreements with the United States.

Addressing Real Sources of Insecurity

Building a safer world also means looking at the real sources of insecurity from which millions of people suffer. Promoting security is not just about fighting a war against terrorism. It is about looking at threats more broadly and understanding them in the context not of state but people's security.

For many people the threat to personal security does not lie in terrorist attacks but in the failure to eradicate extreme poverty and preventable diseases, to arrest and treat the spread of HIV/AIDS, or to halt the flow of small arms. For many women, life will continue to be insecure as long as they are unprotected from violence in their homes and communities. For many people, real security will remain illusory as long as police, courts, and state institutions in their country remain inept or corrupt.

A war was fought to rid the world of weapons of mass destruction. Yet the real weapons of mass destruction are small arms and conventional weapons, which kill almost four hundred thousand people a year. The uncontrollable proliferation of light weapons makes it easier to recruit children to fight wars. The world is awash with small arms: there is one weapon for every ten people and there are enough bullets produced each year to shoot every man, woman and child on this planet, twice. Developing countries spend about $22 billion a year on weapons. For $10 billion, they could achieve universal primary education.

The uncontrolled trade in arms puts the world at risk. In the name of combating the so-called war on terror, many governments, led by the United States, have relaxed controls on exports to governments that are known to have appalling human rights records, among them Colombia, Indonesia, Pakistan, and Israel.

A global problem needs a global solution. An arms control treaty has been in the making in the UN for many years. The permanent members of the UN Security Council are the main producers and traders of weapons. Whether or not an effective treaty will be adopted eventually depends on their willingness to address this problem. Their failure to do so will call into question not only their commitment to human rights but also their responsibility as guardians of international security.

Directly as well as indirectly, women's rights have suffered under a narrow security agenda. For many women, gender violence is the greatest threat to security that they face. In many countries there are no laws to protect women. Even where there are laws, police and the judiciary fail to apply them properly. In some countries discrimination against women is severe, creating an environment in which women are routinely suppressed and attacked. Poor women are more exposed to violence and less able to escape it than women of wealthier means.

All women have the right to be free from violence by state or private actors. Governments need to introduce legislative and judicial changes to protect women's human rights. More support must be given to women's groups to organize themselves against violence. More investment must be made in education for girls and employment for women.

Extreme poverty is a major source of insecurity for millions of people. In a world where globalization has brought unbelievable affluence and wealth to many, absolute poverty has persisted and inequality has grown. The Universal Declaration of Human Rights proclaims that people have the right not only to liberty and freedom of expression but also to a standard of living adequate for their health and well-being, including food, housing, and medical care. Reorienting the security agenda in favor of human security and human rights will require enormous commitment and investment by governments and the international community, financial institutions and business leaders, and civil society. It will require a new approach to aid and trade. New funds must be found to meet the social needs of poor and marginalized communities. New money must be found to help countries build fair and effective justice and policing systems, so that legal justice can go hand in hand with social and economic justice.

Globalizing Human Rights

Global insecurity, far from diminishing the value of human rights, has actually heightened the need to respect them. The failure of the international community to effectively uphold those rights only underlines the importance of human rights defenders and activists in bringing about change.

Local human rights groups, social movements, and activists are the real lifeblood for change around the world, opening up societies, and fighting for international standards of human rights and good governance. They are also an important antidote to attacks on human rights by governments, armed groups, or others. Together with international human rights organizations they form a global civil society that exposes abuse, challenges injustice, and strives for greater accountability.

The challenges facing human rights activists today are stark: to confront the threat posed by callous, cruel, and criminal acts of armed groups and individuals;

to resist the backlash against human rights created by the single-minded pursuit of a global security doctrine that has deeply divided the world; and to redress the failure of governments and the international community to deliver on social and economic justice.

The power of people to bring about human rights change should not be under-estimated. Human rights provide a tool to human rights defenders. They give voice to the powerless: the prisoner of conscience, the prisoner of violence, the prisoner of poverty. They bring hope to millions. Human rights are a banner to mobilize people globally in the cause of justice and truth. They provide a fractured world with a glue to bind people in favor of equality, freedom, and justice, and against violence and abuse. They offer a powerful and compelling vision of a better and fairer world for all men, women, and children, and provide a concrete plan of how to get there. That is why a sustainable agenda for global security is an agenda for human rights.

PART III

Evolving Norms

Over the tumultuous half-century I have been involved in international humanitarian assistance, there have been, not surprisingly, shifting parameters and standards to help guide our actions. This section offers four important views of both positive and negative adaptation to the harsh realities and challenges of complex humanitarian crises. A focus on the limits of state sovereignty or on education for children in conflict areas has only recently been considered by those providing relief assistance. The need to clearly define—and preserve—humanitarian space is presented here, and it is an essential theme that runs throughout the book. So also in humanitarian work is the need for constant review and analysis; the relevant observations of an experienced scholar, and known skeptic, add leaven to our understanding and appreciation of our noble discipline.

The Limits of Sovereignty

Francis Deng

Displacement in all its manifestations, internal and external, has become a global crisis of grave and escalating magnitude. Since the end of the Cold War, the number of people displaced within the borders of their own countries has soared to an estimated twenty to twenty-five million, and the number of refugees is now estimated at over eleven million. Statistics indicate that although the number of refugees appears to be declining, the internally displaced populations worldwide seem to be increasing, a trend that suggests a correlation: As governments restrict the right of asylum, potential refugees join the ranks of the internally displaced. These are people who have been forced or obliged to flee or to leave their homes or places of habitual residence, in particular as a result of or in order to avoid the effects of armed conflict, situations of generalized violence, violations of human rights, or natural or human-made disasters.[1]

Nearly always, internally displaced persons suffer from conditions of insecurity and destitution, and they are acutely in need of protection and survival services. Whereas refugees have an established system of international protection and assistance, those who are displaced internally fall within the domestic jurisdiction and, therefore, under the sovereignty of the state concerned, without established legal or institutional bases for their protection and assistance.

Displacement is not the disease, but a symptom of a public health epidemic with deep-rooted causes. Treating the symptoms or easing the pain through humanitarian assistance is only a first step toward the challenge of diagnosing the disease and attacking it from its root causes. A comprehensive strategy in response to the crisis of displacement must build on the three phases of the problem—causes, consequences, and solutions. Addressing the causes requires going beyond the mere fact of conflicts, communal violence, or human rights violations to appreciate the even deeper root causes. These are often reflected in the traumas of nation-building, involving crises of identity, historical denial of democratic liberties and fundamental human rights, and the deprivations of poverty and severe underdevelopment. Consequences relate to the humanitarian tragedies that result from violent conflicts, gross violations of human rights, and the sudden and massive displacement they generate. Remedies envisage both a response to the emergency needs of the situation and a search for lasting solutions. In other words, the corresponding themes of response would be prevention, protection and assistance, and a secure process of return or permanent settlement in another area, rehabilitation, reintegration, and sustainable development. Action at these three phases must aim at balancing sovereignty, responsibility, and international accountability.

Discharging the preventive responsibilities of sovereignty must begin with addressing the root causes of displacement. As Mrs. Sadako Ogata, former UN High Commissioner for Refugees, has correctly observed, "Whether we speak of refugees or of internally displaced persons, it is clear that there will be no end to their plight until the international community has found ways to deal effectively with the root causes of forced displacement, so as to prevent or alleviate conditions before people flee."[2] Recent years have witnessed a strategic shift in the operational principles of the UNHCR. The new approach "is proactive and preventive, rather than reactive. Instead of focusing purely on countries of asylum, it is equally concerned with conditions in actual and potential refugee-producing states. And as well as providing protection and assistance to refugees, it seeks to reinforce the security and freedom enjoyed by several other groups: internally displaced people; refugees who have returned to their own country; war-affected communities and those who are at risk of being uprooted."[3]

Once displacement has occurred, priority then shifts to providing the affected population with protection and assistance. These functions should normally fall under the responsibilities of sovereignty, but in conflict situations the state often lacks the political will to discharge those responsibilities. Involving the international community to fill the vacuum of state responsibility means negotiating access against the obstacles of defensive state sovereignty. As Mrs. Ogata remarked in 1992, "How to secure the protection of the internally displaced and ensure their access to humanitarian assistance is one of the most important challenges facing the international community. Meeting this challenge will require the development of institutional and practical mechanisms."[4] There have since been important developments in both these areas, which will be highlighted in the course of this chapter.

Magnitude of the Crisis

Displacement is generally a consequence of conflict, which, in turn, is a symptom of deeper societal problems. Conflict occurs when two or more parties interact in pursuit of incompatible objectives, which may involve material or immaterial values. Various forms and degrees of conflict are pervasive features of normal life and, for the most part, are negotiated and resolved by the parties or by third-party mediators. Governance is primarily a function of preventing, managing, and resolving conflicts. The kinds of conflicts that generate internal displacement, however, are generally of a more severe nature, involving deadly violence. As a result of these conflicts, much destruction to life and property is pervasive throughout the world; governments have disintegrated and entire regions have been destabilized, with devastating humanitarian consequences; masses of uprooted populations in the affected countries survive on emergency relief supplies, displaced within their own countries or forced across international borders as refugees.

It is often argued that the internally displaced should be considered and treated like refugees who have not crossed international borders. The analogy is compelling. And yet, the border factor is crucial in legal and institutional terms to qualify one as a refugee who is thereby entitled to receive international protection and assistance. Even more significantly, while the refugee is outside the national framework of conflict and political persecution, the internally displaced, who would be a refugee if he or she had crossed international borders remains trapped within those borders, a potential victim not only of conflict, but also of the persecution emanating from it and alienated from the government that is supposed to be a source of protection and support for citizens.

Overwhelmingly, such persons live in a hostile environment, often deprived of such survival needs as food, shelter, and medicine, frequently subjected to round-ups, forced resettlement, arbitrary detentions or arrests, forced conscription, and sexual assaults. Some of the highest mortality rates ever recorded during humanitarian emergencies have come from situations involving internally displaced persons. According to surveys conducted by the U.S. Center for Disease Control, the death rates among internally displaced have been as much as sixty times higher than those of nondisplaced within the same country.[5]

Compounding the crisis is the nature of the conflicts in which the population is often caught up. Internal conflicts are frequently marked by few or no accepted ground rules. These wars, as former UN Secretary-General Boutros Boutros-Ghali observed in his Supplement to an Agenda for Peace, are "often of a religious or ethnic character and often involving unusual violence and cruelty."[6]

They are usually fought not only by regular armies but also by militias and armed civilians with little discipline and with ill-defined chains of command. They are often guerilla wars without clear front lines. Civilians are the main victims and often the main targets. Humanitarian emergencies are commonplace and the combatant authorities, in so far as they can be called authorities, lack the capacity to cope with them. The number of refugees registered with the Office of the United Nations High Commissioner for Refugees (UNHCR) has increased from 13 million at the end of 1987 to 26 million at the end of 1994. The number of internally displaced persons has increased even more dramatically.[7]

"Today's belligerents," a Foreign Policy Association study points out, "are more and more willing to use humanitarian access, life-saving assistance, and even civilians themselves as weapons in their political-military struggles."[8] The challenge posed by the situation of internally displaced persons and refugees is both to allow them to flee from danger and to ensure their right to remain. As Mrs. Ogata observed, "We must prevent refugee flows, not by building barriers or border controls but by defending the right of people to remain in peace in their own homes and their own countries."[9] The mere fact that people are forced to leave their homes to escape from conflict or persecution implies the violation of fundamental human rights, among them "the right to life, liberty and security of person, the right not to be subjected to torture or other degrading treatment, the right to privacy and family life, the right to freedom of movement and residence, and the right not to be subjected to arbitrary exile."[10] Curative prevention, which means securing the right to remain at home in peace, the right to protection and assistance during displacement, and the right to return home safely and reintegrate into a secure life therefore requires ensuring respect for the human rights of every person. This depends on the willingness of states to accept responsibility for their own citizens and the role of the international community "to foster responsibility as well as accountability of states as regards the treatment of their own citizens."[11]

Much has been written and said about the need for early warning and preventive measures. It is also increasingly acknowledged that most conflicts that have resulted in gruesome humanitarian tragedies have not been the result of lack of early warning, but rather because of lack of the political will on the part of the international community to act in appropriate time. As the former UN Secretary-General Boutros Boutros-Ghali noted in his Supplement to an Agenda for Peace, "Experience has shown that the greatest obstacle to success in these endeavors is not, as is widely supposed, lack of information, analytical capacity or ideas for the United Nations initiative. Success is often blocked at the outset by the reluctance of one or other of the parties to accept United Nations help."[12]

Early warning and prevention essentially mean understanding the sources of potential conflicts and addressing them in time to abort their explosion into violent confrontation. Once a conflict has actually broken out, there is then the immediate need to address its humanitarian consequences while also seeking an end to the hostilities by addressing the issues that led to the conflict in the first place. The success of the effort means restoring peace and creating conducive conditions for reconstruction and development. These are essentially functions of governance that normally fall within the purview of domestic jurisdiction and therefore national sovereignty.

Although the response of governments to displacement generated by natural causes may sometimes be grossly inadequate, on the whole it is sympathetic and supportive of the victims. Likewise, displacement caused by interstate conflicts generally elicits supportive responses from the government of the affected population. In contrast, response to a displacement caused by internal conflicts, communal violence, and systematic violations of human rights is nearly always complicated by the cleavages involved. These cleavages often take the form of an identity crisis, whether based on race, ethnicity, religion, culture, or class. What this means is that the government or any other controlling authority concerned and the affected population identify themselves in divisive terms that undermine solidarity and support. The government or the controlling authority, rather than view the victim population as citizens for whom there is a moral and legal duty to protect and assist, tend to see them as enemies, or part of the enemy, with whom they are at war. In such a situation, which reflects a national identity crisis, the victim population falls into a vacuum of the moral and legal responsibility normally associated with sovereignty. It is to fill this vacuum that the international community is often called upon to step in and provide the needed protection and assistance.

It must be noted, however, that although this notion of identity crisis is pervasive, the degree varies from country to country. And so does the response of governments and other controlling authorities. There are situations of ethnic conflict in which the government still identifies the victim population as their people to whom they indeed provide food and medical supplies, sometimes in cooperation with rebel forces with whom the affected population is ethnically identified. Unfortunately, this appears to be the exception; the pattern is tragically one of denial of solidarity with the victim population on the basis of exclusive identity symbols.

The Challenge of Sovereignty

There are two aspects to the challenges posed by internal conflicts for sovereignty. One is to establish and apply an effective system of conflict prevention, management and resolution; the other is to provide protection and assistance to those affected by conflict. In both cases, the state may not be capable or willing to provide adequate solutions or remedies, especially because the government is nearly always a party to the conflict. And because it is partisan, the government often acts as a barrier to access by the international community to provide protection and assistance to the needy and to help in the search for peace. Such resistance to outside involvement is justified by the invocation of national sovereignty.

Since its inception, sovereignty has developed through several overlapping phases, which may not be neatly delineated historically, but which nonetheless signify an evolution. The first, represented by the Treaty of Westphalia in 1648, is the initial phase when the sovereign reigned supreme domestically and in relations with the outside world. The second, following World War II, marks the erosion of sovereignty with the development of democratic values and institutions internally and with international accountability on the basis of human rights and humanitarian standards. With the greater promotion of these values following the end of the Cold War, the third phase emerged as a reactive assertion of sovereignty by governments whose domestic performance renders them vulnerable to international scrutiny. The fourth is the current pragmatic attempt at reconciling state sovereignty with responsibility.

Genesis of Sovereignty

Sovereignty in legal and political theory was initially conceived in Europe as an instrument of authoritative control by the monarch over feudal princes in the construction of modern territorial states. It was believed that instability and disorder, seen as obstacles to a stable society, could only be overcome by viable governments capable of establishing firm and effective control over territory and populations.[13] The sovereign, as the lawmaker, was considered to be above the law. Indeed, law, according to the "command theory" of the leading positivist jurist, John Austin, is "a rule laid down for the guidance of an intelligent being by an intelligent being having power over him."[14] Law is thus considered the command of the sovereign who is habitually obeyed by his subjects. The power of the sovereign is supposedly not limited by justice or any ideas of good and bad, right or wrong.[15] "For Austin . . . any legal limit on the highest lawmaking power was an absurdity and an impossibility."[16] Even in contemporary literature, it is still argued that "sovereignty is a characteristic of power that relegates its holder to a place above the law. A sovereign is immune from law and only subject to self-imposed restrictions."[17] Although the form of government might vary from monarchy to aristocracy or democracy, it is considered essential that governments maintain order through an effective exercise of sovereignty.

On the other hand, the basic proposition of international human rights law is that "to qualify for the name of government, a government . . . has to meet certain standards, all of which involve restraints on the use of power; no torture; no brutalization; no seizure of property; no state terror; no discrimination on the basis of race, religion, or sex; no prevention of people leaving a particular country, and so on."[18] The limits of the "tyrannical" concept of sovereignty postulates three major premises: (a) "'humanity'—is the *raison d'etre* of any legal system"; (b) "the international system . . . since the Peace of Westphalia, has not been fulfilling what should be its primary function, namely, the protection and development of the human dignity of the individual": (c) "any proposed 'new world order' should be structured so as to maximize benefits not for States but for individuals living within the States, all the way from freedom of speech and elections, on the one hand, to freedom from hunger and the right to education on the other hand."[19]

These principles impose on the international community a correlative responsibility for their enforcement. Herein lies the paradox of the international order. That paradox was indeed inherent in the settlement of Westphalia, from which time "sovereignty created both the territorial state and the international system."[20]

Erosion of Sovereignty

The post–World War II era represents the second phase of the erosion of sovereignty. The application of the right to self-determination, which provided the basis for the process of decolonization, expanded the process of erosion. One of the effective measures in contravention of the narrow concepts of absolute sovereignty was that of international sanctions against South Africa. It was undoubtedly the combination of internal and external pressures that eventually culminated in the collapse of apartheid. The increasing internalization of the human rights agenda and the wave of democratization that is sweeping the world are among the contemporary challenges to sovereignty.

The demands for democratic values, institutions, and practices have devolved the classic notion of sovereign will and authority to the people who are increasingly intolerant of the dictatorship of unaccountable government. More and more, it is recognized that it is the will of the people, democratically invested in the leaders they elect freely or otherwise accept as their representatives, that entitle authorities to value and uphold the sovereignty of a nation. As Michael Reisman has written,

> It should not take a great deal of imagination to grasp what an awful violation of the integrity of the self it is when men with guns evict your government,

dismiss your law, kill and destroy wantonly and control you and those you love by intimidation and terror. When that happens, all other human rights that depend on the lawful institutions of government become matters for the discretion of the dictators. And when that happens, those rights cease. Military coups are terrible violations of the political rights of all the members of the collectivity, and they invariably bring in their wake the violation of all other rights. Violations of the right to popular government are not secondary or less important. They are very, very serious human rights violations.[2]

In the context of international intervention in Haiti, Reisman argues that "in modern international law, what counts is the sovereignty of the people and not a metaphysical abstraction called the state. If the de jure government, which was elected by the people, wants military assistance, how is its sovereignty violated? And if the purpose of the coercion is to reinstate a de jure government elected in a free and fair election after it was ousted by a renegade military, whose sovereignty is being violated? The military's?"[22]

The area of humanitarian intervention has witnessed the greatest erosion of sovereignty, mostly with the consent of the states, but at times through forceful enforcement. Nevertheless, mechanisms and procedures of implementation of the wide array of human rights and humanitarian standards remain undeveloped and grossly inadequate.

Reassertion of Sovereignty

The more the international community has been assertive, the more vulnerably governments have reacted defensively against erosion of state sovereignty. This indeed marks the third phase of the evolution of sovereignty. Governments that are threatened by the erosion of narrow concepts of sovereignty and are defensively trying to reassert it use the argument of cultural relativity and characterize the universality concept as a Western ploy for interfering in the internal affairs of other countries.

Even among the supporters of a more liberal interpretation of sovereignty, its erosion has been viewed with ambivalence. Former United Nations Secretary-General Javier Perez de Cuellar, while acknowledging "what is probably an irresistible shift in public attitudes towards the belief that the defense of the oppressed in the name of morality should prevail over frontiers and legal documents," added the questions, "Does intervention not call into question one of the cardinal principles of international law, one diametrically opposed to it, namely, the obligation of non-interference in the internal affairs of the States?"[23] In his 1991 annual report, he wrote, "The case for not impinging on the sovereignty, territorial integrity and political independence of States is by itself indubitably strong. But it would only be weakened if it were to carry the implication that sovereignty, even in this day and age, includes the right of mass slaughter or of launching systematic campaigns of decimation or forced exodus of civilian populations in the name of controlling civil strife or insurrection."[24]

In place of exclusionary notions of sovereignty, de Cuellar called for a "higher degree of cooperation and a combination of common sense and compassion," arguing that "we need not impale ourselves on the horns of a dilemma between respect for sovereignty and the protection of human rights. . . . What is involved is not the right of intervention but the collective obligation of States to bring relief and redress in human rights emergencies."[25]

Reconciling Sovereignty with Responsibility

Reconciling sovereignty with responsibility, the fourth phase of the evolution, has become the operative principle. Former Secretary-General Boutros Boutros-Ghali, in *An Agenda for Peace*, wrote that "the time of absolute and exclusive sovereignty . . . has passed"; that "its theory was never matched by reality"; and that it is necessary for leaders of states "to find a balance between the needs of good internal governance and the requirements of an ever more interdependent world."[26]

In another context, Boutros-Ghali elaborated his views on sovereignty by highlighting the need to rethink the concept in contemporary global context, "not to weaken its essence, which is crucial to international security and cooperation, but to recognize that it may take more than one form and perform more than one function." Boutros-Ghali goes on to postulate an intriguing concept of universal sovereignty of individuals and peoples: "Underlying the rights of the individual and the rights of the peoples is a dimension of universal sovereignty that resides in all humanity and provides all peoples with legitimate involvement in issues affecting the world as a whole. It is a sense that increasingly finds expression in the gradual expansion of international law."[27]

Living up to the responsibilities of sovereignty becomes in effect the best guarantee for sovereignty. As one observer commented, "Governments could best avoid intervention by meeting their obligations not only to other states, but also to their own citizens. If they failed, they might invite intervention."[28]

This was indeed the point made by the Secretary-General of the Organization of African Unity, Salim Ahmed Salim, in his bold proposals for an OAU mechanism for conflict prevention and resolution. "If the OAU, first through the Secretary-

General and then the Bureau of the Summit, is to play the lead role in any African conflict," he said, "it should be enabled to intervene swiftly, otherwise it cannot be ensured that whoever (apart from African regional organizations) acts will do so in accordance with African interests."[29]

Criticizing the tendency to respond only to worst-case scenarios, Salim emphasized the need for preemptive intervention: "Preemptive involvement should be permitted even in situations where tensions evolve to such a pitch that it becomes apparent that a conflict is in the making." He even suggested that the OAU should take the lead in transcending the traditional view of sovereignty, building on the African values of kinship, solidarity and the notion that "every African is his brother's keeper." Considering that "our borders are at best artificial," Salim argued, "we in Africa need to use our own cultural and social relationships to interpret the principle of non-interference in such a way that we are enabled to apply it to our advantage in conflict prevention and resolution."[30]

It is most significant that the Security Council, in its continued examination of the Secretary-General's report, An Agenda for Peace, "[noted] with concern the incidents of humanitarian crises, including mass displacements of population becoming or aggravating threats to international peace and security and concluded that under certain circumstances, there may be a close relationship between acute needs for humanitarian assistance and threats to international peace and security, which trigger international involvement."[31]

The crisis of internal displacement fits into this model in that it combines human rights with humanitarian concerns, and protection with assistance. Internal displacement is also a challenge to sovereignty in that providing the citizens with physical security and their basic survival needs are among the prerequisites for legitimacy and therefore recognizable sovereignty in the framework of international relations. These are among the principles that have guided the implementation of my mandate as Representative of the Secretary-General for Internally Displaced Persons.

The normative principles of my dialogue with governments are built on the premise that national sovereignty carries with it responsibility for the security and welfare of the citizens. When a state lacks the capacity to ensure the protection and welfare of its people, it is expected to call on the international community to supplement its efforts. The essence of the state responsibility, however, is accountability, both domestically and internationally. If states fail to live up to their obligations toward their citizens with the result that large numbers of people fall victim, their physical and social integrity violated or threatened and their very survival endangered, then the international community has the commensurate responsibility to hold the states accountable and obtain access to provide the needed protection and assistance and help in the search for remedies to the conditions that had caused the violent confrontation in order to restore a just and lasting peace.

International Responses

The plight of the internally displaced has begun to receive significant attention from the international community. Because of the magnitude of the crisis, the inadequacy of the response system, and the urgent need for international remedies, a number of nongovernmental organizations, supported by concerned governments, urged the Commission on Human Rights to take action. Concerted action began with the consideration by the Commission of a report prepared by the Secretariat on the subject of internal displacement.[32] It was then that the Commission requested the Secretary-General to appoint a representative to study the problems. The study was to cover the root causes of internal displacement, the relevant international legal standards, the mechanisms for their enforcement, and any additional measures the United Nations might take to improve the situation of the internally displaced. In preparing the study, I undertook field visits to five countries and engaged in a dialogue with the governments. Since then, in-depth studies of the legal and institutional dimensions of international protection and assistance for the internally displaced, and dialogue with governments have been the core activities of the mandate. As we shall see in the following sections, these have brought about a number of tangible results.

Institutional Arrangements

On the issue of institutional arrangements, it is widely acknowledged that there is a gap in the coverage because there is no one organization, or collection of organizations, mandated to take responsibility for the internally displaced. At the same time, there is no political will to create a new organization with that mandate. Nor is it likely that an existing institution will be mandated to assume full responsibility for the internally displaced. Under the present circumstances, the residual option is that of a collaborative arrangement among a wide variety of agencies and organizations whose mandates and activities are relevant to the problems of internal displacement.[33]

Correlative to the increased involvement of various agencies and organizations is the urgent need for coordination or a central point to assign institutional responsibility in emergency situations. In the last few years some institutional progress has been made in this area. There now exist coordinating mechanisms that promise to bring coherence into the international system. The focal points in these structural arrangements are the Emergency Relief Coordinator (designed as the reference point in the United Nations system for requests for assistance and protection for internally displaced persons), and the Inter-Agency Standing Committee, its working group. A similar coordinating structure is reflected at the field level through the Resident Representatives of UNDP or, in cases of complex emergencies, the Resident Coordinators or Humanitarian Coordinators who chair Disaster Management Teams (DMTs) composed of UN operational agencies and sometimes NGOs and coordinate humanitarian assistance for internally displaced persons.

The High Commissioner for Refugees has observed that the success of international involvement will depend on three key factors: "The first is a well structured division of work, on which coordination must proceed among organizations and institutions with the required expertise and ability to avoid duplication of efforts and fill gaps instead, the second is the ability of the international effort to mobilize and develop local capacities and responsibilities. The third . . . is their firm foundation in common and consistent human rights standards."[34]

Nor should the institutional challenge be seen merely in the context of the displacement that has already occurred. Human rights violations are a major factor in causing displacement as well as an obstacle to safe and voluntary return home. Safeguarding human rights in countries of origin is therefore critical, both for prevention and for the solution of refugee and internally displaced persons problems. If the increasing problem of internal displacement is to be contained and reduced, preventive strategies are critical.

United Nations human rights bodies have an important role to play in this regard. Preventive measures currently relied upon include dialogue with governments, urgent appeals, public statements, emergency meetings, the deployment of human rights field staff, machinery for the protection of minorities, and the extension of technical assistance. Commission reports addressing the root causes of mass exoduses also exemplify efforts at prevention. Human rights treaty bodies, moreover, have been requested to examine measures they might take to prevent human rights violations, and several have adopted emergency procedures and undertaken missions to countries for preventative purposes. The establishment of the post of United Nations High Commissioner for Human Rights has added momentum to the development of preventative strategies. Human rights field staff deployed under her auspices are playing a valuable preventative role. Human rights advisory services and education projects are valuable tools for the promotion of human rights and prevention of violations.

All of these measures, however, are at an early stage of development and human rights bodies should be encouraged to increase their capacities for prevention. Mechanisms for minority protection in particular need to be strengthened, since many displaced persons are members of minority groups who have been subjected to forcible expulsion, resettlement, and other persecution because of their ethnic or other origin. Promising initiatives include the adoption by the United Nations of the Declaration on the Rights of Persons Belonging to National or Ethnic, Religious and Linguistic Minorities and the establishment of a working group by the Submission on Prevention of Discrimination and Protection of Minorities to develop strategies for minority protection and to prevent conflict.

At the national level, promotion and protection of human rights through the establishment of effective national institutions to monitor and promote them is the safest guarantee against involuntary displacement. My country mission reports as Representative of the Secretary-General have emphasized the importance of supporting preventative techniques aimed at empowering the population at the grassroots level. Very often, local communities have built up effective strategies for mitigating the impact of displacement. The coping strategies that displaced populations themselves have developed should be carefully examined by NGOs and international agencies, because such mechanisms are essential elements of prevention and protection.

Irrespective of the level at which preventive strategies are pursued, efforts must be made to ensure that they do not interfere with the freedom of movement. There is a need to reconcile strategies that encourage people to remain within their own countries with those that safeguard the right to leave and seek asylum from persecution. Under no circumstances should the desire to forestall large-scale populations displacements take precedence over assuring the security of displaced populations.

The Quest for Strategy

In virtually all dialogues with the governments and relevant actors, effort is made to link the immediate challenges of protection and assistance with the need to find lasting solutions, which in time draws attention to the causes generating the conflict that triggered displacement. This is, of course, a sensitive area in which reactions from governments are mixed. There are those who claim that it is outside the mandate of the Representative and those who acknowledge the need for peace as the real solution to the humanitarian tragedies of war. Objectively, there is no way the circular link between war, its human tragedies, and the need for solutions that address the root causes can be avoided.

In view of these anomalies and uncertainties, there is still a need for developing a strategy that would address effectively and comprehensively the crisis of internal displacement, both generically and contextually. As argued at the outset of this chapter, such a strategy should approach the displacement problem in its three manifest phases: causes, consequences, and remedies. The corresponding responses would be to develop measures for preempting and preceding displacement, to provide adequate means of protection and relief assistance during displacement, and to seek durable solutions through voluntary and safe return, resettlement, rehabilitation, reconstruction, and self-reliant development.

Ultimately, because conflict is at the core of displacement, emphasis needs to be placed on conflict prevention, management, and resolution in that order of priority. It should also be acknowledged that not only is displacement a consequence and, therefore, a symptom of conflict, but conflict itself is a symptom of deeper societal ills, generally rooted in ethnic, religious, and cultural diversities, disparities, and gross inequities or injustices. It is in the fertile soil of understandable and justified grievances that the virus of violence incubates and eventually explodes. Unless checked in time, this can turn into a chronic condition in the body politic and, as recent developments have shown, can be even terminal to the survival of nations.

Among the characteristics of the soil in which the virus incubates are poverty, scarcity of resources, maldistribution of the little there is, politics repressive of legitimate demands, gross violations of human rights and fundamental liberties, and a sense of hopelessness and despair. Under those conditions, governments or dominant authorities become perceived as tantamount to foreign bodies, implanted into a resistant body politic that is eventually forced to reject them.

To the extent that conflict represents a symptomatic warning of underlying and potentially more serious problems, it can play a positive role if constructively responded to. Indeed, the upsurge in violent conflicts following the end of the Cold War indicates that many latent conflicts were repressed through the awesome power of the bipolar control mechanisms of the two superpowers, driven not so much by the ideals of right and wrong as by ideological alignments and strategic considerations. Repressive, unrepresentative governments and regimes were backed and supported by the superpowers because of their strategic or ideological stand with little or no regard to their domestic legitimacy. With the withdrawal of this support following the end of the Cold War, governments or regimes with the propensity to repress, oppress, and plunder became exposed to internal and external scrutiny and a more determined opposition that they can no longer contain, because they lack the capacity to exercise effective and decisive control over the situation.

This chaotic and often tragic conflict situation paradoxically offers countries and the international community the opportunity to review the normative and operational principles governing domestic jurisdiction and international relations. Foremost of these should be the stipulation of the normative standards of responsibility associated with sovereignty. Rather than a means of barricading governments and regimes against international scrutiny, sovereignty should be recast in response to its contemporary challenges as embodying the will of the people, represented by those they choose through free and fair elections or otherwise accept as their legitimate representatives. Sovereignty must also be viewed as an instrument for ensuring the protection and welfare of all those under its jurisdiction.

A concept that provides the core for formulating such a normative framework remains the human dignity of the individual and the group within the domestic jurisdiction. This concept is provided for in the charter of the United Nations, the International Bill of Rights, and all the human rights and humanitarian principles enunciated in many legally and morally binding documents, including now the Guiding Principles on Internal Displacement. Rather than a means of barricading governments and regimes against international scrutiny, sovereignty should be normatively postulated as an embodiment of the democratic will of the people and a tool for ensuring the protection and welfare of all those under domestic jurisdiction. The incorporation and embodiment of these human rights and humanitarian norms into the Guiding Principles on Internal Displacement is both a preventive and curative prescription. Governments and other custodians of national sovereignty should see the standards not only as a guide, but also as a yardstick for evaluating their own performance.

Conflict prevention, management, and resolution clearly pose paradoxical challenges for both change and stability. The gross inequities of the status quo need to be scrutinized and moderated, if not eliminated. But preserving a legal order that is protective of and responsive to reasonable standards of human dignity must be seen as an overriding goal. It is with these normative principles in mind that governments and the international community are called upon to address the mounting crisis of international displacement, to prevent it by addressing its root causes, to respond to its human rights and humanitarian tragedies when they occur, and to strive to end it by creating appropriate conditions for safe return or alternative resettlement and restoring normal life in the community and the nation at large.

In conclusion, it should be reiterated that the international community has made considerable progress in responding to displacement, in particular with the development of the normative framework, in the form of the Guiding Principles, and enhancements of institutional arrangements at both the international and regional levels. However, much more remains to be done to give these legal and institutional developments meaningful impact on the ground, and above all, to make governments more responsive to the responsibilities of sovereignty for protecting and assisting their own citizens or else risk undermining their legitimacy both domestically and internationally. The glass is half-full, but that implies that it is also half-empty.

The Child Protection Viewpoint

Alec Wargo

I offer personal, field-based perspectives on the often fraught relationship between education[1] and child protection in armed conflict. This personal perspective, garnered from years working in the protection field, will remove us from the world of guidelines and policies and return us to the flesh-and-bone realities around the globe, where students, their teachers, and their communities often find themselves in the midst of armed conflict.

When Education Protects

At the start of my career in child protection with UNHCR in Central Africa, I was only "theoretically" aware of the role of education in protecting children from harm and abuse during conflict and post-conflict situations, and that education personnel could serve as a linchpin in a community's ability to protect its children.[2] Perhaps I still held a somewhat jaded American view of education as sets of buildings with teachers who tried to fill our heads with bits of information in order to pass a series of exams that would place us later in life into a particular skill or field. Sometimes school challenged us, often it bored us, but it was always there, taken for granted.

It was only after I began to work in refugee camps in the early 1990s, and later with UN Peacekeeping in the field, that I began to truly realize that education—when children do have access to it—is at the heart of many efforts at documenting violations perpetrated against children during wartime. It is also, on many occasions, the primary interface for a human rights worker—the locus and the focus of child rights monitors and advocates' efforts to protect children from violence and abuse in times of utter chaos. This can be broken down into three categories of interest for the protection advocate: (1) education as an alert and as a bridge to response, (2) education and protection from recruitment, and (3) education and rehabilitation and reintegration.

Education as an Alert and a Bridge to Response

Rights advocates who monitor and advocate for protection of children have long recognized that alerts from affected communities are the most efficient way to identify violations against their children. In many cases it is the educationalist who alerts us to these grave violations. In many places, education authorities and teachers are among the most highly respected community members, and education itself has high value and prestige. Common practice has been that education personnel are often trained in the rights children have to freedom from harm, often a simplified version of the Convention on the Rights of the Child (CRC) and/or aspects of the Refugee Convention or other applicable legal instruments. The training is done with the expectation that it forms a base upon which action for proactive protection of children's rights can be grounded. This is a worthy exercise and has resulted in a number of interesting dialogues with education and community leaders in affected locales. Many of these dialogues have centered on the ability of the child to partake in decisions of his or her life choices, and, of course, a considerable amount of dialogue has been on the rights of girls and women in their societies.

Let us assume for the purposes of this chapter that child rights and their protection in wartime, especially against grave rights violations, are more or less agreed upon across time and cultures. The question then becomes how can we translate this knowledge, this "rights-based" approach, into action that responds to those violations? This action can be difficult, and sometimes almost impossible, in most conflict situations. When a violation has occurred, protection staff are asked by children's families or community leaders to undertake specific interventions. In the large majority of cases, these interventions fall into one of two general categories of action: (1) corrective response and/or (2) accountability response.

For example, in 2002, while serving as a child protection adviser to the UN peacekeeping mission to the Congo (MONUC), I was approached through the local Catholic Bishop about a case brought to his attention by a group of teachers in a village some three days distant. The case concerned an impoverished single mother's only child, a fifteen-year-old boy who had been excelling against all odds at school. A rebel group active in the area had forcibly abducted him while on his way to school some weeks earlier. The immediate request was to remedy the situation: to assist in finding and advocating for the release of the boy as soon as possible. It was felt that an accountability response was not practicable at the time, because the rebel group in question was in complete control of the area and there were no NGO or UN staff based in the vicinity to prevent repercussions against the family.

In another example, from a similarly isolated community, a rebel soldier had raped an eight-year-old girl in front of her home. The headmaster of the community's primary school brought the case to the attention of a local human rights group, and subsequently the members of that group passed it on to me. In this case, the parents sought both a response to the girl's condition and an accountability response. The girl, along with her mother, was referred to a rape response center for treatment, HIV screening, and psychosocial recovery. The soldier was later tried for the crime, found guilty, and sentenced by a military court.

Teachers and education administrators can, and do, serve as protection alerts with human rights and child rights agencies. However, the crucial factor is whether or not that educator is not only aware of the violations and the child rights perspective but also alert to the need for both a response to and, in some cases, a remedy for those violations. In my experience, these protection alerts can only work if educators are linked meaningfully to advocates and actors who can assist them in accessing services and/or an accountability response. Additionally, a large majority of violations in wartime happen far from major cities and towns, where these actors are normally based. Most might assume that national or provincial education authorities serve as a link from the village to the central or provincial level. But, alas, education authorities are the first to suffer rupture when state control is lost and are often sorely underresourced in conflict-affected states.

The outlook would be bleak if we took such a restrictive view of "education." However, in most cases educationalists do succeed in making these links from far-flung regions. When we reexamine these links from the deep field to urban centers, it becomes clear that when we step back and take a broader view of the "education establishment," it is much larger than most would realize. When we take into account the nontraditional education actors in these countries, we see that communities of faith, NGOs, and civil society are all highly active actors in a network of educational activities, both traditional and nontraditional.

The educational establishment should be viewed not only as the remnants of a Western-influenced Ministry of Education apparatus, but also as the communities of faith, as well as local and international NGOs and UN partners that offer one of the most resilient and widespread monitoring and alert mechanisms available to child-protection actors today. These education networks are also one of the best organized and widespread "bridges" to response. While in many places these networks are engaged as major partners for community-based protection, they are unfortunately not always utilized in a systematic fashion by the international community, including the UN system and donors. More must be done to support and more deeply engage this wider educational establishment as a key partner in protection response.

Education and Protection from Recruitment

Though much has been written about how education can serve as a preventative measure against everything from domestic abuse to gender-based violence, most of my personal experience with prevention of grave violations against children in times of conflict centers around the recruitment of children. It is estimated that approximately 250,000 children, boys and girls, serve as child soldiers around the world at any given time, and their identification and release continues to be a major field of activity for UN, NGO, and civil-society actors.[3]

Educational staff are instrumental in alerting communities to the fact that underage recruitment is a violation of children's rights and can result in untold harm. They are also often an essential first line of defense in preventing recruitment. Schoolgoing children are much less likely to be recruited than those children who are not undertaking some kind of formal or informal education. Why are children who go to school much less likely to be recruited on the whole? Most analyses suggest that children who have access to school, in the large majority of conflict situations where there is no state-guaranteed access to primary or secondary education, are often from less vulnerable families. These are families who have the wherewithal to resist or avoid situations where their children might be directly exposed to armed actors. Their children generally spend the large part of their days in a structured environment, and the link between educationalist community and family can be quite strong. These families, when they do receive warning of impending danger, are often able to move away or use other coping mechanisms to reduce the risk of recruitment of their children.

More vulnerable families either have no means to move or are so destitute that movement would expose them to the direct risk of starvation, or other dangers equal to or greater than the threat of recruitment. Therefore, when we examine the risk of recruitment for school-going children, we appreciate that they are often less vulnerable socially and economically, are able to be alerted through educationalist/community/family lines of communication of impending troubles more readily and, when subject to danger, are often able to move to safety.

School often serves as a community's barometer for trouble, and educationalists are often among the persons in the community consulted on how best to avoid danger. For example, in the South Kivu province of the Democratic Republic of the Congo (DRC), in 2002–2003, the Congolese armed group *Rassemblement Congolaise pour la Democratie-Goma* (RCD-G) began to move its recruitment and training centers farther from urban areas to the isolated island of Idjwi in the middle of Lake Kivu to avoid human rights scrutiny of its child recruitment. The first message I received as the MONUC child protection officer of those recruitments was sent through a human rights worker from a group of teachers on the island. Though the teachers had sent many of their students to the relative safety of the provincial capital of Bukavu to avoid this fate, many children from inaccessible areas were forcibly taken to the island, and a large number of families who could not afford to move from the area or send their children away were recruited. Most were not enrolled in school at the time of their recruitment.

In similar circumstances we ran into hundreds of children, some as young as ten years of age, associated with the *Conseil National pour la Defense de la Democratie/Forces pour la Defense de la Democratie* (CNDD-FDD) rebel group of Burundi, which had migrated from their training camps on the Burundi border with Tanzania to the Uvira/Fizi area of the DRC, where the group maintained a rear base. Most had spent at most only one to two years in primary school and recounted how the CNDD-FDD targeted them for recruitment because "they had nothing else to do." Most of the children came from broken or extremely poor households with no means to send them to school. Many were forced to work to support the family from the age of eight or nine years old. Almost none of them could read or write.

This socioeconomic argument is important to appreciate fully the direct relationship between access to education and the consequent access to protection from grave abuses. Indeed, the other end of this reality is that vulnerable children with no access to schooling sometimes seek out armed groups for various reasons. It is largely true that most child soldiers are unwilling or forced recruits. However, I have run into a not inconsiderable number of child recruits who willingly "volunteered" to fight with armed forces or groups.[4] In my experience speaking with hundreds of these child soldiers over the years, only a very few were enrolled in school at the time of their recruitment. As mentioned earlier, many stated that they had "nothing to do" and were often in dire economic straits or had suffered estrangement from their parents or caregivers. The deceptive offers of a monthly salary (rarely, if ever, paid) or the chance to feed themselves through pillage or extortion was attractive; and lacking any other alternative, many did "volunteer."

Unfortunately, it took these children little time to realize that their decision was not in their best interest—and months or years of suffering, exposure, and disappointment followed. Many lamented never going to school or not being able to finish school, and the promise of schooling under child demobilization programs led more than one child soldier to walk considerable distances to the nearest UN office or outpost to seek release. Making education, formal and informal, more widely available in communities at risk for underage recruitment should be more seriously considered. Education has a worth as a sign of opportunity and status among children in conflict-affected communities, and that value can, and must, be more deftly employed to prevent underage recruitment in the future.

Rehabilitation and Reintegration

In the area of children affected by armed conflict, the advancement of an educational response for children separated or demobilized from armed forces and groups is probably the most developed to date. Most children desire either formal or informal education or skills training upon release from armed groups, although access remains slow and patchy. The high value most former child soldiers place on education is an end or good in itself, but especially for the older children, it also forms part of their desire to "bring something back home" to their families and communities. My experience speaking with demobilized child soldiers about their next steps has always centered on aspects of what they can now do to become productive members of their family and society.

For the former child soldier returning to his or her community, well-structured education programs can mean a lifeline to "normalcy," a future and, in many cases, a hoped-for wage. The structure and community integrated aspect of these programs, if undertaken properly, can provide a good grounding for efforts to prevent re-recruitment or other abuses, either during the conflict or in the post-conflict phase. These challenges are now even more complex when we consider that the numbers of children demobilized *during* a conflict or immediate post-conflict phase are rising relative to those demobilized only after the conflict has come to a halt and stability has returned. This trend for release of children during conflict is welcome but it comes with its own problems and challenges. Chief among these is the re-recruitment of children who have been reintegrated, in some instances on multiple occasions, back into their communities. Education, the structure and alert functions for protection advocates and actors, remains of high value for successful reintegration and protection of children demobilized while conflict continues.

Educationalists also play a key role in managing the fears and expectations of communities who receive demobilized child soldiers. While many parents and communities naturally welcome their sons and daughters back with open arms, some armed groups use children against their own communities and this can cause deep-seated distrust and fear. The UN and its NGO partners have gone a long way to involve community members, including educational staff, in perceiving former child combatants primarily as victims and to convince fearful parents and neighbors that it is a child's right to benefit from reintegration assistance and that this cannot be done without the active acceptance and participation of the community

itself. Alas, each situation is unique, and the work of educationalists and their partners in war-torn communities is different depending on the circumstances prevailing prior to or during release. This only points out that much research and analysis
are required to further strengthen this approach.

To some extent, victims of sexual violence follow similar trajectories during
their reintegration, though often their interface with education is concealed or is
purposefully blurred to prevent the labeling of these boys and girls as sexual victims. This is not to say that educationalists do not undertake or have the potential to lend their support to these children. Indeed, in a number of circumstances
known to me, these staff members have been a crucial support to these children
and their families.

When Education Fails to Protect

Education is at the forefront in preventing, or responding to, abuses against children in wartime. However, in modern warfare there is a palpable trend in which
the educational personnel themselves, and/or the buildings in which that education
takes place, become the objects of abuse or play a role in the abuse of children.

Attacks Against Schools

Most rights monitors would identify the 1990s as the watershed epoch, when
attacks against schools gained the notice of child protection staff. We saw this in
the activities of the Lord's Resistance Army (LRA) in northern Uganda and in
southern Sudan, during the Rwandan genocide, and certainly in Liberia and Sierra
Leone. We currently witness these attacks in places as varied as Nepal, Afghanistan,
Pakistan, the DRC, Somalia, Palestine, and southern Thailand, as well as in the
Syrian conflict.

It is easy to oversimplify the commonalities of these attacks. Some were related
to wider crimes, such as the genocide in Rwanda, where children and educated
men and women, including teachers, were brutally murdered by gangs, many
times in schools and churches. The perpetrators were intent on the destruction of
a minority community and its perceived sympathizers or, later on, in revenge killings against those who were presumed complicit in the killings due to their ethnic
affiliation. It is here that we find education personnel complicit in killings based
on ethnic identity. Similar stories were recounted to me when I served as human
rights officer with the Organization for Security and Cooperation (OSCE) mission
in postwar Bosnia. Sadly, the very pillars of a community, who can give voice to

protection and reconciliation, can also stoke the embers of ethnic hatred. This is a constant danger in societies in conflict where ethnic identity is a key factor, and the educational system, in both its personnel and as a packaged set of ideals and perceptions of the world, often stand at the very heart of it.

There are other instances when education and identity politics have led to massive rights violations and where schools themselves have become a central battleground. I think of the recent conflict in Nepal and the politicization of Nepali education, which will haunt that country for some time to come. During that insurgency, the Maoist youth wing concentrated its recruitment efforts on rural schools throughout the country, abducting whole schools for days of Maoist "cultural" programs. These programs funneled healthy recruits as young as fifteen years of age to fighting units and struck fear into the hearts of teachers and education administrators—who had no choice but to look on or risk harm to themselves and others.

In the post-conflict phase in Nepal, the Maoist youth continue to engage in violent acts, both in schools and in their communities. Currently other political parties have followed suit and created their own youth wings, the largest of which is the Communist Party of Nepal–United Marxist-Leninist (CPN-UML). These youth wings are nominally under the control of the parties, and continue to be a source of interfactional violent acts and killings. Their presence and propagation in schools across the country remain of deep concern to those assisting the peace process in Nepal.

Likewise, in southern Thailand, identity politics in the traditionally Malay areas has taken on a violent character. The instruction of Thai language and culture has become a lighting rod for local resistance by armed actors. Students and teachers in these schools, many of them of Malay identity, have been killed in shootings, bombings, and other attacks by armed groups. More worrisome is the effort on the part of Thai authorities to protect these schools by sending military forces to guard them. Though it may be well intentioned, one must question the wisdom of deploying military personnel into schools, effectively making them targets and removing the civilian nature that such centers of learning must display.

Increasingly, there are also the depressing ideological battles fought over the very fundamentals of education. The questions of what can be taught and who can attend school have generated some of the most gruesome attacks against schools and students in recent history. The worst example of this is the current situation prevailing in the insurgent-controlled areas of Afghanistan, and the neighboring border areas of Pakistan, where the Taliban and their allies have wreaked havoc. The crux of the battle concerns two types of ideological issues: (1) are girls fit to attend school at all, especially in the company of boys? and (2) should children be taught anything beyond Taliban-approved interpretations of religious texts? It has now become commonplace for the Taliban or associated leaders to leave "night letters" threatening attacks on schools if they do not cease allowing girls to attend school or alter the school curriculum to reflect their conservative interpretation for educating young people. Girls' schools in particular have been attacked with bombs, poison gas, and a barrage of threats, and there is little one can do in the more isolated areas until some semblance of security prevails. Add to this the depressing fact that a significant number of madrasas in the border areas appear to be training children to undertake armed conflict as fighters or, worse, as suicide bombers.

Finally, the wholesale attack on schools in the Syrian conflict is extreme. Since the popular uprising against the regime there, schools have variously been used by government forces as bases, machine gun emplacements, detention centers and even places where adults and children are subjected to torture. Many children I met while taking testimonies on abuses against children in that conflict had not been able to attend school for over a year. Teachers as well stated that schools in areas that the government had identified as antiregime were targeted, as were teachers. Many stated that they had witnessed government forces burning or looting schools for what they described as reprisal for perceived sympathy with political change. This reminds us that international efforts to protect schools and students during armed conflict are in their infancy and that much more focus has to be brought to this crucial area.

Infiltration of Education by Armed Groups

When we survey the challenges presented when armed groups attack schools and the difficulties these acts present for protection of education, they pale in comparison to the infiltration of education by armed groups. This does not refer to the abduction or harassment of students and teachers described earlier, but the much more pernicious infiltration of education by armed group cadres and their sympathizers. The latest example of this is the *Palipehutu–Forces Nationales pour la Liberation* (FNL) in Burundi, which, in the period prior to the final peace settlement, demonstrated its hold over sympathizers in the educational establishment, resulting in teachers actively recruiting children for the FNL. It is believed that the recruitment was aimed at securing these FNL sympathizers a demobilization package, which, in turn was promised to the children, although children have been purposely excluded from such schemes in the peace process. Many of these children were exposed to militarized camps for fairly long stretches of time, up to two years, before the FNL agreed to their disqualification. We can also not discount the fact that, if the FNL had not come to an agreement with the government of Burundi, these children would have had a very real chance of taking up arms.

Similarly, in the Congolese refugee camps in Rwanda in the latter half of the 1990s and until quite recently, teachers and community leaders in those camps, sympathetic to Rwandan-backed rebel groups operating in the Kivu provinces of the DRC, actively recruited children to fight the Congolese government forces. As the child-protection focal point for UNHCR at the time, I was amazed that our data showed that an entire portion of the camps' population (boys aged from thirteen to early adulthood) had effectively disappeared. We knew from the data and corroborating evidence that the boys had been sent for military training or other support roles to either the RCD-G, the Banyamulenge (an ethnic Tutsi group residing in the mountains of South Kivu Province of the DRC) forces, or, latterly, the *Congres National Pour la Defense du Peuple* (CNDP). In this instance, teachers and community leaders were either complicit or were too frightened to give evidence. This recruitment is a worry in a number of refugee camps, where similar pressures exist, and more must be done to monitor and halt such practices.

Finally, testimonies from community members and students in Syria point to a disturbing trend of government intelligence personnel utilizing teachers or school administrators to gather evidence from school children on their political beliefs and attitudes and beliefs of their parents, with sometimes dangerous consequences for those parents. Utilizing trusted educational personnel to gather intelligence is a new and worrisome trend in some anti-insurgency efforts around the world.

The Missing Children

Children missing due to recruitment, either "voluntary" or forced, are a much smaller number than the very real problem of the thousands of children, the most vulnerable, who will never have the opportunity to go to school. In most "failed" or "failing" states, the number of out-of-school children can reach 50 percent and more in the most isolated and poor regions, where conflict usually flourishes. These are the children whom the education establishment certainly fails to protect.

We have shown that education can work as an effective monitor and alert for human rights workers and as a bridge to response. But that very same system falls absolutely flat for these "missing" children, because education never sees their faces. It was not surprising, then, that the majority of the children whom I interviewed upon release from one armed group or another recount how they were not able to attend school; how their impoverished parents were powerless to flee or to bribe their children's recruiters to allow their children to remain; and who are also unable or unaware of the alert function that many educationalists can play. In any case, many of these families live days away from the nearest school or do not feel they are able to share their problems with unfamiliar persons.

If education is to protect all children, and the CRC, the most widely adopted piece of international legislation, states that it should, then the international community must do much more to find ways to expand the education safety net during times of conflict. This could be achieved through the establishment of a range of formal to informal educational outreach and community sensitization programs. It should most certainly be prioritized in failed and failing states that are in crisis or conflict.

When Education Itself Needs Protection

From the perspective of the Office of the Special Representative for Children and Armed Conflict (SRSG-CAC), one overwhelming question has to be addressed that is of a different nature from the technical discussions on how to ameliorate the condition or respond to violations against children: How do we stop these attacks? How do we break the cycle of violence against children and their teachers in classrooms during conflict?

Former Special Representative Radhika Coomaraswamy has noted the "changing nature of conflict." And, unfortunately, its trajectory is not favorable to children. In the past children were considered peripheral to the conflict. Now they are often at its very center. Though many experts on this matter may argue why and exactly when this phenomenon of targeting of children and education first appeared, it is undeniable that it is now a fact and that these attacks are not abating. In fact, they are becoming more commonplace.

Again, what to do? One word: accountability. Ninety percent of the armed actors cited in the Secretary General's Annual Report on children and armed conflict are nonstate actors. Some of these nonstate actors have proxies that represent their interests on the sidelines of UN events such as the Human Rights Council and the Committee on the Rights of the Child. But the weight of the UN's state-oriented system is generally not sufficient to engender compliance by these parties.

Security Council Engagement

It was with this in mind that the former SRSG-CAC, Olara Otunnu, began a process in 1999 of engagement with reporting to the UN Security Council, positioning children and armed conflict directly on its peace and security agenda. This was the first "thematic" protection mandate to be entertained by the Council in such a way. Things progressed slowly at first, with Annual Reports of the Secretary General speaking of a vague set of violations against children in times of conflict but without a systematized information gathering network to backstop claims of abuse.

The next breakthrough came in 2001 with Security Council Resolution (SCR) 1379 asking the Secretary General to prepare an annual list of parties to armed conflict who recruited and used children under the age of eighteen years in armed conflict, the "list of shame." After this point the Secretary General also began to call, in a more focused way, for compliance and, when lacking progress, for the possibility of the Council using its power to take measures, including sanctions, against groups and individuals who recruit children.

Actual compliance, however, was slow. This was, first, because the UN system was slow to engage in a concerted campaign in a unified fashion. Second, the information available to the Security Council at the time did not meet the rigorous requirements usually associated with the application of sanctions. Third, compliance work lacked a recognized and agreed format. This was rectified over the next two Resolutions agreed upon by the Council. SCR 1539 of 2004 established the concept of a concrete timebound "action plan" to halt the recruitment and use of children. These action plans called upon the UN country teams to engage with both state and nonstate actors to agree to a set of measurable and timebound activities to prevent recruitment, release children associated with those groups and verify compliance. Failing this, the Security Council reiterated its intention to consider the use of measures, including sanctions, against violating parties. At the same time the Council asked the SRSG-CAC to develop a system-wide plan to strengthen monitoring and reporting on grave violations against children in times of conflict. This was aimed at establishing a more solid basis of information in which the Council might deliberate before exercising its power.

Information Is Power

The Secretary General's plan to provide "timely accurate, reliable and objective information" to the Security Council was unveiled in his report (S/2005/72) of 2005. The plan is important because it defines the way in which reliable information should be collected, verified, and packaged for the Security Council and also identified the six grave violations—including recruitment and attacks on schools—enumerated earlier in this chapter. It also reiterated a call for action plans and an intention to utilize all tools at its disposal to engender compliance among parties engaged in grave violations against children in armed conflict. Most importantly, it also set in place a Working Group of the Security Council that would deliberate throughout the year on specialized reports of children affected by armed conflict, in situations listed in the Secretary General's Annual Report, and make recommendations to the parties concerned, as well as to the Council sanctions committees.

This plan, as set forth by the Secretary General and endorsed by the Security Council, resulted in the first systematic monitoring, reporting and verification mechanisms on child protection. It identified headquarters responsibilities, but it also mandated UN country teams to put in place task forces to undertake systematic monitoring and reporting at the country level. Since that time, the Office of the SRSG-CAC has worked to mainstream monitoring and reporting throughout the UN system and technically backstop the work of UN country task forces on the design and implementation of action plans. It should be noted, however, that though the Council endorsed the monitoring of six grave violations, including attacks on schools, the action plans remained limited to the halt of recruitment and use of children as soldiers. Both monitoring and reporting (MRM) and the implementation of action plans advanced slowly but have now accelerated to the point where knowledge and expertise on MRM and the design and implementation of action plans to halt recruitment and use are widespread.

At the same time, the Council recognized the need to respond, with a recommendation to parties on the other five grave violations listed in SCR 1612. The crucial lesson learned was that more could be expected of the Security Council Working Group regarding concrete recommendations when more in-depth analysis of the violations were available to them. Information is power, and it can and should be used by protection actors to great effect with this mechanism.

However, with a few notable exceptions, the information available on attacks against schools is largely spotty or absent in the Secretary General's reports on country situations to the Working Group. Circumstantial evidence suggests that protection partners have not spent as much time examining the issue and empowering their partners to report and make suggestions on how to better protect schools and students during armed conflict. Without the information and analysis needed, attacks against schools and students and the power of the Security Council to compel parties to respect and protect education in conflict will remain woefully underdeveloped. Other violations have similarly languished, but advances *have* been made that might prove useful for partners wishing to strengthen the protection of education in conflict through this mechanism.

In July 2011, in its Resolution 1998, the Security Council expanded the listing criteria to include those parties to conflict who perpetrate or threaten to perpetrate attacks against schools or school personnel. This is important for the additional attention and focus it will generate for country teams dealing with attacks against schools and students, and it will also result in mandatory action plans to cover this violation. Much work remains to be done, both at headquarters and in the field, in response to these new challenges for protection, and it must include reaching out in a more concerted way to UNESCO, educationalists, and human rights partners in the field.

As stated earlier, it is expected that, when violations are identified, country teams can suggest Security Council interventions as well as actions the parties should take under applicable national and international law. For genuine protection of education and students in armed conflict to become a reality on the ground, UN specialized agencies and their partners must sustain efforts at better monitoring and reporting on attacks against education. Additionally, joint MRM task forces should utilize monitoring and reporting on attacks on education to strengthen their advocacy and recommendations to the Security Council Working Group on Children and Armed Conflict (CAAC). Information is power. Its efficient delivery to those who can hold violators accountable is an opportunity that we can no longer afford to ignore.

Conclusion

I wish to reiterate that more can be done to protect education from attack in all its manifestations, to improve the ability of education to protect children, and to strengthen MRM to protect education in armed conflict.

With this in mind, I would make the following recommendations to the UN system, protection partners, educationalists and donors:

Education is a key stabilizer and must be a part of any emergency planning in conflict prone or conflict-affected areas. Education's role in protecting children from abuse and harm through either direct action or alerts to protection personnel cannot be overstated.

Protection should be seen as a crucial part of education in conflict-affected countries, and funding and training for protection should be built into any programs for these states.

SCR 1612 and 1998-mandated monitoring and reporting can serve to better protect education during conflict, and UNESCO, educational agencies, and NGOs involved in education can and should join country task forces to better monitor attacks on education and to advocate with the Council on appropriate actions as well as action plan engagement with concerned armed forces and groups.

Education outreach for vulnerable communities pre- and post-conflict is an important protection tool. Donors and agencies planning for child protection must seek to ensure broader coverage of disadvantaged communities.

Preserving Humanitarian Space in Long-Term Conflict

Peter Hansen

With very few exceptions, it has been considered self-evident among those in the humanitarian community that to achieve a reasonable measure of success humanitarian action in conflict zones should be predicated upon notions of neutrality and impartiality. In recent years, particularly following the outbreak of numerous local and regional armed conflicts in places such as Angola, Afghanistan, the Balkans, Iraq, Sierra Leone, Burundi, Ethiopia and Eritrea, Chechnya, Colombia, and East Timor, an increasing number of observers have challenged this traditional presumption of humanitarian action, arguing that "humanitarian actors are deeply involved in the political sphere."[1]

For anyone familiar with the humanitarian imperative that has come to define so much of what the United Nations (UN) has stood for since its founding, the implications of this challenge are great. If humanitarian space is purposefully compromised by assuming a political character, the risk of that space collapsing altogether becomes all too real. Some have suggested that the attack on UN headquarters in Baghdad in August 2003 was the result of "a dangerous blurring of the lines between humanitarian and political action" and "the consequent erosion of the core humanitarian principles of neutrality, impartiality and independence" of the UN humanitarian mission.[2] This line of thought maintains that the gradual erosion of humanitarian space in Iraq has been the result of the "choices made" (i.e., policy choices) by the international community through the UN since 1991, beginning with years of hard-hitting sanctions imposed by the Security Council, followed by "the lack of a clear UN mandate" in the aftermath of the US invasion and occupation of Iraq in 2003.[3] The conceptual dilemma it presents is something that would seem to require the careful consideration of all who find themselves on the front-line of humanitarian action in conflict zones, particularly at this critical juncture in the history of the humanitarian enterprise.

This chapter examines what is meant by the concept of humanitarian space, and how such space is best maintained in conflict zones while taking into account divergent views on the subject. To this end, I explore how the largest humanitarian actor in the Middle East—the United Nations Relief and Works Agency for Palestine Refugees in the Near East (UNRWA)—has struggled to maintain its humanitarian space in a particularly volatile conflict zone for over five decades.

Humanitarian Space: Principles, Challenges, and UNRWA's Experience

In his 1995 Annual Report, former Secretary-General Boutros Boutros-Ghali noted that "safeguarding both the concept and the reality of 'humanitarian space' remains one of the most significant challenges facing the humanitarian community."[4] But what exactly is meant by the term humanitarian space? It has been variously described, *inter alia*, as follows:

> "Humanitarian space is more than a physical area; it is a concept in and through which impartiality and non-partisanship govern the whole of humanitarian action . . . in moral terms""; [it is] "a space that is not delimited, that is made up of tolerance and respect for each and every individual once they are wounded or captive, and displaced persons or refugees, no matter to which side they belong."[5]
>
> "If we assume that war and violence are extensions of the political, then we understand the traditional description of humanitarian space as an area separate from the political."[6]
>
> "Humanitarian space is a dynamic term. Far from being like a walled room of fixed dimensions, humanitarian space . . . expands or contracts depending on circumstances. It may be circumscribed—or expanded—by the actions of political and military authorities; it also may be enlarged—or contracted—by humanitarian actors themselves. In short, humanitarian space is neither durable nor transferable but elastic."[7]
>
> "Humanitarian space is that space where humanitarian assistance is provided on the basis of need and is delivered with impartiality. Humanitarian space is 'owned' by humanitarian agencies and actors and extends from their inherent values of independence and impartiality. Military forces must minimize any movement into 'humanitarian space.' Any such movement serves to blur the distinction between humanitarian and military actors."[8]

It is apparent from the preceding characterizations that humanitarian space is based upon two central assumptions. First, it exists simultaneously on both a physical and moral plane. Accordingly, medical relief convoys and hospitals are as much a part of humanitarian space as the awareness by military and paramilitary actors that refugee camps must be respected as violence-free civilian areas. Second, humanitarian space is predicated on the need to maintain designated areas that are neutral and impartial within larger spaces that are inherently political. For example, in the heat of a military conflict between two or more combatants, the provision of medical aid to civilians and other noncombatants in designated health clinics must be protected and respected as inviolable by all parties. Historically, especially over the course of the twentieth century, the concept of humanitarian space has evolved in response to the increasing level of violence experienced by and directed towards civilians and other noncombatants in times of war. In answer to the need to provide protection and assistance to such vulnerable populations in conflict zones, neutral and humanitarian institutions such as the International Committee of the Red Cross (ICRC) and the UN were established, and the international community promulgated an extensive body of international humanitarian law,[9] central tenets of which have been the concepts of humanitarian action and humanitarian space. In the context of the Arab-Israeli conflict, UNRWA has maintained a humanitarian space over its fifty-three-year history that is unique in the UN system. From focusing in its very early years on refugee reintegration activities, UNRWA has developed into a multifaceted organization that provides essential education, health, relief and social services, and microcredit to more than four million Palestine refugees throughout its areas of operations. In addition, the vast majority of the over 300,000 agency staff are Palestinian refugees themselves, which itself uniquely marks the humanitarian space that UNRWA occupies.

Because of the highly volatile and prolonged nature of the conflict in which it operates, UNRWA has been compelled to maintain its humanitarian space in a wide variety of "conflict" situations, including periods of war (1956, 1967, 1973, and 1982), periods of limited and prolonged occupation (1950–1966, 1967–present in the West Bank and Gaza Strip; 1982–2000 in Lebanon) and periods of insurrection or closure (1970 in Jordan; 1987–93, 2000–present in the West Bank and Gaza Strip). In each of these periods, UNRWA has faced numerous challenges to its humanitarian space, including: threats to the physical safety and security of its staff and beneficiaries; the detention without charge or trial of its staff; curtailment of the freedom of movement of its vehicles, goods, and staff; the misuse, damage, and/or demolition of its installations and premises; and the damage and/or destruction of refugee shelters.

While UNRWA has exerted great efforts to maintain its humanitarian space over the years, the period since September 2000—the month in which the current intifada in the Occupied Palestinian Territory (OPT) began—has presented some of the most difficult challenges in its history. Limitations enforced on UNRWA's humanitarian space have been numerous, and have included severe access restrictions and armed attacks on its personnel and installations.

Many of these limitations on UNRWA's humanitarian space have contravened applicable principles of international law, including the Charter of the United Nations, the 1946 Convention on the Privileges and Immunities of the United Nations, the Fourth Geneva Convention and the 1967 bilateral exchange of letters between UNRWA and the Government of the State of Israel (known as the Comay-Michelmore Agreement).

In addition to the Arab-Israeli conflict, armed conflicts in other regions in recent years have given rise to a debate as to whether humanitarian action must be neutral and impartial in order to be effective in meeting its goals. According to Weiss, a number of developments in the 1990s—including "the complete disregard for international humanitarian law" in conflict zones, "the direct targeting of civilians and relief personnel," and "the protracted nature of many so-called emergencies that in fact last for decades"—has split the humanitarian community into two groups.[10] On the one hand are the traditionalists who "believe that humanitarian action can and should be strictly insulated from politics," and on the other are the "political humanitarians, who believe that political and humanitarian action cannot and should not be disassociated."[11] This split has been exacerbated by the international community's increasing willingness to deal with humanitarian crises as threats to international peace and security, most particularly in high profile cases, allowing for the simultaneous and at times combined deployment of military and humanitarian personnel in conflict zones.[12] This incremental integration of the military with the humanitarian witnessed in recent years has brought into sharp relief the dilemmas of humanitarian action and the maintenance of humanitarian space in the contemporary period, and "carries crucial policy and institutional implications for the humanitarian enterprise."[13]

A good example of a conflict that captured the essence of the debate and the resulting dilemma is the war in Kosovo. For the traditionalists, the widespread reference to that war as "humanitarian" was regarded as a particularly striking, if not offensive, oxymoron. As noted by one traditionalist,

How can a war—essentially something that causes destruction, losses and unspeakable suffering—be 'humanitarian'? Even if the motives are of a humanitarian nature—defending the basic rights of any human being—war itself cannot be 'humanitarian.' This most inappropriate libel . . . has been very detrimental to the humanitarian concept itself, and to humanitarian action as such.

The 'merging' of military and humanitarian operations has been facilitated by this gross contradiction in terms, and the ensuing confusion has grown exponentially.[14]

For the "political humanitarians," such "confusion" was a welcome development. In their view, the simultaneous bombardment of Serb forces along with the provision of relief assistance to Kosovar refugees made it possible to stop even greater atrocities before they took place, thereby saving more lives as well as bringing about conditions for a relatively quick political settlement. In this sense, the resort to force was the lesser of two evils, and one that better served the ultimate objectives of humanitarian action.

To the traditionalists, because humanitarian space is neutral and impartial, its proper maintenance depends upon its separation from the political and violent. Because such space is viewed as finite, traditionalists hold that if it is increased there is necessarily less space available for the political/violent and vice versa.[15] Warner has noted that this "zero-sum" relationship has particular "implications for the occupation of a bounded area,"[16] such as during a state of belligerent occupation. For example, if a legal aid center run by a humanitarian agency is raided and shut down by an occupying power, or the protection afforded to refugee camps is violated by military or paramilitary actors, the total area of political/violent space has increased at the direct expense of the humanitarian space formerly maintained by the humanitarian actor. Such has been the case on a number of occasions where UNRWA installations in the OPT, schools and health clinics among them, have been forcibly commandeered by Israeli military forces for use in military operations, or when both the Israeli military and Palestinian militants violated the humanitarian space of the refugee camps in the OPT by conducting armed activities in them.[16]

For political humanitarians, on the other hand, humanitarian space and the political/violent do not operate in a zero-sum context. They argue that the expansion of humanitarian space allows for the parties to the conflict to avoid having to reach a swift political settlement, ultimately resulting in greater civilian suffering. As Warner notes:

> The recent rise in interest in humanitarian affairs is an abnegation of responsibility by those in power. That is, instead of admitting that civil wars or outbreaks of violence . . . are very political activities, these outbreaks are termed humanitarian crises in order to avoid hard decisions about what to do . . . In this sense, upholding humanitarian principles is a *political* move that may undercut the ethical basis of the [humanitarian] organization's activities [emphasis added].[17]

The maintenance of humanitarian space is therefore seen by political humanitarians as an act that effectively shifts "attention away from the politics at the heart"
of a conflict, thereby allowing it to continue interminably while humanitarian
agencies scramble for limited budgets to dole out "Band-Aid" operations on an
ostensibly "temporary" basis.[18] UNRWA has been subjected to such criticism over
the years by both parties to the conflict.

On one hand, Israelis and other supporters of Israel have accused the UNRWA
of "keeping the refugee issue alive" by reaffirming Palestine refugee identity and
rights, thereby rendering a political settlement of the problem in their view far more
difficult to achieve. On the other hand, some Arabs and Palestinians have accused
the UNRWA (as well as other international organizations) of providing a "humanitarian cover" for the Israeli occupation, thereby relieving Israel of its humanitarian
obligations under international law and enabling what in law is meant only as a
temporary condition to remain prolonged and without a final political settlement.

Is the divide between traditionalist and political humanitarian approaches
unbridgeable? Is there a more nuanced and less polarized way to approach the
maintenance of humanitarian space in conflict zones? It would seem that "humanitarians cannot deny political realties,"[19] and that political actors in a conflict must
acknowledge that they too have a vested interest in opening and helping to maintain humanitarian space that is neutral and impartial. As noted by Mary Anderson,
the key factor that must be accepted by all humanitarian actors is that, irrespective
of motives, the aid they provide has multiple political impacts and can either exacerbate or ease the conflicts amid which they work.[20] For instance, "to the extent that
international aid agencies assume responsibility for civilian survival in war zones,
the aid they provide can serve to release whatever internal resources exist for the
pursuit of the conflict."[21] In this way, it can be said that humanitarian aid carries
with it certain "substitution effects."[22] As noted above, in the context of UNRWA's
work, the Agency has been accused by the Palestinians that its vast array of humanitarian and human development aid has effectively underwritten the Israeli occupation, relieving the occupying power of the tremendous financial burden of administering the occupation and enabling it to divert precious resources toward con-
solidating its military control over the OPT. Similarly, international aid can have
"legitimization effects," in the sense that the recipients of such aid may regard the
fact of their receiving it as a legitimization of their political cause or struggle. This
is particularly true if the recipients are a distinct group belonging to or overlapping with a party to the conflict. Again, in the UNRWA context, it is widely known
that the Palestine refugees consider the Agency not merely as an international aid
agency providing for their essential needs, but also as the physical/institutional

embodiment of the international community's commitment to their welfare. In this way, UNRWA can be said to be perceived by its beneficiaries as "humanitarian plus" in both its role and identity.

Humanitarian aid can also have certain "distribution effects," essentially referring to the divisions that necessarily result among people in a conflict zone when aid is provided to one group to the exclusion of others. As a humanitarian actor charged with the task of assisting the Palestine refugees in areas that include considerable numbers of Palestinians who are nonrefugees (in the UNRWA definition of the term), UNRWA has come under the criticism that its humanitarian aid has actually increased divisions among the Palestinians and done relatively little to assist a large sector of the Palestinian population that, in many cases, is as needy as the Palestine refugees themselves.

Although Anderson's analysis treats politics as forming an integral part of the role of humanitarian actors, adopting it is not inimical to the core principles of humanitarian space as neutral and impartial. On the contrary, this approach actually demands that neutrality and impartiality continue to form the cornerstone upon which humanitarian space is maintained. Neutrality, in this sense, cannot be understood merely as not taking sides in hostilities or engaging in controversies of a political or ideological nature, as defined by the ICRC, for instance.[23] Rather, neutrality should be the principle by which a humanitarian actor provides assistance in conflict situations where such assistance is objectively required, having no regard to the dictates or political positions of the parties to the conflict. Neutrality cannot mean equidistance between the parties to the conflict, and a humanitarian actor must position himself based on an ethical compass of justice and fairness. Likewise, impartiality must be understood as making no other discrimination in the provision of humanitarian aid other than on the basis of need, giving priority to those most needy. In this sense, identification or sympathy with race, religion, nationality, and other such characteristics must have no bearing on the provision of aid. In essence then, the efficient and effective humanitarian actor must continually act, and be seen to be acting, as making a good faith effort to remain neutral and impartial in situations that are inherently political. This is not an easy task, by any objective account, but it seems to be one that is required if humanitarian space is to be maintained in a world where the tragic effects of war and conflict are increasingly being borne by civilians. As noted by Weiss:

> In today's world, humanitarians must ask themselves how to weigh the political consequences of their action or inaction; and politicians must ask themselves how to gauge the humanitarian costs of their action or inaction. The calcula-

tions are tortuous, and the mathematics far from exact. However, there is no longer any need to ask whether politics and humanitarian action intersect. The real question is how this intersection can be managed to ensure more humanized politics and more effective humanitarian action. To this end, humanitarians should be neither blindly principled nor blindly pragmatic.[24]

In addition to the effects of resource transfers on conflict zones listed earlier, Anderson identifies a number of "implicit ethical messages" in humanitarian activity that also affect conflict. One of these messages is the idea of "impunity" of humanitarian staff who control scarce resources, such as vehicles and fuel, and sometimes "use them for [their] own pleasure without accountability to the people for whom the resources were intended, even when their needs are great."[25] Another such message is the idea of valuing lives differently,[26] highlighted when international aid agencies furnish expatriate staff with supplemental "hazard" pay for serving in particularly harsh duty stations, while failing or being unable to extend similar benefits to local staff. While humanitarian action carries with it a number of other implicit ethical messages, these few examples highlight the difficulty inherent in maintaining humanitarian space without attracting criticism from those who are affected by it. Like many other humanitarian actors, UNRWA has faced criticisms of an ethical nature while seeking to maintain its humanitarian space. For example, funding constraints have prevented UNRWA from extending "hazard pay" to its area staff on a continuous basis, though expatriate staff receive the same.

As noted earlier, humanitarian space is elastic and its contours are continually defined by the parties to the conflict and the humanitarian actors involved in the situation. Special attention must be given to those occasions where a political actor's perceptions impel it to limit humanitarian space to the point where the continued maintenance of that space becomes virtually untenable. Such cases often occur where a party to the conflict enjoys a preponderance of power in a given conflict zone, such that any limitation of humanitarian space by that party is justified under the doctrine of "military necessity" or "national security." Resort to "security" interests provides the disproportionately powerful party to the conflict with a discretion that effectively trumps the efforts of the humanitarian actor to maintain humanitarian space. This problem is compounded by two factors. First, the notion of "military necessity" or "national security" is itself so nebulous as to allow the claimant very wide latitude vis-à-vis the humanitarian actor. Second, the claimant enjoys such overwhelming control over the physical space in which the humanitarian actor operates, that there is usually little that the latter can do to actually reverse developments on the ground. In the OPT, the Israeli authorities often state that the restrictions on UNRWA's humanitarian space are necessary due to considerations of military security or are justified under Israel's inherent right of self-defense. One of the bases upon which this claim is advanced is the Comay-Michelmore Agreement, which requires the government of Israel to "facilitate the task of UNRWA to the best of its ability, subject only to regulations or arrangements which may be necessitated by considerations of military security." At no time have the Israeli authorities and UNRWA been able to agree on the scope or application of the language relating to "military security." While UNRWA has taken the position that the term can only be construed narrowly in the specific emergency context of the immediate postwar period in June 1967, and is in any event not applicable by virtue of Article 103 of the UN Charter,[27] Israel has taken the position that the term continues to apply to its operations in the OPT, more than 5 decades after the close of the 1967 hostilities, and has traditionally construed it very liberally. This has resulted in greater limitations on humanitarian space in the OPT than UNRWA believes are reasonably necessary.

When one party to the conflict is so powerful as to enjoy overwhelming control over the physical space in which the humanitarian actor operates, it is useful to consider the options available to maintain humanitarian space. One of the more obvious options is for the humanitarian actor to engage the powerful party in negotiations/discussions on issues of concern, including reference to relevant provisions of international law, status agreements which the humanitarian actor may have with the powerful party, and general appeals to the humanitarian imperative and practicalities. Here, skills of persuasion and diplomacy must be employed in convincing the powerful party that the maintenance of humanitarian space in the conflict zone is ultimately in its own interests, not only military, political, and economic, but moral as well.

When such negotiations/discussions are exhausted, another mechanism that is available is to attempt to persuade the powerful party to cease its limitations on humanitarian space through public pronouncements, either in the media or otherwise. This has been put to good use in many conflict zones in defense of human rights and protection of civilian persons and refugees, among many others. It is a widely accepted form of conflict management and moral suasion that can, if employed properly, be utilized to great effect. This is particularly so in the current information age, where sources of information are unprecedented and knowledge can be transferred around the world, quite literally, at the click of a button. What must be stressed, however, is that publicity must not be used in a frivolous manner nor resolved to in haste. As in negotiations, good judgment is required in making the decision to "go public" and reticence in doing so is generally to be advised, if only for the sake of maintaining credibility and guarding against any backlash that may result from alienating the powerful party to the conflict. Should publicity fail to render a result, however, the humanitarian actor may look to regional and ultimately international intervention to help maintain its humanitarian space. The increasing number of times the international community has resorted to the use of sanctions and even military force since the early 1990s is well documented. Suffice it to say, that both the Security Council and regional bodies, such as NATO, have been employed in various conflict zones around the world in the name of humanitarian assistance, which itself has increasingly allowed the concept of "humanitarian intervention" to be debated by policy makers, academics, and commentators alike. Of course, humanitarian intervention is a matter that only states—and then only a very limited number of states at that—may initiate, but there have been precedents where humanitarian actors have played a central role in the intervention effort once underway. Examples include the UNHCR's role in repatriating and providing humanitarian aid to refugees in Iraq, Bosnia-Herzegovina, Kosovo, East Timor, and Afghanistan.

For its part, UNRWA has not accepted limitations on its operations and has sought to engage the parties to the conflict in a dialog, at times resorting to publicity in an effort to maintain its humanitarian space. Thus, it has continued to make representations to the Israeli authorities at all levels, including meetings with the Israeli Ministries of Foreign Affairs and Defence, to have constraints on UNRWA's humanitarian space removed or alleviated. As a matter of policy, UNRWA has agreed, without prejudice to its positions of principle under international law, to consider pragmatic solutions that attempt to meet legitimate Israeli security concerns, while easing the movement of its staff members and other such restrictions on its humanitarian space. On other, far more limited occasions, UNRWA has issued public statements on the situation of the refugees (for instance with regard to the demolition of refugee shelters) casting light on the practices of various parties to the conflict and calling upon them to change their behavior. Finally, on an even more limited number of occasions, UNRWA has relied for support of its humanitarian activities on the international community through the General Assembly and the Security Council, albeit not through economic sanctions and military force, but through the reaffirmation of the need to support UNRWA in ensuring "the safety of civilians" in the OPT and calling on all parties to "respect the universally accepted norms of international humanitarian law" as stated for example in Security Council Resolution 1405 of 19 April 2003. Overall, UNRWA's efforts to engage the Israelis on these issues has been unrelenting and principled in its commitment to core humanitarian values. Nevertheless, the responses of the Israeli government have been grossly inadequate to address these issues. According to a November 2003 status report issued by the Task Force on Project Implementation in the OPT, the "multiple assurances" given by the Israeli government that "humanitarian aid will be fully facilitated . . . contrast dramatically with the facts on the ground," and the "operational environment" has "deteriorated to a degree which many donors consider both unmanageable and unacceptable."

Nevertheless, very serious limitations continue to be imposed on UNRWA's humanitarian space in the OPT, primarily, though not exclusively, by the occupying power. Israeli soldiers throughout the OPT have on many occasions failed to show respect for UNRWA personnel, their vehicles, or their identification cards, as required under international law. On-duty staff members also have been verbally abused, physically assaulted, threatened at gunpoint, and shot at. Since March 2002, eight UNRWA staff members have been shot and killed by Israeli troops, and agency ambulances have been shot at by Israeli soldiers. In addition, there have been many instances where UNRWA installations, particularly schools, have been shot at by Israeli troops, resulting in a number of deaths of and numerous injuries to both school staff and pupils. For their part, the Israeli authorities insist that such shooting incidents occur only because Palestinian militants fire on Israeli positions and settlements from within UNRWA school compounds. While there have been a very limited number of such incidents at the beginning of the current intifada, UNRWA moved to provide twenty-four-hour unarmed guards for all of its facilities and called on the Palestinian Authority for greater police protection. In addition to violating UNRWA's privileges and immunities, even the search and inspection procedures imposed by the Israeli authorities on agency staff in the OPT can pose a threat to their safety and well-being. Such was the case in the Gaza Strip where UNRWA staff and vehicles are required to be searched prior to being allowed to enter the Al Mawasi area. Accessibility to health service installations in the OPT has been hindered for both patients and staff, including those being transported in ambulances and requiring critical care.

In the face of such seemingly overwhelming obstacles, the humanitarian actor must make every effort to engage parties to a conflict that resort to "military necessity" and "national security" grounds on their own terms. As noted, the humanitarian actor must challenge, wherever reasonable, the logic upon which such claims are based. An effort must be made to convince the disproportionately powerful party that its "security" may not reasonably be under threat and that its overall national interests may in fact be better served by helping maintain humanitarian space intact. Such efforts require a good understanding of basic international humanitarian law doctrine such as military necessity and proportionality, and a willingness to engage the political actor on these terms. They also require an acknowledgment on the part of the humanitarian actor that the neutrality and impartiality of the space it aims to maintain sometimes depends on actively engaging with political players, and that given the balance of power on the ground, their efforts may often produce little or no results. Such are some of the pitfalls of maintaining humanitarian space in conflict zones that have been marked by protracted political disputes.

UNRWA's efforts in actively defending and maintaining its humanitarian space in the OPT have encompassed a wide array of activities and programs. Foremost among them has been its Refugee Affairs Officer (RAO) Program initiated during the intifada of 1987–1993. Following the request of the Secretary-General to enhance its "general assistance" capacity in the OPT, the RAO program was launched in 1988 to facilitate UNRWA operations in the difficult circumstances of the intifada and to provide a degree of passive protection to the refugee and nonrefugee population of the OPT. The program included a "legal aid scheme" run by UNRWA for the benefit of the refugees. Following the conclusion of the Declaration of Principles of Interim Self-Government Arrangements (DOP) in 1993, the RAO program was phased out.

In 2001, UNRWA launched the Operations Support Officer (OSO) Program to reinforce its existing operations in the OPT and to help deal with the increasingly severe access restrictions faced by the UNRWA. Like the RAO program before it, the OSO program aims to maintain the humanitarian space in which UNRWA operates. It has accomplished this by, *inter alia*, helping to facilitate access of staff members and UNRWA vehicles, reporting on the developing humanitarian crisis in the OPT, and in monitoring and inspecting all UNRWA installations on a regular basis to ensure that they are not being used for any unauthorized or improper purposes.

Another important policy of UNRWA that has helped it maintain its humanitarian space has been the standard requirement of its staff to remain at arms length from all activity, particularly political, that may call into question the neutrality and impartiality of its humanitarian mission. Among other things, agency staff have been instructed to conduct themselves in accordance with established principles and practices of the UN and of the need to refrain from engaging in any activity that is incompatible with their status as independent and impartial UN civil servants. In particular, staff have been informed that they must be scrupulous about the protection of UNRWA installations against any kind of abuse or unauthorized use which may reflect negatively on the agency's position as an independent and neutral body of the UN, including ensuring that political meetings are not held in UNRWA installations, that posters of a political nature are not affixed to the premises, and that UNRWA property, including vehicles, is not in any way used for any purpose unconnected with UNRWA operations. UNRWA staff have been informed that any misuse of their position will—in addition to creating legitimate apprehensions in host countries, in the occupying power, and in donor states, regarding the confidence to be reposed in the agency—result in disciplinary measures being taken against the staff member, including the possibility of dismissal. Although these statements of UNRWA's commitment to neutrality and impartiality have been accepted by its staff, some criticism has been levied by staff members and the wider Palestinian community accusing the agency of attempting to infringe upon the right to free speech of its staff members. This is demonstrative of the tension that exists in the process of maintaining humanitarian space not only in the OPT, but in any conflict zone where local staff strongly identify with one or the other party to the conflict.

What of the future of humanitarian space? Lincoln Chen has noted that "the ultimate shape" of humanitarian space "is being contested by public policies and action on-the-ground," and "will be determined, in part, by new issues, new ideas and new players."[28] One such idea is the concept of comprehensive "human security" which he identifies as having "four basic principles": first, that human security is "people-centered," as opposed to state-centered; second, human security comprehensively promotes freedom "from both violence and poverty"; third, human security is strategically based on protection from the state and empowerment at the grassroots level; and fourth, human security is interdependent in the sense that the security of one can never be achieved at the expense of another.[29] The idea of comprehensive human security meshes neatly with global developments on every score, from the social-scientific to the political, from the economic to the technological.

As noted earlier, the information age has played a significant role in helping expand and maintain humanitarian space in conflict zones. All signs indicate that the role of media and information in this regard will only intensify as technology and access to it develops. A good example of the use of technology and information to expand and maintain humanitarian space are the specialty websites devoted to the topic of humanitarian intervention and activism, such as the OCHA-run Relief-Web. This is in addition, of course, to the growing body of academic and specialty journals on humanitarian action, refugees, and other such subjects with a humanitarian focus. For its part, UNRWA has its own website and has regularly made use of the media (through press releases, interviews, and periodic newspaper articles) to help promote its mission among its stakeholders and the international community at large, all of which has enhanced its ability to maintain its humanitarian space.

In conclusion, it can be said that the decade since the end of the Cold War has been an immense challenge for all humanitarian actors. The marked increase in interstate and intrastate conflict, low-intensity conflict, and the rapid proliferation of nonstate actors in conflict situations has caused untold suffering to innocent civilians around the world. These events have posed considerable challenges to the maintenance of humanitarian space in conflict zones. The humanitarian community today has to tread a fine line while adhering to principles of neutrality and impartiality in areas that are inherently political and usually violent. While UNRWA is unique in the UN System by virtue of its organizational status, beneficiary base, and evolution of its mandate, it has faced and continues to face the same challenges in maintaining its humanitarian space that all humanitarian actors now have to deal with. UNRWA's experience with multiple conflict situations, in the OPT in particular, provides a useful example for other humanitarian actors to follow. It goes without saying that the contours of humanitarian space will continue to be shaped by those who are actually engaged in the activity of humanitarian intervention—states, multilateral organizations, and civil society actors. As such, new measures to promote the idea of humanitarianism all over the world, most particularly in conflict zones, should be developed in a manner that highlights the great importance of the values that lie at the core of humanitarian action and space, including neutrality and impartiality, but also encompassing core principles of justice, fairness, equality, and liberty.

Humanitarian Action in a New Barbarian Age

David Rieff

If the hope for human progress and for a better world can be said to rest on any-thing, it rests on the great documents of international law that have been promul-gated since the end of the Second World War. These include, first and foremost, the United Nations Charter and the Universal Declaration of Human Rights. But while these documents offer a global vision of what the world might become if humanity is lucky, they remain more hope than reality. In contrast, the corpus of international humanitarian law, that is, the rules governing armed conflict, have actually proved its utility again and again over the course of the past half-century. The four Geneva Conventions and their Additional Protocols, the Genocide Convention, and, more recently, such initiatives as the Rome Treaty banning landmines, are no mere pious sentiments. They have saved innumerable human lives. Think, for example, of the fact that since the adoption of the international treaty that banned the use of poison gas as a weapon of war, gas, so ubiquitous in the trenches of the Western Front dur-ing World War I, has probably only been used a handful of times since. Norms, it seems, can sometimes influence realities.

That said, it would be a misreading of history, and, perhaps, a culpable exercise in self-flattery as well, to make a fetish of the law and imagine that realities will invariably or inevitably migrate toward norms. Despite the more grandiose claims of human rights activists, as well as of distinguished philosophers such as Jürgen Habermas, the record is more mixed: Over the course of the past half-century, there are examples where they have and examples where they have not. The full legal emancipation of African Americans in the US civil rights movement of the 1950s, 1960s, and 1970s is an example of a law-based reform or, to put it differently, a nor-mative transformation that did end up transforming American social reality even though at least a significant minority and possibly even a majority of Americans were against such decisions as *Brown v. Board of Education* when they were first handed down. And yet, in contrast, normative changes related to the status and treatment of children encapsulated in the UN Convention on the Rights of the

Child have had limited impact outside the developed world despite the best efforts of many dedicated activists and political figures.

In other words, the record is mixed. Those who believe that human progress is inevitable often describe this as a matter of "two steps forward, one step back," as the former head of Human Rights Watch, Aryeh Neier, did in his history of the human rights movement. This is not to say that no progress has been made or that it is unreasonable to expect that more will be made in the future. To the contrary, even among those of us for whom the Classical Greek vision of history as cyclical seems to conform better to the realities of our sad world than the Christian, Marxist, or, indeed, liberal expectation that progress in the moral order of the world is as bound to take place as progress in scientific understanding, would hardly want to do away with the notion of progress altogether. As the great liberal realist, Raymond Aron, once put it, "if one is not [an advocate of progress], what is left?" Humanity, he added, had no hope for survival "outside of reason and science."[1]

Aron's conclusion in large measure amounted to insisting that one had to be optimistic in spite of what one knew—"despite the twentieth century, I remain an advocate of progress," was the way he put it. This is not to be confused with the more self-congratulatory fables that have captured the imagination of far too many decent people in the contemporary world, and that revolve around the notion that a "revolution of moral concern"—the phrase is that of the Canadian writer and erstwhile politician, Michael Ignatieff— began in the aftermath of World War II, gave rise to the United Nations system as well as to the transformation of both the concept of state sovereignty and the reach of international law. For those who believe in its reality, this revolution has no downside, no tragic element to it (unlike all previous revolutions in human history, whether economic, like the Industrial Revolution, or political, like the American Revolution). Instead, it promises to usher in a better world in which the worst human cruelties and historical tragedies—another World War I, Shoah, or Gulag Archipelago—will not be permitted to unfold and whose perpetrators will not enjoy the impunity that they have throughout most, if not all, of human history.

Aron was not an optimist. Nor, lest it be forgotten, were the founders of the United Nations. To the contrary, many of them had been soldiers and all of them anguished observers of the most terrible war the world had ever known. They were idealists, not utopians, and steely idealists at that. But if an Eleanor Roosevelt or a Gladwyn Jebb viewed the nascent world body as a means of preventing the kind of descent into the inferno that the Nazi experience had revealed to be a constant human possibility rather than as a means of inducing any ideal world order, their successors gradually became more optimistic. A document like Secretary General

Boutros Boutros-Ghali's 1991 "An Agenda for Peace" described a world that really might be perfectible. And the final documents that accompanied the decade-long extravaganzas of UN conferences of the 1990s, culminating in the formulation of the so-called Millennium Development Goals, had a similarly utopian tinge to them. Poverty would be halved by a date certain; States that abused their own populations would be forced to desist because the Westphalian order, with its culture of impunity, was fading and we were entering the age of rights. War would be limited in scope, with limitations on what weapons could be employed when and where, steadily expanding protections for noncombatants, property, and cultural and religious sites growing in scope.

This would happen, activists often argued, because of the transformation and expansion of legal norms and the campaigning of civil society groups. The context for the change would be the UN, which was viewed (and, indeed, for all its faults continues to be viewed in this way by many people throughout the world) as the sole legitimate authority for international rules that could apply to all of humankind. The fact that the UN was an institution without much real power and that the term civil society is so nebulous as to be more a sociopolitical Rorschach blot for campaigners and activists than a term that has any real specific gravity passed largely unnoticed during the 1990s—that "silly season" of the inflated expectations. (Otherwise, why is Human Rights Watch, which has no democratic accountability, viewed as an emblematic institution of civil society while the US National Rifle Association, with four million members, is viewed as something else?)

Instead, there was the very real expectation that the world was becoming a more civilized place. Again, why the same decade that witnessed the Balkan catastrophe and the Rwandan genocide could interpret itself as a period of enormous promise is a question for psychiatrists, not political analysts. But that optimism was real. And the creation of the International Criminal Court, which was heralded as the first institution that promised to genuinely promise an end to impunity for war criminals, served as the capstone for these generous and well-intended expectations of decent people around the world.

As Undersecretary General for Peacekeeping, Kofi Annan had presided over the two worst failures of the United Nations during the first post–Cold War decade. But as Secretary General, Annan not only acknowledged the UN's failures—however belatedly, and, in the case of Rwanda, not until 2004 on the eve of the tenth anniversary of the genocide, and then only quite ambivalently—but made the UN Secretariat a bully pulpit for this "revolution of moral concern" and for individual human rights as finally "trumping" state sovereignty. Annan's UN was a place in which international law, above all international humanitarian law—that is, the laws of war—was viewed as the essential component for building a more decent world order. And in speech after speech and document after document, UN officials from the Secretary General himself on down emphasized the need for States to comply with the obligations they had under the various international treaties and conventions to which they had signed on. The problem, UN officials repeated, was no longer one of first principles; the transformation of the normative environment had seen to that. Rather, the question was now one of making these norms binding—in short, of enforcement.

In retrospect, this approach begged at least as many questions as it answered. To begin with, there was the uncomfortable matter of why, if the norms were so terrific, the reality of the world was so dire? But at least that objection could be answered by saying that just as it had taken a great deal of time and struggle and false starts to get the norms right, so it would take a long period before effective modalities of enforcement were arrived at. And activists could point to studies ranging from the report on UN peacekeeping by the former Algerian foreign minister, Lakhdar Brahimi, to the Canadian government-sponsored document on humanitarian intervention, "The Responsibility to Protect," as examples of serious efforts to think about implementing the new norms and of, in effect, institutionalizing and reifying that "revolution of moral concern."

More difficult was the issue of what possible motivation could impel States to act out of essentially altruistic motives, which, however much they had been weakened by the realities of globalization, were still the fundamental constitutive elements of world order. That is, why would great powers intervene to prevent genocide in places of little economic or geostrategic significance to themselves except very rarely and inconsistently? One did not have to be a Kissingerian realist, or the reincarnation of Lord Palmerston, to conclude that States had never behaved in this way in the past. For all of history until the post–World War II era, the conduct of States had largely been determined by interests, rather than ideals. The question was what, if anything, had changed? Was Ignatieff's idealist template of the human rights revolution of the second half of the twentieth century really that compelling? Or, as the British diplomat Robert Cooper argues in an influential book, *The Breaking of Nations: Order and Chaos in the Twenty-First Century*, did the fact that a successful global economy required a rules-based order really imply a commitment to a human rights rule as well?

On the face of things, that appeared unlikely. Africa, where most of the crises that might require so-called humanitarian intervention were occurring, was by the turn of the millennium almost irrelevant to the world economy except for certain key resources like oil that could be extracted even during civil wars and famines. At a generous estimate, it accounted for some 3 percent of world trade. The Balkans, East Timor, Haiti: they were similarly marginal in geoeconomic terms. This reality, which is as undeniable as its elaboration is unpalatable, tends to confirm Ignatieff's thesis, not Cooper's. At the very least, it threw the debate back into the context of morality. And if the 1990s had proved anything, it was that where morality was concerned the so-called international community was highly selective in its commitments. The British might decide to do something about their ex-colony, Sierra Leone, but even the highly interventionist Blair government was at pains to point out that its deployment was not to be construed as the first of many. There would be no British troops sent to Zimbabwe on human rights grounds although the tyranny of Robert Mugabe was almost as destructive to its own people as the Revolutionary United Front had been in Sierra Leone (the Mugabe government simply used hunger and internal displacement as its principle weapons, rather than the mutilations that were the monstrous hallmark of the Revolutionary United Front). The Clinton administration made the same point after the United States–led war in Kosovo in 1999.

Of course, had the great powers been willing to give the UN a standing force and the authority to deploy it, as the UN's own Sir Brian Urquhart had once suggested, the dilemma might not have been so acute. But the great powers found a weak UN exactly to their liking, while, in much of the developing world, the critique of absolute state sovereignty that Kofi Annan had pursued was viewed as a way of legitimizing neocolonialism rather than guaranteeing or helping to secure people's human rights. Inevitably, instead of being narrowed, the gap between the new norms of international humanitarian law and realities on the ground began to widen. The fact that some humanitarian interventions, notably the one in Kosovo, were undertaken without UN approval only increased skepticism in the developing world about possible hidden agendas in the revolution of moral concern.

Perhaps, had the September 11 attacks not taken place, some consensus might have been arrived at. Possible, but not likely. While the attacks on the World Trade Center and the Pentagon did transform the landscape of international relations, many of the contradictions between norms and realities that September 11 put in such sharp relief were already part of the geostrategic landscape. It is just that, like icebergs in the North Atlantic, they lay largely submerged and out of view.

So many factors militated against norms becoming reality. First and foremost, the UN had no real power to set the agenda anywhere except where the great powers had no great interest in setting one themselves. Thus, before September 11, the UN view on Tajikistan carried some weight, but once the US decided to invade Afghanistan the UN was relegated to the sidelines. Second, there was no appetite in the rich world for the kind of redistributive justice that would have begun to address the underlying inequities that were at the root of so many so-called humanitarian or human rights crises. The refusal of the European Union nations to radically overhaul their policies of massively subsidizing their own agricultural sector was one illustration of this. The comparative failure of the debt relief movement to sway Washington in any truly significant way was another. Third, despite what Third World intellectuals might imagine, there was no appetite in Western Europe, Japan, or the United States, to "recolonize" the world. The logic of Secretary General Annan's speeches might sometimes seem to imply endless wars of altruism, but neither Washington nor Brussels was prepared to make any such commitment or to facilitate and subsidize a UN force that would.

The September 11 attacks only exacerbated these trends. But they exacerbated them to a remarkable degree. Confronted by terrorism, whether or not it was appropriate to call the necessary response to it a "war" as the Bush administration did, it was the politics of that most profound and essential interest—existential security—that was at the fore of policymakers' calculations, not elective wars in the name of humanitarianism and human rights. At the same time, much as had been the case during the Cold War, States threatened by terrorism were not only immediately engaged in curtailing domestic civil liberties but tended to be more willing to overlook human rights violations, even on a massive scale, by States that might play a strategic role in the antiterrorist campaign.

The American government's volte-face on Uzbekistan—surely one of the most abusive regimes on the face of the earth—because the Karimov dictatorship had facilitated US operations during the invasion of Afghanistan was a case in point. In fairness, human rights concerns have always been ignored—as much if not more so in Europe as in the United States—when major commercial interests were at stake, as the case of China has demonstrated all too vividly. It is true that, during the so-called Arab Spring, the French government proved itself to be willing to take the lead in the international intervention to overthrow the Gaddafi dictatorship in Libya, with which it had strong commercial ties. But the Western response to the Arab Spring generally is something of an outlier, and are best understood as Western governments believing change in the Arab Middle East is inevitable and, for once, attempting to help shape events rather than react to them.

Senior UN officials are perfectly well aware of these trends. But since it has little real power (to use Joseph Nye's categories, it has no hard power and only a small amount of soft power), and since its legitimacy is derived so importantly from its commitment to the primacy of international law, the world organization was hard-pressed to shift gears to somehow respond to or at least accommodate these new realities. Perhaps, had it done so, it would have destroyed its own raison d'etre. But by not adjusting, the UN found itself wrong-footed by the new world disorder that the rise of Islamic terrorism and the international response to that terrorism had brought into being. In effect, it believed it could remain a noncombatant in that struggle. But neither the terrorists, nor, for that matter, the Bush administration were prepared to concede the UN the right to maintain such a stance.

Sergio Vieira de Mello was without question the most brilliant UN diplomat of his generation, a throwback, in terms of charisma, dedication, intelligence, and drive, to such figures as Folke Bernadotte and Brian Urquhart. But when he reluctantly accepted Secretary General Annan's plea to becoming the UN's special representative in Baghdad after the overthrow of Saddam Hussein, de Mello never seems to have imagined that the anti-US insurgents and terrorists would view the UN as aligned with the US invasion. In a sense, he was right: Institutionally, the UN had opposed the war. As de Mello saw it, he was trying to help the Iraqi people, not serve the US occupation authorities. As the UN report on his death concluded, neither de Mello nor his colleagues seem to have fully taken in the fact that to the Iraqi guerrillas, the UN was just as much the enemy as the US was. And de Mello was not so much wrong—what else could he have done? To have hunkered down in a bunker, as the Americans did, would have been to betray everything the UN and he personally stood for—as overtaken by a colder world. Faithful to his ideals, he died for his belief in the UN, which, whether one shares it or not, ennobles his sacrifice. But it is by no means clear that those ideals can be held on to.

The ways in which the United States has turned the international order on its head in the aftermath of September 11 are obvious. By eschewing any serious commitment to the multilateralism that lies at the heart of international law, the future of any viable world system, however embryonic, in any usable time frame, is open to question. But terrorism also throws that future into question. For terrorism, by definition, challenges the state's monopoly on force, which must lie at the heart of any international system worthy of the name. It also deforms, if it does not negate entirely, the soldier-civilian distinction that lies at the heart of international humanitarian law. To be sure, that distinction was already under threat from the revolution in military technology of the last decade. A guerrilla force cannot fight a modern army equipped with night vision equipment (this has deprived guerrilla forces of their strongest traditional advantage, the night), thermal imaging, GPS, smart weapons, drones, and satellites. Or, rather, it cannot fight such an army while obeying the laws of war. To the contrary, it must employ perfidy, pretending until the moment it attacks that its fighters are noncombatants, and it must employ terror, because while it cannot hope to challenge a modern army on the battlefield, it can hope to demoralize that modern army's citizens back home.

The idea that guerrilla forces would simply bow to the superior technology of modern armies from developed countries is as utopian as the expectation that war itself has been superseded. An American judge once remarked famously that the US Constitution was not a suicide pact. By the same token, for the guerrilla fighter, neither are the laws of war. And from Gaza to Iraq, the force of that reality is becoming pOf course, where this leaves an international system (a sounder concept than international community) that is law-based is very much an open question. And it is hard not to feel that, notwithstanding the Arab Spring, and the success of democratization in Burma, that a new barbarian age is upon us. One of the first victims of that age was Sergio Vieira de Mello. He will, of course, not be the last.

PART IV

Actors

The ultimate challenge early in humanitarian crises is to maintain a necessary equanimity in the face of terrible disorder, so that one can forge an effective response. One must channel the skills and energies of the multiple actors that are required to change, at first, chaos into a semblance of stability, and later, hopefully, into peace. As a physician, I have been accustomed to employing the tools of public health in dealing with epidemics. The logic, and even the terminology, of preventive medicine, is understandable to politicians, diplomats, military, journalists, and academics, as well as the medical profession. A number of the contributors in this section have employed medical analogies in fashioning their texts.

One of the supreme creations of the human spirit is the idea of prevention. Like liberty and equality, it is a seminal concept drawn from a reservoir of optimism that centuries of epidemics, famines, and wars have failed to deplete. It is an amalgam of hope and possibility, which assumes that misery is not an undefiable mandate of fate, a punishment only redeemable in a later life, but a condition that can be treated like a disease, and sometimes cured or even prevented.

Such optimism is essential for those who choose disaster relief work as a profession. This section includes profound reflections by realists who have seen the devastation of conflicts and disasters, yet know there is also beauty and hope in our profession. I have selected two UN Secretary Generals, a university President, a long-term UN humanitarian relief leader, two renowned diplomat/scholars, a military-civilian authority, and a journalist to represent the many actors I have met on a journey of healing and solidarity in disaster areas. In several chapters I have purposely maintained the tense used by the authors at the time of writing in order to demonstrate the urgency and dilemmas faced by senior decision makers.

The Challenges of Preventive Diplomacy

The Role of the United Nations and Its Secretary-General

Boutros Boutros-Ghali

> One system of metaphors that I have recently used extensively is the comparison between peace and health. . . . Peace research and health research are metaphors for each other, each can learn from the other. Similarly, both peace theory and medical science emphasize the role of consciousness and mobilization in healing.
>
> —Johan Galtung[1]

Introduction and Definitions

In matters of peace and security, as in medicine, prevention is self-evidently better than cure. It saves lives and money and it forestalls suffering. Since the end of the Cold War, preventive action has become a top priority for the United Nations.

From the beginning, a preventive role had been envisaged for the Organization. Article 1 of its Charter had stated that one of the purposes of the United Nations was "to take effective collective measures for *prevention* and removal of threats to the peace" (emphasis added). But the Cold War reduced almost to zero the Organization's capacity to take such measures collectively.

When the Cold War began to thaw in the mid-1980s, two consequences followed. First, it became possible at last for the Member States to act collectively in matters of peace and security. Second, the need for preventive action was made brutally clear to them. The Cold War might have been over, but the world was still plagued by a number of wars that it had spawned, almost all of them wars within states. These were the so-called proxy wars in which each of the protagonists was backed, politically and in *materiel*, by one of the Cold War power blocs. The United Nations Security Council was now able to take effective action to end most of them. But the cost was high. Major peacekeeping operations had to be established in Namibia, Angola, and Mozambique, between Iran and Iraq, in Afghanistan, in Cambodia, and in Central America. At the same time, the collapse of communism in the Soviet Union and Eastern Europe was creating a new set of conflicts, one of which was to bring about the deployment in the former Yugoslavia of the UN's largest-ever peacekeeping operation.

It is not surprising that the Member States began to look for more economical ways of maintaining peace and security. On December 5, 1988, the General Assembly adopted a "Declaration on the Prevention and Removal of Disputes and Situations Which May Threaten International Peace and Security and on the Role of the United Nations in this Field." Through that instrument, the General Assembly declared that States should act so as to prevent in their international relations the emergence or aggravation of disputes or situations. It encouraged the Secretary-General to approach the States directly concerned with a dispute in an effort to prevent it from becoming a threat to the maintenance of international peace and security; to respond swiftly by offering his good offices if he were approached by a State directly concerned with a dispute; to make full use of fact-finding capabilities; and to use at an early stage the right accorded to him under Article 99 of the Charter (namely to bring to the attention of the Security Council any matter that in his opinion may threaten the maintenance of international peace and security). This decision represented a marked departure from the Cold War culture, in which the legitimacy of a political initiative by the Secretary-General had usually been challenged if not taken explicitly under Article 99.

On January 31, 1992, at the end of the first-ever meeting of the Security Council at the level of Heads of State and Government, the Council adopted a statement that *inter alia* invited me to prepare an analysis and recommendations on ways of strengthening and making more efficient the capacity of the United Nations for preventive diplomacy, for peacemaking and for peacekeeping. As I worked on the resulting report, which was later published as "An Agenda for Peace,"[2] it quickly became clear that preventive diplomacy is in fact a portmanteau for a range of prophylactic measures that can be taken by States, groups of States, or international organizations to help maintain peace and security between and within States. Since that report was published, the United Nations has gained experience not only in preventive diplomacy, strictly defined, but also in preventive peacekeeping, preventive humanitarian action and preventive peace-building. Let me define these four main types of preventive action.

Preventive diplomacy is the use of diplomatic techniques to prevent disputes from arising, or from escalating in armed conflict if they do arise, and, if that fails, to prevent the armed conflict from spreading. Article 33 of the Charter requires parties to disputes that could endanger peace and security to seek a solution by negotiation, inquiry, mediation, conciliation, arbitration, judicial settlement, resort to regional agencies or arrangements, or other peaceful means the protagonists may choose. To those techniques can be added confidence-building measures, a therapy that can produce good results if the patients, i.e., the hostile parties, will accept it. Central to the idea of preventive diplomacy is the assumption that the protagonists are not making effective use of these techniques on their own initiative and that the help of a third party is needed if the threatened conflict is to be prevented by diplomatic means.

The techniques employed in preventive diplomacy are the same as those employed in *peacemaking* (which, in United Nations parlance, is a diplomatic activity, not the restoration of peace by forceful means). The only real difference between preventive diplomacy and peacemaking is that the former is applied before armed conflict has broken out, while the latter is applied thereafter. But in the world today there are many endemic situations where the causes of conflict are deeply rooted and chronic tension is punctuated from time to time by acute outbreaks of virulent fighting. Examples of such situations are those arising from the conflict between India and Pakistan over Kashmir, Israel's occupation of parts of southern Lebanon, and the conflict in southern Sudan. In such cases it may be artificial to make a distinction between preventive diplomacy and peacemaking or indeed between preventive and postconflict peace-building. Those who want to help control and cure such chronic maladies need to maintain their efforts over a long period of time, varying the therapies they prescribe as the patients' condition improves or deteriorates.

One is sometimes asked to give examples of successful preventive diplomacy. It is not always easy to do so. Confidentiality is usually essential in such endeavors. Time may have to pass before one can say with such confidence that success has been achieved. Many different peacemakers may have been at work, and it can sound presumptuous for just one of them to claim the credit.

A conspicuous success, which history now permits us to claim for the United Nations, was the Good Offices Mission undertaken in great secrecy in 1969/1970 by Under-Secretary-General Ralph Bunche, on behalf of U Thant, to resolve an Iranian claim to Bahrain before that country achieved full independence. U Thant said of it: "the perfect Good Offices operation is one which is not heard of until it is successfully concluded or even never heard of at all."

Preventive peacekeeping involves the deployment of international military and police personnel to perform a variety of possible functions: to deter aggression, to help maintain security, to build confidence, to create conditions favorable to negotiations and/or to assist in the provision of humanitarian relief. As with all peacekeeping, a wide range of tasks can be considered, but it is essential that each mandate should specify with absolute precision which tasks the force will actually perform.

Preventive humanitarian action is action that, in addition to its humanitarian purpose of bringing relief to those who suffer, has the *political* purpose of correcting situations, which, if left unattended, could increase the risk of conflict. A wide range of measures may be required. They may include planning for the humanitarian action that will be required if a crisis breaks, e.g., the stockpiling of relief goods in certain places. But they may also include creating conditions that will help to persuade refugees or displaced persons to return to their homes, e.g., improvements in security and gender, greater respect for human rights, and creation of jobs, etc. One example is the efforts of the international community to facilitate the return to their homes of the Rwandese refugees in Zaire and thereby alleviate the tensions that their presence has created between the Governments of Rwanda and Zaire.

Preventive peace-building is the application to potential conflict situations of the idea of postconflict peace-building, which I set out in "An Agenda for Peace." Like its postconflict cousin, preventive peace-building is especially useful in internal conflicts and can involve a wide variety of activities in the institutional, economic, and social fields. These activities usually have an intrinsic value of their own because of the contribution they make to democratization, respect for human rights, and economic and social development. What defines them as peace-building activities is that they additionally have the political value of reducing the risk of outbreak of a new conflict, or the recrudescence of an old one.

An example in the context of potential interstate conflict is the offer in 1951 by the then International Bank for Reconstruction and Development (now the World Bank) to provide its Good Offices to India and Pakistan to help both countries resolve their dispute over the waters of the Indus River by approaching it as a technical and engineering problem rather than a legal and political one. The Bank's offer was accepted and after nine years of negotiation, the parties signed the Indus Waters Treaty, which became the basis of the biggest waterpower and irrigation project in the world at the time. In due course it made the two countries independent of each other in the operation of their water supplies, thereby removing the risk of conflict on that set of issues.

The Secretary-General's Role in Diagnosis and Prescribing Preventive Therapy

None of these preventive treatments need exclude use of any of the others. Indeed, a fully integrated international response to an impending conflict could prescribe them all. Nor does the United Nations have—nor claim—an exclusive right to prescribe and administer these treatments. The most effective prophylaxis may be achieved through coordinated team work by the United Nations, various of its specialized agencies, one or more regional organizations, individual Member States and nongovernmental organizations.

There are five generic conditions that have to be fulfilled if the Secretary-General of the United Nations is to be able to apply the preventive treatments effectively. They are discussed in the following paragraphs with particular reference to the most pressing situations, which, at the time this chapter was written, demanded preventive action by the international community. That was the internal crisis in Burundi. It is worth recording in this context that, in the week this chapter was finalized, the Minister of Human Rights of Burundi, in a statement to the United Nations Human Rights Commission, described her country as being "a patient on the operation table" and appealed to the international community to help in finding "a permanent cure."

Fulfillment of the conditions becomes more difficult when, as is so often the case, the potential conflict is an internal one. More than 60 percent of the actual or potential conflicts in which the United Nations played an active peacemaking or peacekeeping role related to disputes within states, though several of them also had a significant international dimension too. As is well known, Article 2(7) of the United Nations Charter provides that the United Nations should not intervene in matters that are essentially within the jurisdiction of a State or require its Members to submit such matters to settlement under the Charter. The General Assembly's declaration of December 5, 1988, to which I have already referred, provided that, "States should act so as to prevent *in their international relations* the emergency of aggravation of disputes or situations" (emphasis added).

Since the end of the Cold War, however, there has been a growing readiness by the Member States to accept, or even insist, that the United Nations' preventive, peacemaking, peacekeeping and peace-building services should not be denied to a conflict simply because it is a conflict within a State and not one between States. At the same time, Member States have continued to insist on the inviolability of their sovereignty and strict respect for Article 2(7). Because the sovereign state is the basic building block of the international system and will so remain, it is not possible to resolve this contradiction on a generic basis; Member States will continue to defend their sovereign rights. But in practice the contradiction will continue to be resolved on a pragmatic basis in certain situations where there is broad agreement within the international community that an internal conflict is so dangerous and/ or cruel that international efforts have to be made to control and resolve it.

As a result, however, the United Nations cannot take preventive action without a specific request from, or at least the consent of, the Member State or States concerned. From the Secretary-General's point of view, the ideal is that he should receive a request from the government. But sometimes, when the threat of imminent conflict is evident, he feels compelled by his general mandate for preventive action to take the initiative in suggesting a course of preventive therapy. Even when such an idea is put forward tentatively and confidentially, it can be taken as a slight to the sovereignty of the state concerned and the Secretary-General is blocked from further action.

The Secretary-General also has to be ready to propose preventive action in cases where a country no longer has a government capable of exercising sovereignty in an effective way, the so-called failed state syndrome epitomized by Somalia. In such cases, the Security Council may decide that the state of war is so threatening to the country's neighbors or is causing so much suffering that the Council is obliged to establish a UN operation to bring it under control without seeking governmental consent. But the United Nations will still need the consent and cooperation of those who actually control the situation on the ground in the various parts of the country. As has been demonstrated in Somalia and Bosnia, the lack of such consent and cooperation can prevent the United Nations operation from carrying out the tasks entrusted to it by the Security Council, even when the Council's decision has been taken under Chapter VII of the Charter.

The first of the five conditions for preventive action is that the Secretary-General should have the necessary capacity for the collection and analysis of information. One of the main reasons for my decision in 1992 to bring all the Secretariat's political work into a single Department of Political Affairs was to create this early warning capacity. That department, working with the Department of Humanitarian Affairs, has its own early warning system to detect impending humanitarian emergencies. With the Department of Peacekeeping Operations, it has created a "Framework for Coordination," which is essentially a set of procedures for ensuring that the three departments review at regular intervals all information relevant to a potentially threatening situation and institute timely consultations with other elements in the United Nations system that may have information to contribute and/or a role to play in a concerted preventive action.

It is sometimes said that the United Nations is handicapped in its peace efforts by the lack of an intelligence service of its own. I do not believe that this need be the case. Much information is available to the Secretariat from the media and from academics and nongovernmental organizations, which often contribute their own interesting perspectives to the analysis. Above all, Member States have responded generously to my request in "An Agenda for Peace," which asked that Member States be ready to provide me with the information needed for effective preventive diplomacy. Of course, the information they provide may sometimes reflect their own national interests and their own preferences for action by the United Nations. But if information on the same situation is sought from several States, it is not difficult to form an accurate picture.

That said, the United Nations, like the rest of the international community, was caught unaware by the assassination of the President of Burundi in October 1993, as it was by the shooting down of the aircraft carrying the Presidents of Burundi and Rwanda in Kigali six months later, and by the horrors that followed both incidents. There will always be acts of extreme political violence that cannot be predicted with precision. But the United Nations needs both to be sensitive to the conditions that can lead to such acts and able to contribute to contingency planning for an adequate response by the international community when they occur.

The second condition is that the Secretary-General should have the clinical capacity to prescribe the correct treatment for the condition diagnosed. To fulfill this condition, he needs to be able to assess both the factors that have created the risk of conflict and the likely impact of the various preventive treatments available. Making those judgments in an interstate situation is easier than in an internal one. In the first case, much can be learned from consultation with the States involved and their neighbors, friends, and allies. In the second, the crisis is often due to ethnic or economic and social issues of an entirely internal nature and of great political sensitivity, in which the potential protagonists may include nonstate entities of questionable legitimacy and with shadowy chains of command. If in such circumstances the Secretary-General probes for the information needed to identify the right treatment, he can find himself accused of professional misconduct by infringing the sovereignty of the country concerned.

Another potential source of difficulty for the Secretary-General at this stage of the process is the need for triage. His analysis of the symptoms may lead him to conclude that there is no preventive action that the United Nations can usefully take. This could be because he judges that, contrary to the general impression, conflict is not actually imminent and that what is being observed is posturing or shadow-boxing rather than serious preparations for war. Or he may judge that there is no effective treatment that would be accepted by the parties, or even that there is no effective treatment at all. Such conclusions will not always be welcome to the Member States. They rightly want the Secretary-General to do everything possible to prevent conflicts. But the reality is that not all—perhaps not even many— actual or potential conflicts are susceptible to the United Nations treatment at all times. Selectivity and careful timing are necessary, especially when Member States are so reluctant to make resources available for the Organization's peace efforts.

In Burundi, the ethnic massacres of October 1993, to which reference has already been made, led me to dispatch a Special Representative to that country with instruction to inform himself about the situation, to help prevent it from deteriorating further, to facilitate national reconciliation and to recommend to me further preventive measures that the United Nations could take. His initial advice was that the situation was so threatening that the United Nations' efforts should be concentrated on stabilizing the patient and that, for the moment, the modalities for longer-term treatment were a matter of second priority.

After my Special Representative's efforts and those of other peacemakers had brought about a certain stabilization, notably through the signatures of almost all the political parties of a "Convention of Government" in September 1994, attention was turned to longer-term therapy. This required action on two fronts: promotion of a political dialogue and national reconciliation, for which a country-wide "National Debate" was the chosen remedy; and measures to improve security. For the latter, I had already proposed to the Security Council at various times a number of possible remedies. These had included the establishment of a humanitarian base, manned by the United Nations troops, at Bujumbura Airport; the maintenance in a neighboring country of a military presence capable of intervening rapidly if the situation in Burundi should deteriorate rapidly; and the deployment of a contingent of United Nations guards to protect humanitarian activities. However, these ideas had not found favor either with the government of Burundi, whose armed forced were strongly opposed to the stationing of any foreign troops in the country, or with the members of the Security Council.

The situation in Burundi began to deteriorate further. I warned its leaders and parliamentarians that they could not count on continuing support from the international community unless they produced convincing evidence that they were ready to reconcile their differences. In other words, I told them that unless the patients took their physicians' advice seriously, the physicians would turn elsewhere. The country's condition did not improve, and I reaffirmed to the Security Council my conviction that the international community should prepare for the possibility of a humanitarian emergency so severe that foreign forces would have to intervene. I again put forward the ideas of the United Nations guards and/or preventive deployment of foreign forces in a neighboring country. This proposal again proved unacceptable to the government of Burundi and to the Security Council. Then, I urged that Member States should at least undertake contingency planning so that troops could be quickly deployed to Burundi if the worst happened and a humanitarian intervention became imperative. The Security Council responded by inviting me to pursue consultations with Member States to this end.

The third condition for preventive action is that the parties to the potential conflict (the patients) should accept the action proposed by the Secretary-General. This is a *sine qua non* because he has no power to impose any remedy on them and can act only with their consent. In any case the remedy will have no effect unless the patients have confidence in it. Sadly, this is usually the most difficult condition to fulfill. There are, of course, at least two patients in every potential conflict. Usually one of them is more favorable than the other to international involvement; indeed, the very fact that Party A wants international involvement is often cause enough for Party B to oppose it. Sometimes also there exists earlier agreements committing the governments involved to give priority to bilateral means. An example of this is the Simla Agreement of July 1972, in which India and Pakistan agreed "to settle their differences by peaceful means through bilateral negotiations or by any other peaceful means mutually agreed between them." At other times, powerful countries in the region concerned may object to United Nations involvement and may insist that the parties have recourse to regional mediators.

In internal conflicts, sovereignty is an added complication. A government faced with an opposition that is threatening to take up arms is understandably reluctant for an international organization to come on stage, professing its impartiality and apparently treating government and opposition as equals. The Secretary-General has to proceed with great delicacy and finesse in such circumstances if he is to succeed in persuading both patients to consult the doctor and to take the medicine he prescribes.

Returning to the example of Burundi, the parties have very different views about the desirability of United Nations—or any other foreign—intervention. The main political party representing the Hutu majority has welcomed proposals for contingency planning for a possible humanitarian intervention. But the main party representing the Tutsi minority has reacted very negatively, as have the Burundi Armed Forces, which are largely recruited from the minority.

The fourth condition for action is that the Secretary-General, having prescribed a preventive treatment and got the patients to accept it, must persuade the other Member States, and especially the members of the Security Council, to give him steady political support. Unless they are ready to use their influence in a concerted effort by the international community as a whole, the efforts of the Secretary-General alone are unlikely to produce the desired results. The reactions of the Security Council to my various proposals for preventive action in Burundi have already been described.

The Secretary-General must also—and this is the fifth and final condition for success—persuade the Member States to provide the necessary resources to finance the agreed preventive action. The mandates given to him by Article 99 of the Charter, by the Security Council statement of January 31, 1992, and by the Resolutions and Statements adopted by the General Assembly and the Security Council, respectively, in response to "An Agenda for Peace," provide the Secretary-General with considerable freedom of maneuver in diagnosis and prescription, as will be evident from the foregoing description of my own initiatives related to Burundi. But he has no power to commit funds without the authority of the General Assembly, which will have to be convinced of the legitimacy, feasibility, and likely efficacy of the prescribed treatment. If it includes the deployment of military personnel, more than financial authority will be needed. The political authority of the Security Council will also be necessary, as well as a readiness on the part of Member States to contribute the troops and equipment required, whether as a UN peacekeeping operation or as a multinational force authorized by the Security Council but under national command.

To sum up, the salient fact that emerges from this analysis is that the Secretary-General's ability to take effective preventive action depends most critically on the political will of the parties to the potential conflict. In international politics, as in human medicine, the physician cannot impose treatment that the patient is not prepared to accept. Important improvements have been made in the Secretary-General's capacity to diagnose and prescribe. Failure to take effective preventive action is, in any case, only rarely due to lack of early warning; the symptoms are usually there for all to see. What is too often lacking at present is a predisposition by the parties to accept third-party assistance in resolving their dispute. Ways have to be found to persuade them, without infringing on their sovereignty or other rights, that it is in their own interests to accept the help of the United Nations and other international players, rather than to allow their dispute to turn into armed conflict. And the Member States of the United Nations have to be persuaded to pay the costs of providing that help.

The Secretary-General's Role in the Application of Preventive Therapy

Once a course of therapy has been defined and agreed upon by all concerned, decisions have to be taken on the modalities for its application. There is no fixed pattern. Specific modalities have to be worked out for each case. The Secretary-General's role can take many different forms. He can do the work himself, directly or through his Secretariat. He can refer the patients to specialists, such as specialized agencies of the United Nations system, regional organizations, individual Member States, or nongovernmental organizations, and work with them to apply the therapy. He can coordinate the work of others or simply provide them with political and moral support.

The Secretary-General often performs his role through a senior United Nations official or outside personality, appointed as his Special Representative or Special Envoy, who takes up residence in the country or region concerned or visits it on a regular basis. The mere appointment of a Special Representative or Envoy can have a political impact. It alerts the Member States of the United Nations to a possible new conflict and alerts the potential protagonists to the international community's concern. There are other conspicuous actions available to the Secretary-General that can achieve similar results—the dispatch of goodwill or fact-finding missions, a public offer of his good offices, briefing of the media, a report to the General Assembly or Security Council, or a formal notification to the Council under Article 99 of the Charter.

Such public manifestations of the Secretary-General's concern can sometimes have a useful therapeutic effect. But more often he will prefer to provide his good offices quietly, especially where the looming conflict is an internal one. Quite apart from sovereignty-related sensitivities, it is easier for parties to make concessions when it is not publically known that they are being urged to do so by the Secretary-General of the United Nations, who can guarantee little or nothing in return. As already mentioned, preventive diplomacy is usually best done behind closed doors, which can make difficulties for the Secretary General if the world is clamoring for the United Nations to do something but he knows that to reveal what he is actually doing would impair his chances of success, as well as being the diplomatic equivalent of violating the Hippocratic oath.

Where preventive peacekeeping takes the form of a United Nations operation, the Secretary-General's role is more clearly defined and more exclusive. It is he who designs the operation; obtains the Security Council's authority to establish it; assembles the necessary troops and equipment from Member States; deploys, commands, and manages the operation; and reports on it to the Council. But even in this situation the Secretary-General can find himself exposed to considerable pressure from countries directly or indirectly involved in the conflict.

It is not, however, to be assumed that preventive peacekeeping will always be done through a United Nations operation. In the case of Burundi, I believe that the peacekeeping therapy would be so demanding militarily that it could be provided only by Member States capable of responding with the necessary rapidity to a crisis in a distant theater, and that the correct prescription would, therefore, be a multinational force authorized by the Security Council under Chapter VII of the

Charter. In such a case the Secretary-General's role is likely to be less than if the operation were under United Nations command.

In the case of preventive humanitarian action, one aspect of the Secretary-General's role is to establish adequate arrangements for the coordination of relief activities. Another is to take, or support, the political action required to persuade the governments concerned to create the conditions that will permit resolution of the humanitarian crisis. As already noted, these can include a wide range of measures in the fields of security, law and order, human rights, institution building, reconstruction, restoration of economic activity and social programs, and may, therefore, require the Secretary-General to play a coordinating role in this field also.

Peace-building is perhaps the preventive therapy where the Secretary-General's role is least well defined. In the case of preventive diplomacy and humanitarian action he has the necessary authority to administer the therapy that he has agreed upon with the parties. For preventive peacekeeping he has to obtain the authority of the Security Council, but well-established procedures exist for him to do so, and for the operation to be deployed once authority has been obtained.

But peace-building is more complicated. It can require a wide range and variety of actions, not all of which will fall under the direct executive responsibility of the Secretary-General. His functions in this context are essentially those of a general practitioner. He can diagnose the patients' condition and advise them that certain general measures of a political, economic, or social nature will help reduce the risk of conflict. Such therapies can include confidence-building measures, increased respect for human rights, more just law enforcement, strengthening democratic institutions, improving social services, addressing gross economic injustices, sharing natural resources more fairly, and so on. But for a detailed prescription and for help in administering the therapy, the general practitioner will have to refer the patients to various specialists inside and outside the United Nations system, including nongovernmental specialists.

This gives the Secretary-General three roles in the implementation of preventive peace-building, all of them delicate. The first is to persuade the specialists to apply the therapy that he has prescribed and the patients have accepted. The best way of doing this, of course, is to associate the specialists with the earlier consultations and make them a part of the diplomatic process, through which the parties are brought to accept the desirability of preventive action and the nature it should take.

The Secretary-General's second role is to coordinate implementation of all the agreed upon peace-building actions. In some cases this can be done through the standard arrangements for coordinating the United Nations system's operational activities for development through a United Nations Resident Coordinator. But usually wider coordination will be necessary, especially if the overall prescription includes diplomatic, peacekeeping, and/or humanitarian elements. In that case, the normal arrangement is for the Secretary-General to appoint a resident Special Representative, who should have not only diplomatic skills but also sufficient experience in the economic and social fields to give him or her credibility with the specialists in those fields.

The Secretary-General's third role is to monitor the political impact of the agreed peace-building measures, so that he can assess how well the patients, i.e. the parties to the potential conflict, are responding to the therapy and whether the prescription needs to be modified—or, of course, discontinued if the risk of conflict has been sufficiently alleviated. Obviously, the Secretary-General will depend, to a considerable extent, upon the advice of his Special Representative; but this is an area where visits by the Secretary-General himself or by his senior officials to the country or region concerned, and direct contacts with their leaders, can be of great value.

Epilogue

Prevention is indeed better than cure. I hope that this chapter demonstrates the high priority that my colleagues in the Secretariat and I attach to improving the United Nations' capacity in the preventive field, as desired by the Member States for well-founded political, humanitarian, and financial reasons. But the chapter should also have shown that preventing the malady of conflict is even more difficult than preventing the diseases that afflict the mind and the body of human beings.

There are no guaranteed vaccinations to prevent conflicts from starting and no miracle cures to end them once they have started. The best prevention is for the region or country concerned to follow a strict and healthy regimen of democratization, human rights, equitable development, confidence-building measures, and respect for international law, while eschewing indulgence in such unhealthy practices as nationalism, fanaticism, demagoguery, excessive armament, and aggressive behavior. Most of the elements of such a regimen are prescribed in the United Nations Charter and in the corpus of international law.

The difficulties of prevention in the field of peace and security do not arise because the warning signs of conflict are more difficult to detect than those of human disease; on the contrary, they are usually more obvious. Nor is it that the therapies are less effective; many effective therapies have been devised over the years. The United Nations dispensary is well stocked and many experienced consultants and specialists are on call.

The problem is with the patients and with the friends and enemies of the patients. Human beings may be full of phobias and superstition about disease but they can usually be relied upon to respond fairly rationally to the diagnoses and prescriptions of their physicians. The same cannot, alas, be said of governments and other parties to political conflicts. Many general practitioners would have been tempted to retire in despair long ago if their advice had been disregarded by those to whom they prescribed therapies. But the Secretary-General of the United Nations cannot abandon his principal duty to avert imminent conflict any more than a conscientious physician can abandon a difficult case. The Secretary-General's duty is to use all the means available to him, be they political, military, economic, social, or humanitarian, to help the peoples and governments of the United Nations to achieve the goal, emblazoned in the first paragraph of its Charter, of saving succeeding generations from the scourge of war.

Initial Response to Complex Emergencies and Natural Disasters

Ed Tsui

On January 17, 2002, one of Africa's most active volcanoes unexpectedly erupted in the Democratic Republic of Congo (DRC). As lava rapidly advanced toward the lakeside city below, fuel depots erupted into slow burning fires, tremors and shocks crumbled buildings and collapsed houses, heat and lava flows destroyed water and electrical systems, ash covered the landscape and lava-turned-to-rock covered parts of the lake.

As a result, about 400,000 of Goma's 500,000 habitants were forced to flee to unstable areas of the DRC and Rwanda, where rebel elements remained active. Nine died, and one hundred were wounded. About 40 percent of the town's infrastructure was destroyed, leaving thousands without electricity or potable water.

If ever there were a typical natural disaster, the eruption of Mount Nyirangongo was not it. Its location on a contentious border in an area plagued by armed conflicted placed it squarely in the middle of a long-standing, regional, complex emergency, where state and nonstate actors compete for control, misinformation is rampant, and humanitarian access is limited.

A number of other factors added to the complexity of the response including the many actors involved; the threat of further eruptions or factures from associated volcanic *and* seismic activity, whose interplay was classified by both vulcanologists and seismologists alike as a new phenomena; and the potential for contamination of Lake Kivu, a primary source of both food and drinking water in an already impoverished area and, ironically, of noxious gases that threatened to ignite.

Yet the international humanitarian response was as quick as it was comprehensive, and, in spite of the complexity of the situation, largely succeed in alleviating the immediate needs of those most affected.

The Office for the Coordination of Humanitarian Affairs (OCHA) was but one of many players who made this response a success. OCHA and its partners over the years have learned a great deal about the types of tools, mechanisms, and processes needed for an effective emergency response. New technologies, increases in the scope and magnitude of both complex emergencies and natural hazards, as well as the need for common tools to address them, and a growing appreciation by the Member States of the importance of humanitarian assistance and the protection of civilian to the achievement of peace, security, and development are only a few of the trends that have shaped the nature of emergency response as we know it today. But despite the growing need for humanitarian interventions in ever more complex operating environments, the key lessons learned by the international humanitarian community regarding emergency response in the last two decades are straightforward. In short, over time we have come to understand that an effective response depends on the following:

1. Solid needs assessments that allow relief agencies to jointly determine who does what where, under the umbrella of a comprehensive humanitarian action plan
2. The proper staff and emergency response tools available at the right time in the right place
3. Common tools for natural disasters and complex emergencies, to be adapted for application
4. Emergency funding mechanisms that ensure money is readily available and easily dispersed
5. Well-developed information management networks through which accurate-as-possible data are immediately available to key decision makers
6. Reviews that draw the lessons learned from each response and help apply them to the next

Each of these lessons was manifested in the Goma response, which included, among other actions, early reinforcements of experienced humanitarian staff, including a senior emergency manager; the provision, through daily updates, of credible and timely information about the crisis at both the field and international levels; the on-site establishment of extraordinary information exchanges and a specialized center to process, analyze, and share humanitarian data; the issuance of an interagency emergency appeal for funds; the rapid dispatch of vulcanologists to the field; and the procurement of emergency nonfood items for the affected population.

As such, this particular response to a sudden onset emergency highlights not only the need for, but also the increasing efforts by, aid actors, in particular OCHA, to ensure that the above elements are consistently at the disposal of the international system, so that each response is timely yet flexible, specialized when needed, and above all, well coordinated.

As an example of how aid can effectively reach it victims also provides a benchmark of comparison to other international emergency responses, where, for whatever reasons, action was neither as swift nor as decisive. Thus, it further highlights the need for greater consistency in the application of the emergency response tools and mechanisms at the disposal of the international humanitarian community.

Before I elaborate on these lessons and themes, it is useful to understand the increasingly challenging and multifaceted backdrop against which aid workers struggle to deliver assistance in the field and that has shaped the formulation of emergency response.

Natural Disaster and Complex Emergencies

In the last two decades alone, more than three million people have died in natural disasters caused by extreme weather resulting from global warming and other related atmospheric changes, as well as by deforestation and soil erosion caused by unsustainable development practices. Combined with poverty and population pressure, growing numbers of people are being forced to live in harm's way, on floodplains, unstable hillsides, and earthquake-prone zones.

Similarly, the end of the Cold War has resulted in profound changes not only in the number but also in the nature of armed, internal conflicts. In the last decade of the twentieth century, regions once thought to be beyond war, such as Europe, became entrenched in it; simmering socioeconomic tensions in many African countries resurfaced; and the war on terrorism gave way to far reaching humanitarian implications in Central Asia and the Middle East. In this period, conflicts have claimed more than five million lives and driven many times that number of people from their homes. At present, it is estimated that more than 40 million people have been displaced by conflict worldwide.

Increasingly, as we saw in Goma, the traditional distinctions between the two types of crises—natural disasters and complex emergencies—are not always so clear. Interplay between the two has become common. This is particularly true in the case of drought, which differs from most natural disasters in that it is slow in onset and may continue for a prolonged period of time, which can lead to a conflict over scarce resources. In ongoing emergencies, drought can also exacerbate existing tensions.

Whatever the cause, the resulting effects of these emergencies are similar. They include extensive violence and loss of life, increasingly among innocent noncombatants and civilians, massive displacements of people, and widespread damage to societies and economies. But despite the similarities, key differences in the immediacy, duration, scope, and political complexity of a crisis have increasingly called for special capacities or services in the initial response.

Immediacy

In the event of a natural disaster, such as an earthquake or volcano, thousands of lives are put at immediate risk. Many can be lost within hours or days of the incident if search and rescue and other life-saving efforts are delayed. In these cases, a rapid initial response is critical, and often more easily applicable, to the goal of saving lives.

Complex emergencies, on the other hand, are characterized by a total or considerable breakdown of authority. They usually involve more deliberate violence— and therefore violations of human rights and international humanitarian law—targeted at civilians, as well as political and military constraints that hinder response and pose more significant and sinister security risks to aid workers.

Duration

As a result of these differences in immediacy, the life-saving stage that follows a natural disaster response may be over within a matter of days or weeks, notwithstanding the reconstruction efforts that may follow.

The chronic humanitarian needs arising from war, however, often continue for months and even years. Additionally, as the nature of an emergency changes—for example, from the immediate aftermath of military action, to a long-simmering standoff between government and militant groups, to a negotiated peace—humanitarian assistance programs may evolve and become more varied, encompassing simultaneous relief programs as well as rehabilitation and reintegration activities. These situations necessitate longer-term initiatives designed to minimize human suffering over time.

Scope

Natural disasters increasingly span several countries. For instance, when successive cyclones hit southeastern Africa in February 2001, rivers and dams overflowed throughout the region, resulting in widespread flooding in Mozambique, Swaziland, Botswana, Malawi, Zimbabwe, and South Africa, affecting more than two million people. But although several neighboring countries can be affected by the same natural disaster, especially in case of drought, their relationships are not always strained, and cooperation is more common.

In complex emergency situations, however, the international and cross-border dimensions are almost always characterized by political differences between those concerned. One need not look further than the former Federal Republic of Yugoslavia, the Great Lakes region of Africa, or the West African subregion for examples of how conflict spreads, displacing thousands in a tangled web of cross-border movements. Responding to such crises requires a higher level of regional coordination and interaction with a greater multiplicity of actors, who are often at odds with each other.

Key Elements of a Successful Response

Against this backdrop, the international community has seen an increasing trend toward more integrated, as well as more standardized, yet flexible, application of initial response procedures, tools, and mechanisms in crises. This versatility entails being able to deal with the full range and potential interplay of crises, from purely complex emergency and natural disasters situations to every possible combination in between, based on common platform of response practices, tools, and mechanisms that consist of the following:

1. *Solid needs assessments that allow relief agencies to determine jointly who does what where, under the umbrella of a comprehensive humanitarian action plan*

When a crisis erupts, the international community—including government, nongovernmental organizations (NGOs), donors, member states, the Red Cross Movement, and the United Nations—is usually alerted by an array of monitoring systems, including individual as well as shared sources of information, ranging from the field reports to earthquake bulletins, weather notices, and press reports. Once alerted to a crisis, the international humanitarian community must gauge the willingness of the affected state to accept assistance. Although the primary responsibility for taking care of the victims of crisis always rests with the affected state, governments whose national capacities are not sufficient to meet the needs may either directly request assistance or pose no objections to humanitarian assistance.

Once the acceptance or nonobjection to aid is established, the humanitarian community focuses its attention on ensuring the impartial and timely interagency assessment of the humanitarian situation on the ground. These assessments, often led by OCHA in its role as a nonoperational and therefore unbiased facilitator of humanitarian response, are vital to ensuring that a wide spectrum of policy and decision makers are well informed from the outset of crisis, when time sensitive decisions regarding funding, deployments of staff and assets, and staff security must be made under enormous pressure. OCHA's experience has shown the importance of striking a balance between the depth and speed of reporting and the accuracy of the initial assessments. In crisis situations, initial assessments often must be updated hourly to reflect new, incoming information resulting from fast-moving events. Emphasis must therefore be placed on conveying what is known at the moment.

They also form the basis for the coordination of assistance in a rapidly evolving situation involving a multiplicity of actors with sometimes overlapping mandates. Especially critical is the prioritization of needs—whether they be in the food, shelter, health, water, sanitation, or protection sectors—and the subsequent assignment of tasks and responsibilities based on the individual mandates, strengths, and comparative advantage of each organization. Thus in response to a sudden onset crisis, initial actions may focus on determining who does what where. OCHA's role is to ensure that, drawing on system-wide capacities, all needs are met without duplication and that often-scarce resources are efficiently used.

Ongoing assessments throughout the crisis will then form the basis of longer-term interagency planning efforts designed to ensure that there is (1) a common understanding of the problems and constraints besetting affected populations, (2) a joint and complementary action plan for addressing them, and finally (3) an effective use of limited resources for those activities that are of mutual concern to all—such as communication, logistics, security, and information management. These are often realized through the development of a Common Humanitarian Action Plan (CHAP), which forms the basis of an inter-agency appeal process, of which OCHA is the custodian. Through this process—known as the Inter-Agency Consolidated Appeals Process (CAP)—national, regional, and international relief organizations jointly develop a common humanitarian programming, strategic planning, and resource mobilization document, which is regularly reviewed and revised. In the event of a sudden deterioration of an existing emergency for which a CAP has already been developed, the plans to respond to the evolving crisis may already have been incorporated in the CAP as possible planning scenarios. If not, the CAP may be rapidly reviewed and revised to reflect the new needs. Similarly, in cases where a natural disaster occurs in a country with a CAP, a revised CAP is usually issued, reflecting the new needs presented by the natural disaster.

In natural disaster settings, needs are determined jointly by the resident agencies on the basis of rapid assessments, which are conveyed along with funding needs in situation reports that are issued within the first twenty-four hours of a crisis and then updated daily.

2. *The proper staff and emergency response tools available at the right time in the right place*

No matter how experienced the first in-country responders to an emergency are, the sudden onset of a crisis is inevitably marked by alarm and confusion as national authorities and their UN and NGO counterparts struggle to assess the situation, often in conditions of extreme danger and limited access. Depending on the type of crisis, the leading humanitarian official on the ground, usually the UN Resident Coordinator (RC), may be forced to deal with many competing concerns, ranging from assessing the situation to evacuating nonessential staff to dealing with the media. Coordination at this stage is especially critical to ensuring that humanitarian assistance is delivered in a targeted, effective, and complementary manner.

OCHA facilitates this process by either rapidly establishing a field presence and coordination structures in country or by providing extra support to actors already in the country in the form of temporary rapid response teams, otherwise known as "surge" capacity.

Usually, existing resident agencies—headed by the RC—will support the government's efforts to respond to a disaster or complex emergency. If new structures are needed, OCHA's head, the Under-Secretary-General for Humanitarian Affairs and the Emergency Relief Coordinator (USG/ERC), in consultation with a range of humanitarian actors, determines—based on analysis of the humanitarian, political, military, and security situation—whether the crisis warrants a country or regional response, and decides which coordination mechanisms best fit, including whether there is a need to appoint a Humanitarian Coordinator (HC) to oversee the coordination of international aid efforts. Often the Resident Coordinator will also serve as the Humanitarian Coordinator (R/HC). These permanent structures help ensure not only the success of the initial response, but the development of common strategic planning and monitoring of humanitarian assistance throughout a crisis.

Either way, quick and decisive leadership from the USG/ERC in the initial phase of an emergency is critical. In consultation with UN agency and Secretariat department heads in New York, the USG/ERC may decide to visit the stricken country personally in order to assess the damage first hand, and then report back to the Secretary-General, the Security Council, donors, agencies, and NGOs on an appropriate course of action. Or she/he may deploy one of OCHA's senior managers or an OCHA Regional Disaster Response Advisor (RDRA) already in the region to the emergency site, in order to support resident UN agencies, the R/HC, and the local government in the initial assessment and response.

It has become clear from numerous evaluations of OCHA's initial response that such senior leadership is a perquisite to success. The presence of these additional senior staff can lend the necessary authority and legitimacy to build consensus for effective coordination; deal with other senior officials, especially in situations requiring access negotiations; and draw worldwide attention and resources to the aid efforts. In East Timor, for instance, despite the lack of a meaningful contingency plan to respond to the outbreak of mass destruction and violence on September 4, 1999, the Assistant Emergency Relief Coordinator managed to fly into Dili by September 6, 1999, where he remained as one of only two international humanitarian representatives in East Timor until the reentry of the humanitarian community on September 20. Under his leadership, coordination was immediately established and a preliminary assessment document begun.

The ERC may also decide to deploy interdisciplinary rapid response teams or "surge capacity" to support the government and/or the R/HC in assessing the situation and coordinating the relief response.

These working-level emergency reinforcements, by providing specialized capacities or boosting existing ones in times of extreme demand, can help take strain off governments, resident UN agencies and other organizations; focus attention on the need for extraordinary levels of coordination and contingency planning; and if necessary reorient resident agencies from their normal development focus to the different demands of disaster response.

Their timely arrival can also be critical to the success of an initial response. In the past decade, OCHA has been increasingly called upon to provide such surge capacity on very short notice to R/HCs at the outset of a new crisis, when an existing emergency intensifies or to relieve temporarily or replace a critical staff member of an existing unit. In Goma, for instance, within thirty-six hours OCHA had fielded a UN Disaster Assessment and Coordination (UNDAC) team and staff with specialized skills from nearby offices in Eritrea and Kenya, as well as from Geneva. The Assistant Emergency Relief Coordination (AERC) was on the ground within forty-eight hours. Within seventy-two hours, OCHA had a total of fourteen staff members on the ground, backed up with support from desk offices in New York and Geneva.

While OCHA in the past has drawn staff on ad hoc basis to respond to a sudden onset or deterioration in a complex emergency, the need for more systematic internal procedures has been recognized. As a result, OCHA, borrowing from the expertise of its more automated initial response to natural disasters, has also built up its own in-house capacity to deploy within twenty-four hours OCHA-trained staff, who are fully conversant with OCHA's mandate and the operational specifics of the organization, in order to establish immediate and effective coordination mechanisms in a sudden-onset emergency. Depending on the crisis, these may include information management and technology, operations, logistics, administration, and communications capacities.

Increasingly, one of their first tasks is to establish what has become known as a Humanitarian Information Center (HIC). By providing a venue for humanitarian exchange, HICs promote communication and cooperation, especially in crises involving a multitude of actors. Typically staffed by information management and data specialists borrowed from humanitarian agencies and international NGOs, HICs offer a range of products and services that make coordination and response possible. These include, but are not limited to, Internet-based data repositories containing baseline information on at-risk countries: Who? What? Where? (3Ws) databases containing vital statistics on population, internal displacement, refugee movement, and needs; country encyclopedias and digital libraries of UN reports and documents; road maps to assist relief convoys and missions; and thematic maps illustrating key sectorial data including housing damage, schools and clinics, and the location of mines. HICs also often provide humanitarian aid workers with accessible, central meeting rooms, common office equipment and announcement boards as well as Internet and fax access.

3. Common tools for natural disasters and complex emergencies, which build on the comparative advantage of the others without losing their ability to be applied in unique situations

The international humanitarian community has increasingly recognized the need to have at its disposal a range of flexible and integrated emergency response tools that can be used in either complex emergency or natural disaster situations. OCHA, based on its experiences over the years and the increasing demands of its partners, is increasingly attempting to provide the international humanitarian community with an integrated menu of emergency response tools, which include the following subjects.

United Nations Disaster Assessment and Coordination (UNDAC)

Originally designed to provide assessment capacity and support for the coordination of incoming relief at the site of sudden-onset natural disaster, UNDAC teams are drawn from a roster of volunteer national emergency managers, who are nominated and funded by more than forty participating countries, together with staff from OCHA, UN agencies, and other international organizations. They can be deployed within twelve to twenty-four hours anywhere in the world and are capable of performing a variety of tasks, including assessment, coordination, and information management, as well as providing experts in specialized fields of disaster management, such as search and rescue, chemical spill management, and infrastructural engineering.

Until very recently UNDAC was used primarily as a natural disaster response mechanism. Since 1993, it has also been deployed in response to complex emergencies, and UNDAC continues to strengthen its capacity to respond to these types of situations.

International Search and Rescue Advisory Group (INSARAG)

At the same time, OCHA recognizes the benefit of retaining the unique nature and purpose of some specialized response mechanisms. To that end, OCHA continues to help mobilize international urban search and rescue (SAR) teams, who specialize in rescuing victims trapped by rubble. They are drawn from a network of government-provided experts known as INSARAG. Additionally, in cooperation with the United Nations Environmental Program (UNEP), OCHA facilitates the deployment of rapid response teams with environmental expertise to coordinate the UN emergency response to environmental emergencies, such as chemical or oil spills and forest fires.

On-Site Operations Coordination Centers (OSOCC)

The rapid establishment—usually by UNDAC or the first international search and rescue team on the ground—of a temporary OSOCC at the site of a disaster can help provide a locus for information management and sharing as well as the coordination of various aid actors, particularly when infrastructure or communication facilities are lacking. But although initially conceived of to assist local authorities of the affected country in managing the disaster, in particular to coordinate international search and rescue teams, OSOCCs have proved valuable in their flexibility and adaptability to various situations and needs.

Internet-based virtual OSOCCs can also be used in both complex emergency and natural disasters to exchange information, identify needs, and plan ongoing responses in real time from anywhere in the world. Virtual OSOCCs proved vital in the initial response to earthquakes in El Salvador, India, and Peru, as well as in Afghanistan.

Civil-Military Cooperation (CIMIC)

In crises in which there is a peacekeeping mission already in place or in which militaries are heavily involved in the humanitarian response, OCHA staff, sometimes based in HICs, will often liaise with CIMIC staff attached to various militaries or peacekeeping operations in order to ensure the complementarity of peacekeeping and humanitarian programming and to share vital security information. They also help facilitate the most effective use of military and civil defense assets in humanitarian operations by promoting interaction between the humanitarian and military cells of a relief operation. In most cases, individual UN agencies and the larger NGOs establish their own links with military cells. However, in some instances, OCHA will serve as the hub for the mobilization and deployment of these assets and act as a direct liaison between humanitarian and military cells during a humanitarian relief operation. In this case, OCHA identifies personnel experienced in civil-military coordination to work closely with the R/HC.

UN Joint Logistics Centers (UNJLC)

OCHA may also assist in the establishment of UNJLCs where logistical information, data about the estimated global need for food and nonfood items, and information about distribution of relief to beneficiaries is exchanged and shared with the humanitarian community. For example, during the response to the flood in Mozambique in early 2001, OCHA's Military and Civil Defense Unit (MCDU) participated in establishing a joint logistics center to coordinate the use of military planes, boats, and communications equipment for rescue, water purification, food distribution, and shelter activities.

Physical Assets

It goes without saying that the rapid deployment of emergency aid items is critical to meeting the needs of the affected population. But when contingency plans are lacking or the emergency is entirely unpredicted, it can take days for relief organizations to reposition stocks. Recognizing the need for instant access to relief supplies, the UN, with support from key donors, has established a permanent renewable stock of donated disaster relief items at the UN Humanitarian Response Depot in Brindisi, Italy, which includes tents, blankets, kitchen sets, generators, water purification/distribution equipment, and tools. Together with the World Food Program (WFP), which administers the depot, OCHA organizes the immediate transport free of charge of these basic nonfood survival items to disaster-affected areas, subject to the donor agreement and availability.

OCHA also maintains a database of relief sources for use by the broader humanitarian community. Designed to function as humanitarian yellow pages, the Central Register includes a list of stockpiles for noncommercial equipment and supplies, directories for search and rescue teams, national emergency response offices, a register of available military and civil defense assets, and a roster of disaster management experts. This enables emergency response staff to identify and approach quickly the potential providers of the required international assistance.

4. Emergency funding mechanisms that ensure money is readily available and easily dispersed

It goes without saying that an effective response to sudden-onset emergencies and disasters depends heavily on the availability of funds to support immediate action. The willingness of donors to fund such response is often high, largely because when compared to protracted emergencies, the immediate needs of an initial response are more easily defined, direct life-saving results are more visible, and public pressure to act is at its greatest. But, in its efforts to capitalize on this fact, the international humanitarian community faces two main challenges.

The first is to provide donors accurately and quickly with interagency funding and needs assessments. In natural disaster situations, this is typically accomplished by including funding needs, determined jointly by the resident agencies on the basis of rapid assessments, in its situation reports, which begin being issued within the first twenty-four hours of a crisis.

In a new complex emergency situation, the mechanisms for immediately communicating needs to donors are less clear. Typically, ad hoc "flash appeals" or "donor alerts" covering needs for one month may be issued within the first few weeks of a new crisis. As the crisis evolves, the initial requirements presented in flash appeals or donor alerts are subsequently incorporated into the more formal CAP.

In support of broader humanitarian objectives, OCHA also provides emergency cash grants of up to $50,000 from its own reserves to meet immediate, specific relief needs, such as the purchase and transport of blanket, tents, and tools; manages a Trust Fund for Disaster Relief for life-saving activities; and often acts as a channel for bilateral donor contributions in sudden-onset natural disasters.

5. Well-developed information management networks through which accurate-as-possible data are immediately available to key decision makers

Although vital to coordination throughout an emergency, the role of information technology and management initial response is increasingly being recognized by a wide spectrum of policy and decision makers as being the most vital at the outset of a crisis, when accurate, timely data are needed to make time-sensitive decisions. Technological advances, as well as the increased expectations they generate among ourselves and the public at large, are in part responsible for this dilemma. As television and satellite transmissions increasingly focus public attention on poverty and suffering through real-time images of the victims of disaster and conflict across the globe, we face greater pressure to respond not within weeks, but within days or hours. Indeed, it is not uncommon for journalists to reach the scene of a disaster and start broadcasting before we do. In short, humanitarian actors must ensure that accurate information rises quickly to top decision makers.

Although the first task of the R/HC, with support from rapid deployment or assessment teams, is to survey the situation quickly and define the needs and type of assistance required, doing so in a both timely and accurate manner can be challenging, especially in the deep field. Information flow in an emergency is often limited by the lack of national information management capacity, limited access, damaged communication systems, insecurity, and poor communication among actors, all of which can lead to isolated decision making on the basis of disparate analysis.

All too often, when a crisis erupts, valuable time is wasted gathering baseline information about an affected area, which is often already available by the internet. Even more troubling are the instances in which our greatest challenge is not the *lack* of information but rather too much of it from too many, sometimes conflicting sources—making it difficult to discern the most critical and relevant data from the not so useful. Just as the uncoordinated arrival of relief supplies can clog a country's logistics and distributions system, the onslaught of unwanted, inappropriate, and unpackaged information can impede decision making and rapid response to an emergency.

These challenges highlight the need for more systematic ways to process and standardize information, as well as to begin information gathering and sharing on vulnerable countries well in advance of crises.

At the most basic level, OCHA does this by issuing situation reports on the overall humanitarian situation in country. These situation reports chronicle information on changes in the humanitarian situation, loss of life, material damage, national response, agency response, relief needs by sector and region, and the resultant funding appeals. Before on-site actors are able to develop or adjust their Common Humanitarian Action Plan and present comprehensive funding needs, these situation reports serve as vital conduit for communicating to donors the scope of the needs. They are ideally informed by the individual or joint assessments, the R/HC typically issues these reports at least daily, and often twice a day, during the first few days of a crisis and then weekly or biweekly as the crisis becomes less acute. The reports are shared with the host government of the affected country, the UN system on the ground, donor embassies, and with the NGO community.

Time-critical documents such as these used to be distributed by fax, telex, and cable. Today they are available to these partners and the public through two OCHA information-sharing platforms, the Integrated Regional Information Network (IRIN, www.irinnews.org) and ReliefWeb (www.reliefweb.int). The former is a humanitarian news service that provides unbiased reporting on humanitarian crises through updates, analysis, and alerts on a range of political, economic, and social issues on forty-six countries in Africa and eight in Central Asia. The latter provides, via the Web, twenty-four-hour coverage of relief, preparedness, and prevention activities for complex emergencies and natural disasters worldwide and acts as a gateway to documents and other sources of information related to humanitarian assistance and relief.

As part of its efforts to provide a more integrated response through all phases of a crisis, OCHA also deploys information specialists to the field as a part of its surge capacity or rapid response teams. Similarly, information management, as opposed to technology, is increasingly being recognized as a core function of UNDAC.

At the more sophisticated level, OCHA information managers also support initial response by working closely with their humanitarian partners to develop information products and tools, such as geographical and thematic maps, databases and digital reference libraries, and virtual coordination centers that improve the coordination of humanitarian assistance. In particular, much work remains to be done in the critical area of identifying cost-effective and simple technologies that work in the deep field, from which information is often most scarce.

6. Reviews that draw the lessons learned from each response and help them apply them to the next

When all is said and done, continued improvements in the initial response to crises depends largely on the extent to which the lessons learned in one situation are both recorded and then applied in similar contexts. To this end, lesson-learning reviews can help identify strengths and weaknesses in international response coordination mechanisms and ensure that lessons identified are integrated into future contingency planning and coordination structures. Given the need for actors to focus on the work at hand, so-called real-time exercises may be less appropriate in the context of an initial response but should be undertaken almost routinely at the end of each emergency activity. These need not be full-fledged and lengthy exercises;

important to their success is a relatively light design, one that uses a method that facilitates joint learning and provides instant feedback.

OCHA is fully committed to such systematic reviews of lessons learned for all its emergency activities and is currently experimenting with different modalities for such reviews—one of the first being lessons review of the 2002 Goma earthquake. Clearly the usefulness of these reviews depends very much on the interest and will of participants—staff and key partners alike—to genuinely reflect on what work and what did not and to identify workable recommendations for future activities. Over time OCHA hopes to distill lessons from these country-specific exercises and review their broad validity for similar activities and complex emergency situations.

Another way to identify lessons are external evaluations undertaken by independent consultants. In 2001, for example, OCHA asked independent evaluators to analyze its performance in response to the 2000 Gujarat earthquake, address some broader issues about the efficacy of the UN system's disaster-response capacity and to identify lessons for future activities. Similarly, OCHA also commissioned an independent evaluation of its response to the East Timor crisis in 2000. Both exercises produced sound and transparent basis for reviewing OCHA's performance.

However, unless such individual activity or country-specific exercises are systematically reviewed for their potential application in similar activities, fully incorporated into institutional memory and applied in policy- and decision making, their usefulness is limited. Recognizing this challenge, OCHA recently created an Evaluation Studies Unit within its Policy and Studies Development Branch and is in the process of putting in place an evaluative framework and strategy, in consultation with its key partners.

The strategy recognizes the evaluation activities provide little added value, if their recommendations and lessons are not applied in current and future programming, as well as policy and decision making. To that end, OCHA's strategy aims also to create and/or improve systems for sharing the results of evaluations and reviews in a meaningful way, and to establish follow-up mechanisms.

Conclusion

Through this combination of shared experience, the international humanitarian community has made great strides in its efforts to create a common platform of response practices and tools. Overall, it is reacting more quickly and in a more coordinated manner to bring relief to the victims of disasters and emergencies. But as the war on terrorism and other sources of conflict continue, we are certain to face ever increasing and perhaps unanticipated challenges in the delivery of humanitarian assistance. To that end, we must look beyond improvements in how we respond to crisis. We must learn to be quicker and detect and prepare for crises before they occur. The earlier we intervene, the more likely we are to have a meaningful impact on the ground. Similarly, we must more consistently enter all crisis situations with a clearly defined and viable exit strategy that guides all of our actions, even in the initial response, toward the ultimate stability and recovery of the affected country.

Greater advocacy efforts before, during, and after an acute crisis can also help us to better harness public and political attention, especially in the early days of the crisis when international attention is the highest. The very fluidity of the situations in which we work has focused us to remain flexible, and that has led to many improvements in our response. In the coming years, we must continue to demonstrate the same level of versatility and ability to learn from our past interventions so that we may ultimately save more lives.

The Peacekeeping Prescription

Kofi A. Annan

If I were a doctor examining the health of the world today, I would be greatly alarmed at the state of my patient. The international community, vibrant in its resolve to achieve a strong, stable, and healthy political environment as the post–Cold War era began, has been drained and weakened by one bout after another of violent conflict during the last decade. In Somalia, Bosnia, Rwanda, Sierra Leone, Kosovo, and elsewhere, it has had to weather the massive displacement of people, extensive loss of life, and irreparable damage, which are conflict's concomitants. Clearly, this is a pattern that must be broken.

Ideally, each of these bouts of conflict would either have been prevented completely or nipped in the bud. Prevention is—and would have been—by far the best medicine. But the practice of prevention, in both medicine and politics, is uneven. Some diseases resist early treatment. Some patients resist treatment until their conditions become critical—or even longer. Because of this, it becomes necessary to address conflict fully blown, to treat the bout of conflict at or near its height.

Even at this stage, the efforts undertaken, while hopefully curative and sometime palliative, also have a preventive aspect to them. They can prevent the escalation of conflict or the resumption of it. As in the case in which a primary tumor is discovered, intervention of this kind can prevent metastasis and hopefully bring the disease into remission. Thus, when we speak here of the "peacekeeping prescription" or the "treatment" it entails, we must always be clear that, while we have one eye on the crisis of the moment, we have the other on protecting the future and preventing the threat now posed against it from becoming a reality. Prevention is a great part of the goal of peacekeeping, and, in many instances, has constituted a large (and often overlooked) part of its success.

Many of the conflicts of the last ten years have had to be treated using the peacekeeping prescription, for various reasons. And, as with any other ailment, the disease has manifested itself differently in each instance, and the treatment has had to be adapted to those variations. Peacekeeping has proved itself a flexible remedy. Since the first edition of *Preventive Diplomacy*, we have deployed new United Nations peacekeeping operations in Haiti, Guatemala, the Balkans, Sierra Leone, the Central African Republic, and the Democratic Republic of Congo. While these have been adapted to differing circumstances, the main themes I enumerated in this volume in 1996 remain valid today. As Secretary-General, I remain committed to enhancing the Organization's capacity to understand conflict and to respond in a meaningful and timely way.

If we are to strengthen the international community, if we are effectively to confront the conflicts before us and those that await, if we are to prevent their spread or resumption, we need to understand three things as clearly as possible: the disease we are addressing, the treatment we are applying, and the changes to both of them that are occurring. It is to those points that I wish to turn here.

Diagnosis

In the context of peacekeeping, how do we define and diagnose the disease of conflict? What are its symptoms? Technically, peacekeeping is prescribed for conflicts that constitute a threat to international peace and security. The civil strife in the former Yugoslavia was identified as constituting this kind of threat, as were the genocide that ravaged Rwanda and the interclan warfare that engulfed Somalia in the early 1990s.

A quick cross section of these conflicts alone can highlight two of the most important characteristics of conflicts for which peacekeeping has been prescribed: most of them are intrastate wars, and many of them have been identified as ethnic conflicts.

Peacekeeping through the first forty years of the more than fifty-five-year history of the United Nations was devoted primarily to the treatment of conflicts between clearly delimited armed forces on either side of a cease-fire line; missions were deployed to separate antagonists, verify cease-fires, and promote accord. Following the fall of the Berlin Wall and the dissolution of the bipolar system, however, a seminal change occurred. Increasingly, the conflicts for which peacekeeping was prescribed were internal in nature. More than two-thirds of the operations deployed since the end of the Cold War—and more than two-thirds of those currently in the field—have been sent to respond to internal conflicts. These recent wars, which include the former Yugoslavia, Somalia, Rwanda, Sierra-Leone, and Kosovo, share other traits. These conflicts have displaced hundreds of thousands or even millions of people, riven entire societies, devastated economies, caused irreparable physical and psychological damage, and risked involving or have actually involved other countries.

Many of them have also been perceived as showing strong symptoms of ethnic conflict. Ethnic conflict as a symptom is, at best, extremely difficult to assess. Looking at any of the internal conflicts we have mentioned, most of us would be hard pressed to say exactly where ethnic differences were the cause of conflict and where they were the result of it. Ethnic differences are not in and of themselves either symptoms or causes of conflict; in societies where they are accepted and respected, people of vastly different backgrounds live peacefully and productively together. Ethnic differences become charged—conflictual—when they are used for political ends, when ethnic groups are intentionally placed in opposition to each other. Of the conflicts we have mentioned, it has been said that they are not really ethnic conflicts, but political conflicts in ethnic clothing. It is a point that we will have to continue to observe and consider.

The broader range of symptoms, which it has become necessary to address, have created what are basically new strains of conflict. Although the kinds of conflict to which peacekeeping traditionally responded are still very active—and even still virulent in certain areas—the kind of conflicts that occupy us principally today (and that will probably do so well into the future) constitute more of a complex or syndrome in nature. They display many different but connected symptoms and usually require multiple medications.

Prescription

In developing and prescribing treatments for these conflicts, the United Nations has attempted to focus upon and reflect the complexity and individuality of the cases before it. We have attempted to better identify and understand both the new strains of conflict appearing and the possible responses to them. We have reconfirmed the necessity of the core elements of the treatment. We have expanded its range of application. And we have improved our understanding of when it should be applied, in what dosages, and when it should be withdrawn.

In response to the symptoms and strains just mentioned, mandates prescribed in the last few years have far exceeded the traditional supervision of truces and separation of antagonists; they have expanded to include elements as diverse as monitoring free and fair elections, guaranteeing the delivery of humanitarian aid, overseeing land reform, observing and reporting on human rights abuses or violations, maintaining presence in towns and villages under attack to prevent loss of life, establishing safe and secure environments, assisting in the strengthening or rebuilding of social and political structures, and even acting to save failed States.

We have found, however, that regardless of the symptoms of the conflict, their variety, or the other elements of our treatment, three core components of the peacekeeping prescription remain crucial: humanitarian, political, and security. The common element of all the cases we have confronted is that each of them has required treatment for the individuals and groups who have suffered the consequences of conflict, for the political structure that has been either shaken or broken, and for the social environment that has been drained of trust, confidence, and any semblance of stability.

We have learned painfully that even in the case of an active civil war, a purely humanitarian response is both dangerous and impractical. The treatment we attempted in Somalia confronted both the international and national communities with the grim reality that it is sometimes not enough to unload aid and expect a problem to right itself. When the United Nations entered Somalia, it faced a situation in which thousands of people were dying daily. As time went on and the effects of the famine were countered, it became patently clear that the continuing high death rate was being caused not so much by the absence of food and the presence of natural disaster as by a group of ambitious armed men who prevented food from reaching the needy.

To allow ourselves the simplistic response of funneling aid into a port, only to have it sequestered and sold on the black market by the men controlling that port, would have been less than inadequate—it would actually have worsened the problem. Alain Destexhe, the former Secretary-General of *Médecins Sans Frontières*, referred to this kind of prescription as "the humanitarian placebo," explaining that, when it is applied, "aid becomes the pretext for political inaction, which leads only to catastrophe."

We have learned that the linkage of the humanitarian, political, and security components, handled well, can ensure a mission's progress. And we have realized that, handled poorly, this linkage created only a vicious cycle. Where security is present, humanitarian aid reaches those who need it, political instability is diminished, and restoration can move forward. Where security is absent, humanitarian aid is blocked, violence increases, political stability is weakened, and the situation is exacerbated. All three elements are essential.

Rwanda, Somalia, and Bosnia have also reinforced the lesson that we must not only prescribe the right elements, but also prescribe them in the right dosages. Because of this, there has been movement, both within the United Nations and outside it, toward peacekeeping with a credible deterrent capacity. The easiest way to see the extent of the change in dosage is to compare the United Nations mission in Bosnia in 1992–95 with two other missions: its NATO-led successor and the UN operation in neighboring Eastern Slavonia.

For nearly four years, the United Nations Protection Force (UNPROFOR) in the former Yugoslavia spanned not only Bosnia and Herzegovina, but Macedonia and parts of Croatia as well. Its mandate included guaranteeing the delivery of humanitarian aid, observing cease-fires, aiding the evacuation of displaced persons, remaining present in towns under siege to deter attacks upon them and prevent loss of life, and keeping Sarajevo Airport open throughout what became the longest humanitarian airlift in history. All this it did with little over thirty thousand people (of which only roughly twenty thousand were in Bosnia and Herzegovina), at an annual cost of roughly $1.7 billion.

The NATO Implementation Force (IFOR), which was deployed in Bosnia and Herzegovina alone, was considered robust in comparison to the UNPROFOR. Within a narrower area, a far more restricted mandate, and with far more equipment, it deployed sixty thousand troops for a period of one year, after which it was replaced by the smaller, but still robust, Stabilization Force (SFOR). This was in addition to the United Nations International Police Task Force, the UN Civil Affairs and Human Rights teams, UNHCR, the OSCE staff present to support the election process, and other international actors who took on various tasks within the mission area. Beyond these, the operation in Macedonia continued to be run by the United Nations until 1999. IFOR, with fewer tasks, a smaller mission area, three times the personnel, at three to five times the cost, constituted a stronger, and no doubt more potent, prescription for peace in the Balkans. Similarly, when the United Nations deployed a multinational peacekeeping operation in Eastern Slovenia, it arrived with a strong, well-equipped force that provided credible deterrence against violations. Partly as a result of this, the operation was able to successfully and peacefully provide protection to the transitional administration in what had been a highly volatile region of the former Yugoslavia. The UN brought another advantage, as well. By deploying a well-integrated, multidimensional operation under sole UN authority, the Organization was able to implement a comprehensive strategy to address the conflict in its various manifestations, thus laying the groundwork for a lasting peace.

The concept of a stronger presence, a critical mass, has in fact long been supported by the United Nations. When the six Safe Areas in Bosnia were being mandated, the United Nations asked for 34,000 troops to "provide deterrence through strength." The Security Council agreed to allow it only 7,600, and the UN's Member States took nearly a year to provide them. There was also concern expressed within the Organization regarding Somalia when UNITAF, the U.S.-backed coalition operation, was replaced by UNOSOM II. UNITAF, a well-armed and well-trained coalition force of 37,000, was deployed in southern Somalia alone, with a mandate limited to the establishment of a secure environment for the delivery of humanitarian assistance. When UNOSOM II, the United Nations Peacekeeping Operation in Somalia, replaced it, it was deployed throughout the country with a nation-building mandate that included pursuing disarmament, repatriating refugees, establishing a national police force, and fostering national reconciliation. But it was given a force of only 28,000 to achieve it. In other missions at other times, the same kind of problem has occurred.

It is important that we realize at this point (and remember as future crises arise) that, if we want an intervention to succeed—if we want to counter the symptoms that are present, halt their spread and prevent their recurrence—two things are necessary. First, its mandate must be practicable. Second, it must be provided resources adequate to achieve its mandate.

These recent years, when internal conflict has been so prevalent, have brought us a number of late, expensive, large-scale operations. But they have also broadened the other end of the spectrum with the first United Nations Preventive Deployment Operation (UNPREDEP). The UNPREDEP in the former Yugoslav Republic of Macedonia, though in the same theater of operations with UNPROFOR, and later IFOR, played a very different role in the treatment of the region. As the Balkan situation worsened, many worried that it would also spread laterally, involving or enveloping one country after another. Those working to address the conflict in 1992 had the conflict of 1914 in the back of their minds. For that reason or others, as the situation in the former Yugoslav Republic of Macedonia grew increasingly unstable and the Balkan conflict threatened to spread through and beyond it, the United Nations' first preventive deployment was mandated. With the strength of 11,225, UNPREDEP monitored activities at the country's border and worked to contribute to the maintenance of peace and security within it. By applying the right elements in the right strength over the right period, the international community created what might well be a paradigm for future preventive deployment missions and what was certainly a highly successful element of its treatment in the Balkans.

In 1999, United Nations peacekeeping missions are treating different variants of the same disease worldwide. A number of them are classical peacekeeping missions, whose mandates consist primarily of observing cease-fires and separating antagonists. The others are, as Cambodia was, more complex and multidimensional in nature, treating the abuse of human rights through the deployment of observers to monitor the human rights situation; treating the presence of mines with the implementation of demining programs; treating the need to return both military and guerillas productively to the civilian sector with demilitarization and demobilization programs; treating the absence of broadly representative, legitimate government with the administration and supervision of fair and free elections; treating the absence of effective administration by building the capacity of newly legitimated authorities and addressing a wide range of other symptoms. In each case, as in the missions just examined, the questions of the proper diagnosis and prescription, correct medication and dosages are essential. So, for all of them, are two other parameters: When should the treatment begin? For how long should it run?

The beginning point of treatment is, perhaps, the most difficult decision of all. We have learned that peace can be neither coerced nor enforced. There must be a genuine desire for peace among the warring parties. No system can achieve peace when leaders use negotiation not to end conflict but merely to prolong it to advantage. And no agreement, however well intentioned, can guarantee peace if those who sign it see greater benefit in war. The patient must embrace the treatment fully and willingly.

Yet, can we always wait for a conflict to ebb and the will for peace to emerge before we intervene? Recent experience has shown us that, if anything, urgent intervention is sometimes necessary at the very height of conflict, even if only to keep the disease and its symptoms from raging completely out of control. It is preferable—and more prudent—to intervene at a moment of relative stability, but situations like Rwanda, and more recently East Timor, have made us realize that emergency measures might first be required simply to stabilize the patient enough so that treatment can be administered. Measures of this kind are not likely to lead to recuperation on their own, but they can help the patient to survive until the tumor of conflict is ripe for removal. And, as we have seen in Rwanda, they are far preferable to the devastation that is their alternative. Along with preventive deployment, it is this kind of intervention that constitutes the preventive element of peacekeeping. It is preventive not in the prophylactic sense, but rather in the sense that, given a conflict in progress, it can help avoid the worst.

Intervention of this kind, however, is risky, costly, and not always effective. Where the will to pursue treatment and cure cannot be mustered, where the patient has not responded—as in Somalia and more recently in Angola—there is, beyond a point, no real alternative to curtailing the treatment and hoping that the body proves capable of treating itself. These are the cases that are most frustrating for us, the cases where we realize that what we have is an imperfect instrument at best, even if the only ones available. They highlight the fact that our approach to violent conflict is very similar to our approach to cancer or AIDS: an incomplete understanding of the nature of the disease means that our response to it will have to follow the law of successive approximations, requiring us to learn from failure as well as success.

But even where a treatment is effective, should it be limited in time? Long-term therapy is never popular with those who have to pay for it. It is often difficult to see progress, and it is nearly always impossible to prove the benefit achieved by avoiding further deterioration. In this context, the call for quick cures and sunset clauses has become nearly clamorous. This is dangerous for a number of reasons. First of all, in situations like Cyprus, where the United Nations has had an operation for over thirty years, political accord has proven frustratingly elusive, but armed conflict has been halted. The dynamics of the situation are such that there is little doubt that conflict could quickly rekindle were the mission withdrawn. With roughly $44 million a year, we are able to keep the Cyprus conflict in check. Is it worth risking having to spend far more in the wake of new devastation and bloodshed to avoid that preventive investment?

Second, the larger missions, the international coalitions, partly because of their large size and cost, usually deployed with very firm and tight deadlines. In each case, however, they went into situations where the problems that plagued the patient were deeply embedded and where more than a symptomatic treatment most probably required more time than they allowed. In this context, the great hazard of an arbitrary deadline is that it can actually subvert the process of reconciliation and recovery rather than move it forward. We need to understand and acknowledge that for a treatment to be effective it must run until it has achieved what it can and needs to do, not just until the insurance coverage runs out.

We have applied this lesson in Kosovo, where no arbitrary time limit has been imposed on the international presence. Furthermore, in 1999, the UN mission in Sierra Leone has been expanded due to the increasing demands of the situation. And a mission has been sent to the Democratic Republic of Congo, following movement in the peace process there. These cases reveal a determination not to be swayed by pressure for quick and conclusive results. Long-running, deeply rooted conflicts cannot be resolved overnight.

The efforts we have made have improved our sense of what we are dealing with and how we must handle it. They have allowed us to respond to the complexities of the crises that have faced us and to broaden the range of our response to them. They have refined our sense of what dosages should be applied when and for how long. And they have reminded us that peacekeeping as a therapy is valuable (sometimes vital) in both its curative and preventive capacities.

Prognosis

Stepping back from all of this, however, we realize that the outcome of our efforts will and must depend upon other things as well. An effective response to conflict, as to cancer, must nourish the body as best it can, giving particular attention to organs within it that are vulnerable. We must ensure that the circulatory system allows nourishment to move throughout every limb; we must prevent and treat blockages and dysfunctions. We must use the presence of peacekeepers like a form of chemotherapy, to contain the spread of the tumor and, hopefully, to reduce it to an operable size. We must do what we can to bring about a remission and move toward a cure. Above all, we must be patient and persistent. We must not allow hope to be lost, and we must not lose it ourselves.

Hope, the desire of the people on the ground to cure the conflict that afflicts them, it the single most essential factor in determining its probable outcome. This becomes eminently clear to us when we reflect upon the definition of an epidemic: an agent that acts literally "against the people." The participation of the people is necessary to mount and sustain conflict. They, ultimately, bear in greatest part its consequences. Without their support it is impossible to bring it to a halt.

A number of other factors, however, are also crucial in developing prognosis. Generally, they fall into two categories: those relating to the patient's general health and will to live and those relating to the level of care received. Strength and hope alone are not enough. Perseverance and dedication to the course of treatment prescribed are vital. Like the diabetic who takes an intentionally liberal interpretation of his dietary restrictions, the government whose commitments to peace are honored more in the breach than in the making, and the group that uses a peace process not so much to end conflict as to prolong it to its own advantage, undermine their own future and perhaps foretell their own doom. The will to sustain life or peace needs to be accompanied by the commitment to do what is necessary to sustain it.

But what of the factors that are not within direct control of the patient? When we consider the level of care received, a number of important criteria come quickly to mind. The most immediate is the rapidity of response. A clear diagnosis and practical prescription are also essential. The presence of a treatment team that is unified in its approach, consulting and working closely, is also vital. Adequate resources, technology, training, and equipment are indispensable.

Rapid response is vital, particularly from a preventive perspective, because in cases like Rwanda, the conflict's worst effects are often felt at the earliest stages. A rapid response is thus essential if we are effectively to limit the range, extent and momentum of a conflict. Of the million lives lost in the Rwandan genocide, the vast majority occurred in the first three months of the conflict between the deaths of the Presidents in an air crash on April 6, 1994, and the installation of the new government on the following July 19. We must be clear, however, that a rapid response means more than simply examining or diagnosing the problem early. It means establishing an adequate presence on the ground as quickly as possible. In the case of Rwanda, Member States of the United Nations passed a resolution in the Security Council five weeks after the crash, authorizing a mission of 5,500 to treat the conflict. Four months later, only 550—ten percent of that number—had been contributed and deployed. The mission did not reach its full strength until October, nearly half a year after the crash and months after the bulk of the killing had occurred. Rwanda is clear proof that, as a number of people have said, "we shouldn't wait until we hear a fire alarm to begin putting a fire department together."

Closely tied to this point is the need for adequate resources, personnel, equipment, and training. In the context of public health and medicine, where the fragility of the organism with which we are dealing is understood, the importance of proper training and equipment should need no emphasis. What could 550 peacekeepers do at the height of the Rwandan genocide, when they were surrounded by armed factions that totaled over fifty thousand? What good can a contingent do when deployed to the Balkans in winter if its government sends it without winter clothes and other supplies, untrained and unprepared? To mount and sustain an effective operation, appropriate resources are required.

Even where we have the will and resources to react rapidly, however, we do not yet have enough. For treatment to be effective in and beyond its initial stages, a clear understanding and unified approach among all involved in the treatment is vital. This means that the mandates passed by the Security Council must be clear, pointed and practicable; that member governments and troop contributors must be willing to provide and sustain the support necessary to implement them; that ongoing consultations between the obstacles and difficulties that arise as the mission pursues its tasks; that unified command must be observed and respected both within the mission and by all who support it from the outside; and that agencies and organizations cooperate maximally. This is no small task, but we are making substantial and encouraging progress toward it. My reform program has placed great emphasis both on clean lines of authority as well as effective mechanisms to ensure that all parts of the UN system that can contribute to the success of a mission can work together in a single, integrated effort.

But if the international community is truly to become more effective, whatever steps we take within the Secretariat must be complemented by corresponding action from Member States. The unfortunate reality up to now has been that the will to act differs greatly from case to case. It is important for the Security Council to respond with consistency and for governments to follow up to those decisions by making troops available, when necessary, to help implement them.

Clear and achievable mandates are also vital if we are to respond adequately to the needs of a situation, present a credible and effective response, and maximize the safety and productivity of those who have gone to serve. Initial international intervention in the former Yugoslavia was hampered by both vague and limited mandates. The Security Council must, thus, identify the right medications and the right dosages. And the "right dosages," in this context, need to be determined not only in the light of the needs on the ground, but also in the light of support that will be available (or be made available) from member governments. The strength and structure of a peacekeeping operation must permit it to do two things: carry out its mandate and defend itself. Determining the right dosage is the first step toward achieving this; ensuring that governments promptly provide adequately trained and equipped troops is the second. Our ability to respond more rapidly, preventively, and effectively depends very much on this.

Further actions will need to be taken if we are to intervene more effectively in either a preventive or curative capacity. We must have adequate information sharing. Many countries possess information facilities far beyond anything available to the United Nations. Enhanced information sharing by those governments could be of significant use in addressing the conflicts that face us. It would have a direct impact upon our capacity to analyze situations and the ways in which they are likely to develop, another factor that is crucial to a rapid and effective response.

Beyond the Secretariat, beyond its Member States, however, there lays one other step to be taken. As we approach each crisis, we must ensure that the public at large has the firmest possible understanding of what lays before us. Strong, sustained support on their part is absolutely vital. For this reason and others, we must above all work to mobilize and optimize understanding. The health profession realized long ago that there were a number of benefits in pursuing this goal: it helps those who are ill better understand what they are dealing with; it helps those who are concerned better understand how they can best contribute; and it helps each of us understand how we can best stave off the disease or recognize it early. The heart disease and breast cancer campaigns are admirable models of this.

We are slowly learning the same lessons in the area of conflict, but there are a number of obstacles impeding our progress. The first of these is that the general public has come to misunderstand to a great degree what peacekeeping missions were meant to do and can do. Second, too few of us are aware of the positive side of the peacekeeping prescription—what it can achieve and has achieved. To take a few examples, what have most of us read of Cambodia, Namibia, Mozambique, or El Salvador? And how many realized, when the UN was under fire from public opinion for failing to stop the fighting in the former Yugoslavia, that our troops had not the mandate, much less the means, to do so? At the same time, the successful facilitation of the delivery of humanitarian aid received precious little coverage. Last, it is true that today we hear, see and read far more of conflicts in various parts of the globe than we did during the Cold War. Full-blown crises are news, nascent conflicts are not. In an age when international intervention is decided by governments, and governments are propelled by public opinion, this means that effective and preventive rapid reaction is remarkably difficult. Neither do ongoing concern the media unless there is a reason for renewed interest. In many countries, the nuclear tests by India and Pakistan were followed by revived media coverage of the Kashmir dispute. Apparently of no direct concern to other parts of the world, the conflict between Eritrea and Ethiopia floats in and out of the media.

When global attention reaches a conflict at its height, a number of problems can occur. Acting at this point is the costliest and most dangerous way to intervene. It is also the least likely to succeed. Without any doubt, media coverage has generated in recent years a degree of attention and response that the conflicts examined here would otherwise never have known. But it also has shown that the public needs to be aware earlier of what is happening and could happen in a conflict area. Technology has made it possible for governments (and often the media) to know about many conflicts very early on, yet this information often takes far too long to reach the public at large. The problem is one of focus, priorities, and, once again, political will. If our efforts are indeed to become more preventive, if they are to limit more tightly the incidence and escalation of violent conflict, that focus must shift.

The steps that we have taken and the problems that we have identified show us that, while we have made substantial progress in developing and applying the peacekeeping prescription, our understanding of both conflict and its cure are far from complete. As with AIDS and cancer, each step brings us closer, but the disease itself changes even as we work, making a cure even more evasive. This, however, must not daunt us. We realize today that peacekeeping is not a wonder drug, that it is not applicable to every situation and not guaranteed to cure every case. But, as we struggle to understand better the disease of conflict, the most intractable that humanity has known, we cannot help but be encouraged by the inroads we are making.

Conclusion

Having looked at the developments of both the disease of violent conflict and the peacekeeping prescription, having examined the prognosis of both the patient and the treatment, we have given a clearer context and direction to our efforts. In closing, I would like to broaden it.

As I reflected on the idea of the peacekeeping prescription, on the concept of peace as an integral and essential component of international public health, I recalled a speech in a similar vein given more than sixty years ago by former U.S. President Franklin Roosevelt. In October 1937, as the first shadows of World War II gathered, President Roosevelt delivered what has since become known as the "Quarantine the Aggressors" speech, in which he warned that the "epidemic of world lawlessness is spreading." Taking the public-health perspective that we have adopted here, he asserted that:

> War is a contagion, whether it be declared or undeclared. It can engulf states and peoples remote from the original scene of hostilities. We are determined to keep out of war, yet we cannot insure ourselves against the disastrous effects of war and the dangers of involvement. . . . We cannot have complete protection in a world of disorder in which confidence and security have broken down. If civilization is to survive . . . the will for peace on the part of peace-loving nations must express itself to the end that nations that may be tempted to violate their agreements and the rights of others will desist from such a cause. There must be positive endeavors to preserve peace.

These words remain both sobering and encouraging. They are sobering because they reemphasize the depth and breadth and length of the challenge before us; they remind us that violent conflict is as old as humankind itself. They are encouraging because they show us very clearly and tangibly the recent progress that we have made in addressing it.

Roosevelt's necessity of quarantining the aggressors is no longer the only option. Even in instances where conflict is advanced, the peacekeeping prescription does not simply quarantine the victim and leave him to his fate. The new tools and approaches that we have developed have allowed us to remedy cases where the patient would otherwise have been lost. As in medicine, we have developed techniques for detecting problems earlier. Through research and experience, we have honed our understanding and our methods. New tools and technologies have made it possible for intervention to be more targeted, separating, identifying, and correcting in treating specific symptoms and improving the prognosis. We have, as Roosevelt urged us, undertaken "positive endeavors to preserve peace."

In doing so we have achieved a great deal. In places like Namibia, Mozambique, El Salvador, and the Aouzou Strip, cures have been achieved. In other areas we have been able to bring the conflict into remission. In yet others we have halted its growth. Some areas—like Somalia—have proven resistant to treatment, and the international presence has had to be withdrawn, with the hope that the body's own defenses would help stabilize it. But these are the exception, not the rule. What will develop in Iraq and Kosovo remains to be seen. In Africa we continue to respond to ever more complicated and distressing situations.

I admitted earlier that, if I were a doctor examining the health of the world today, I would be greatly alarmed at the state of my patient. And indeed I would. But what I did not tell you is that I would not be pessimistic about his prognosis. My work, and particularly those aspects of it which we have had a chance to discuss here, has given me a keen sense of what we can achieve together—and what we should do. I believe that we have made great progress in this treatment. I believe that we will continue to do so. And I believe that the challenges ahead will demand nothing less of us.

Reviving Global Civil Society After September 11

Richard Falk

9/11 challenged the American way of life in a manner that is unprecedented, and it is evolving with a significance of which we are only beginning to grasp. To uphold the blessings of democracy, we must start with the understanding that as members of a constitutional republic, we are citizens and not subjects. Subjects discharge their political responsibilities to society by unconditionally obeying the government. Citizens face a more complex challenge. Their need, especially in periods of crisis, is to strike a balance between loyalty and patriotism on one side and conscience and independent judgment on the other. A passive citizenry forfeits the virtues of democracy as well as betrays a lack of confidence in public debate on controversial issues. Without the benefits of vigorous debate and a genuine political opposition, alternatives to war and militarism tend to be bypassed. The more extreme voices counseling political leaders gain influence, a climate of chauvinistic nationalism is likely to dominate public discussion. This pattern of behavior represents both a general observation and is intended as a critical commentary on the drift of American domestic and foreign policy since 9/11.[1]

This assertion of citizen responsibilities might have seemed too obvious in this country to comment upon only a few years ago. It has suddenly become a matter of some urgency in the aftermath of the mega-terrorist attacks in 2001. Because these attacks caused such great symbolic and substantive harm, and because the adversary was a concealed terrorist network operating by stealth in sixty or more countries in such a manner as to be everywhere and nowhere, there was a tendency on the part of the citizenry to close ranks behind our political leaders, relying on their capacity to fashion an effective response that would restore our sense of security. This call for unity by the government was a natural response to such an unprecedented challenge, but it has had several serious unfortunate side effects, including the disruption of some very positive global developments of a humanitarian character that had been moving forward in the decade after the end of the Cold War.

These developments owed a great deal to the activism of citizens from democratic societies around the world, as well as to their organizations, which often took the shape of voluntary transnational associations.[2]

What makes the present context particularly disturbing is a rediscovery of the fragility of societal reality. Despite American power and wealth, the country has become vulnerable to hostile extremism as a reaction to a presence and policies around the world that are generating intense resentment. Despite the achievements of modernity, existing forms of democratic governance are unable to control either the passions that animate politics or the technologies that are relied upon to establish security. There may be a tragic predicament that is embedded in these realizations. Security for the citizenry is likely to remain elusive despite impressive technological innovations and the greatly intensified efforts of regulatory institutions.[3] We confront a serious possibility that the pursuit of security in our daily lives may prove to be both ineffectual and repressive at the same time, thereby imperiling the quality of democracy without providing protection against these new forms of extremism directed against our nation and people. What is more, which is the relevant point of this essay, the pressures exerted by the challenges of mega-terrorism have diverted energies and resources away from some exceptionally promising developments in the humanitarian sector that were occurring in the 1990s. These developments were exciting in several distinct ways, raising hopes for significant improvement in the human condition, as well as representing encouraging steps from the perspective of global justice. Such initiatives exhibited both the growth of transnational social forces emerging out of civil society, often acting internationally as nongovernmental organizations (NGOs), and an unusual spirit of collaboration between governments and NGOs that was giving rise to a distinct type of diplomacy that could be described as "a new internationalism" motivated by ethical concerns, entirely different from the preoccupations with power and wealth that formed the subject matter of geopolitics as practiced by leading states.

It seems reasonable to maintain that prior to September 11 there was a multifaceted upsurge of humanitarian initiatives that had already within the space of a decade established a rather remarkable record of achievement, with prospects for continuing progress. I have previously described this set of developments as the first global normative revolution in human history, that is, a definite trend in international relations emphasizing the relevance of ethical values and issues of justice that were posing a challenge to the dominant realist paradigm that reduced international relations to calculations of power.[4]

A Global Normative Revolution in the 1990s

The centerpiece of the emergent normative revolution was the genuine rise of human rights from the outer margins of diplomacy and international concern to a position that seemed close to the center of foreign policy, bearing directly on issues of whether or not to seek economic gains in relation with countries whose governments were responsible for repressing their own populations. Some prominent observers of the global scene insisted that human rights had become the secular religion of our era.[5] Such a sweeping generalization undoubtedly reflected wishful thinking, but it was also a historic comment on some extraordinary reversals of expectations that had occurred in the 1990s. The collapse of the Soviet system of internal and regional domination was facilitated by strong grassroots resistance that had long been demanding the implementation of human rights. The amazing surprise transformation that took place in South Africa without bloodshed early in the same decade was definitely hastened by the anti-apartheid movement that was inspired by the global consensus condemning the institutionalized racism of Pretoria as a crime against humanity. Such positive outcomes owed a great deal to pressures exerted by people acting on their own on behalf of human right goals, organized at the level of civil society, and mounting moral outrage that persuaded governments to override material and strategic interests by joining in the struggles to achieve change.

These encouraging initiatives reflected the interplay of many different influences, but in this chapter the focus will be on the distinctive contributions made by the NGO world, and civil society generally. This contribution is particularly evident in relation to the expanding role of human rights in world politics. The domain of human rights as a subject for NGO activism goes back to the period immediately after World War II.[6] It is doubtful that sovereign states in the late 1940s would have assented to an international framework imposing duties to respect human rights if their leaders had thought such standards were meant in any but an aspirational spirit. What made the Universal Declaration of Human Rights (UDHR, 1948) a feasible *political* project was the expectation that the rights set forth would remain internationally unenforceable. This expectation was formalized by calling the document a "declaration" thereby signaling that it lacked the legal stature of a treaty, and hence was not obligatory. It was also evident after World War II that very few countries were governed in accordance with the UDHR, and that their governments would never have lent their approval to an international instrument that gave the UN or other states a legal basis to push for implementation.

Human rights NGOs in the years following 1948 realized that a great opportunity existed to use this aspirational document to promote some desired modifications of behavior by repressive states, and at least to depict persuasively severe human rights abuses. Amnesty International took advantage of their realization that governments increasingly care about their reputation, and that allegations of human rights abuses are black marks when backed up by genuine information and given wide distribution by the world media. Such allegations could not be dismissed as the propaganda of ideological adversaries as was the case in the exchange of Cold War charges and countercharges being made by officials in Washington and Moscow. NGOs put human rights on the world policy map long before the 1990s, and paved the way for many governments to adjust their regulatory policies.[7] To begin with, the UDHA was converted in the mid-1960s into a pair of treaties called "covenants" that were widely ratified by states around the world. It became a matter of political legitimacy for states to commit themselves formally and existentially to the overall goal of conforming their political practices to human rights standards. This evolution, although welcome, was less attributable to changes of heart on the part of governments and more to a combination of sustained pressure by human rights organizations and some parts of the media over the years and a closely related trend toward the democratization of political life. Thus, despite its modest beginnings, human rights NGOs and international institutions increasingly viewed the UDHR as a framework of rights to be seriously implemented, which included the push for treaty-making procedures and for the further elaboration of specific rights that deserved wider recognition (for instance, prohibition of racial discrimination, protection of women and children, prohibition of torture).[8]

This NGO role was then reinforced by historical circumstances that led to opposition groups in authoritarian societies to rely on *international* human rights standards to back up their demands for political reform. This process of opposition was most dramatic in the settings of Eastern Europe and South Africa where the wider struggle for fundamental change showed that human rights would no longer be reduced to a set of pieties but were now a serious dimension of political conflict. The same dynamic was to a degree also visible in the Asian pro-democracy movements of the 1980s, which did not achieve success in all instances, but exhibited the degree to which people everywhere were inspired by growing feelings of entitlement to fundamental human rights.[9]

What happened in the 1990s that was so encouraging was that human rights seemed to become an active ingredient of international public policy, generally exhibiting a sincere concern of the general public about the suffering endured by vulnerable populations, groups, and individuals victimized by governmental wrongdoing.[10] This upgrading of human rights was also institutionally expressed within the United Nations, principally by establishing a High Commissioner for

Human Rights, which in turn led to more prominence being accorded the work of the Geneva-based UN Human Rights Commission.

The second development in the previous decade that formed part of the normative revolution getting underway, even though it remained controversial in some settings, was the willingness of the organized international community, or portions of it, to undertake humanitarian intervention designed to rescue or protect vulnerable populations or minorities from oppressive practices of their government.[11] The idea behind humanitarian intervention is the claim by an *external* political factor that it refuses to respect the supremacy of territorial sovereignty in the face of extreme abuse of human rights. The occasion giving rise to humanitarian intervention in the 1990s was the accusation of ethnic cleaning of a disfavored ethnic or religious component of the territorial population with the goal of expulsion, an abusive policy that was also often coupled with genocidal practices involving massive rape and massacres. Humanitarian intervention generated the sort of debate that was also in the background of discussion about the implementation of human rights generally.[12] There were several issues: Should the obligation to uphold human rights be implemented by force? Were the motives underlying humanitarian intervention truly humanitarian or were those claims masking geopolitical goals? Must the UN Security Council always authorize humanitarian intervention? Did the results of such interventions bring benefits to the vulnerable peoples?

To be sure, there were disappointments and ambiguities associated with purported humanitarian interventions. The Kosovo intervention seemed almost a reward for the violence of the KLA; NATO relied on tactics that caused extensive death among Serbian civilians, while acting to minimize its own; it proceeded without formal mandate from the United Nations; and during its aftermath, insufficient effort was made by occupying forces to protect the Serbian minority against "reverse ethnic cleansing." At the same time, the intervention provided the only available means to ensure that the great majority of the Kosovars would be rescued from a repetition of the ethnic cleansing that had earlier caused so much death and destruction in Bosnia.

Of potentially even greater significance for the future of world order, a consensus seemed to be slowly taking shape among leading states insisting that sovereignty was no longer an absolute grant of authority, and that the moral, political, and legal prerogatives of rulership were conditioned upon adhering to the most basic human rights standards. If a government henceforth severely abused its people, or a portion thereof, respect for its sovereign rights would be diminished, if not ignored, by the international community. Human rights NGOs cannot take the major credit for instances of humanitarian intervention, but it has often been their presence on the ground in the society experiencing, and their credibility validating, oppressive circumstances that leads to media emphasis, which in turn tips the balance toward intervention within governmental circles and at the United Nations.

It is important to recall the 1994 massacre of upwards of 800,000 in Rwanda when the UN refused to respond to urgent calls for humanitarian protection, and in Bosnia during the first half of the 1990s when an overly passive engagement by the UN seemed partly responsible for a particularly brutal enactment of ethnic cleansing, culminating in the 1995 massacre of about 7,000 Muslim males at Srebrenica.[13] This subject matter of humanitarian intervention remained problematic whether the decision is to take positive action or to refrain from doing so. There is no doubt that powerful states use the cover of humanitarian intervention to advance strategic goals, and refuse to allow such responses in comparable situations if their interests so dictated. It is reasonable for smaller states and for ex-colonial states, and the non-Western world generally, to be deeply suspicious of humanitarian intervention as it invariably has involved the Euro-American complex of states imposing its political will with mixed motives on one or another non-Western state. Such suspicions are deepened if, as in Kosovo, the UN is bypassed to avoid a veto of a resolution in the Security Council authorizing force, and if supporters argue that in the future, not even the imprimatur of a regional grouping such as NATO is necessary, but that it is sufficient to enlist "coalitions of the willing."

The third dimension of this focus on the ethical side of international relations that assumed significance in the 1990s were various efforts to obtain redress in various forms for historic grievances.[14] This surge of concern disclosed an increased willingness to treat the crimes of the past as unresolved: the activism of Holocaust survivors; of comfort women in the Japanese setting; of a variety of slave labor initiatives seeking compensation after the Cold War ended; of claims for reparations associated with the institutions of slavery and colonialism; of an array of commissions devoted to "truth and reconciliation"; and of grievances advanced by indigenous people who had been dispossessed from their historic lands and endured humiliations and deprivations.[15] This sense of the obligations of present society for past abuses of state power, most of which were treated as legal and valid at the time of their occurrence, represented an extraordinary recognition that these historic wounds continued to cause suffering to victims and their descendants, and would never be healed without some active curative response. Many of these grievances had persisted without serious notice for decades, if not centuries. Why had these past injustices abruptly generated formal responses and increased activism in the 1990s when they had been ignored for so long? There is no simple response, no single explanation. Certainly, the end of the Cold War removed obstacles that had shielded some governments from accountability. Also relevant were the trends toward upholding human rights and democratization. But perhaps most important was the spreading awareness of civic empowerment. Holocaust survivors and their descendants led the way, but also led others with grievances to push for acknowledgement, compensation, apology, and other types of redress.

In this climate of opinion, the credibility of claimants was greatly enhanced. To be sure, there was also practical and principled resistance. Those accused tended to be defensive, contending that there was no current responsibility for what had been done previously in an atmosphere where values and legalities were different. There was no consistent response from issue to issue, and from country to country. There were some impressive symbolic and substantive steps taken toward reconciliation, and in the direction of reversing past injustice. Swiss banks were induced to return deposits and settle many claims of Holocaust victims valued in the billions. Corporations using slave labor in Germany offered compensation. Apologies were expressed by leaders such as President Bill Clinton for the institution of slavery, and by the British queen for the imposition of colonial rule. The Canadian and Australian governments established education and compensation funds that were dedicated to preserving what traditional remnants of indigenous civilizations remained, and to provide symbolic recompense for past wrongs.

These evidences that the international community and civil society were coming to some sort of acknowledgement of these historic injustices was again, I think, an important element in this unexpected normative revolution that was beginning to take shape in the 1990s. Its essential character was to exhibit the interaction of governments and civil society with respect to a series of issues bearing on the responsibility of the state. The state, as well as other international actors, was being humanized by this process by which injustices, even if in the distant past, were being heeded, and to some extent addressed. Such a process reflected the capacity of NGOs to help generate an ethical climate of accountability that exerted influence on all global actors, including the United Nations.

There was a still further fourth major element of this normative revolution that again exhibited the growing strength of civil society to reshape the role of the state and its institutions with regard to issues of global justice. This element concerned dramatic efforts to make leaders individually accountable for crimes of state committed against their own peoples.[16] The Pinochet litigation, arising out of action taken in Spanish courts leading to an extradition request directed at the British government, came about as a result of tireless efforts by those individuals and their relatives who had been victimized in Chile during the period of dictatorship not giving up on the pursuit of justice when living in exile in Spain. The dramatic fact of Pinochet's 1998 detention in Britain and the series of legal challenges associated with the detention produced some notable achievement. The practice of torture was confirmed by the House of Lords, the highest British judicial tribunal, as an international crime that can be apprehended and punished anywhere in the world, not just in the country where it occurred.[17]

Also significant was the renewal of the Nuremberg idea that even leaders of sovereign states are not exempt from individual criminal accountability for their official deeds, that the shield of sovereign immunity is not available. What happened unexpectedly in the 1990s after a lapse of more than forty-five years—first in relation to the Balkans and Rwanda—was the revival of the radical idea applied to defeated countries after World War II that political and military leaders of sovereign states are not above the law. Of course, the pursuit of Pinochet, which in the end failed because he was found medically unfit to stand trial and returned to Chile, suggested the analogous criminality of a host of other leaders still at large around the world. Some of those accused were linked to powerful states. The most widely discussed instances were Henry Kissinger, especially for his role in the wrongdoing of the Pinochet government, and Ariel Sharon for his alleged responsibility for the massacres that took place in the Palestinian refugee camps of Sabra and Shatila back in 1982. Questions were raised as to whether the world is ready for such criminal accountability, which, given the realities, would lead to very uneven and selective enforcement of such standards of accountability.

The moves to detain and prosecute Pinochet stimulated civil society by suggesting that the rule of law might reach those responsible for the worse excesses of governmental and military authority. The Pinochet controversy, together with the experience of the ad hoc tribunal in The Hague dealing with crimes attributed to individuals associated with managing the breakup of former Yugoslavia, led civil society activists to embark upon an ambitious project to institutionalize the process in some enduring way through the establishment of a permanent international criminal court entrusted with the prosecution of the most serious international crimes. What ensued was an effective collaboration between a transnational coalition of NGOs and a series of moderate governments that generated a political process that led in 1998 to the Treaty of Rome and then to the establishment of the International Criminal Court (ICC) in 2002. Such a major institutional innovation was brought into being with surprising speed, securing more than the required sixty ratifications in a period of a few years.

This experiment in institutionalization is still in its infancy. It is opposed vigorously at present by the United States, and ignored by several other powerful countries, including China and Russia. If it could come later to obtain universal participation (as is the case with the UN), it would likely be viewed as the greatest institutional innovation since the United Nations itself. Its significance, symbolically and substantively, is that it expresses a determination to extend accountability and the rule of law to those who represent the state at the highest level. The creation of procedures by which to impose such accountability is a step forward in the efforts to overcome the impunity, at least on the international level, previously enjoyed by those who control sovereign states. Also, even compared to Nuremberg, the ICC is ambitious. The earlier criminal prosecutions of leaders were linked to a war, and embodied "victors' justice," the winners judging the loser.[18] Here, any leader at any point is, theoretically at least, subject to indictment, whether of a powerful or a weak country. The establishment of the ICC in an interdependent globalizing world could yet become an extraordinary step forward in the struggle to create global democracy as a complement to national democracy, yet to reach this goal there are major obstacles that must be overcome.

The fifth component of the normative revolution involves the rise of the global civil society, which has become a source of lawmaking and global policy formation. Literally thousands of NGOs are now associated with the representation of transnational social forces in a variety of regional and global arenas. Their presence was a robust and influential feature in the first half of the 1990s of such UN conferences as those on population, environment, human rights and women's rights that advanced a people-oriented agenda on these matters of global concern. This agenda clashed with the priorities of leading governments and global corporations and banks.[19] Increasingly, the focus of efforts emanating from global civil society was placed upon the supposed excesses of neoliberal globalization. The emphasis on globalization led to demonstrations around the world that gained major attention from the media, particularly in the aftermath of "the battle of Seattle" in late 1999. The demonstrators and their discussion forums highlighted the antidemocratic operations of the International Monetary Fund (IMF) and the World Trade Organization (WTO), as well as the lending practices of the World Bank.

This antiglobalization movement, although diverse and inchoate, is properly considered as part of the normative revolution that is being described. Its main thrust was to resist some of the capital-driven impacts of globalization that seemed to be producing increasing inequality within and among states, as well as leaving some states that lacked investment trade opportunities out in the cold. This global civil society movement was not opposed to globalization as such. It was insisting on reforms that would lead to what might be described as "humane globalization." These criticisms were increasingly engendering a response from some of those most closely associated with the world economy in its recent globalizing phase. George

Soros and Joseph Stiglitz echoed many of the complaints that were being shouted by the demonstrators about the way the global economy policy was proceeding.[20] As a result, the language associated with globalization began to exhibit more concern with such issues as the reduction of world poverty, the promotion of greater economic equality, the protection of human rights, particularly labor rights, and matters of environmental protection.

The 9/11 Attacks: Detour or Derailment?

Against this background of positive initiatives, I want to raise the question as to whether the 9/11 attacks have resulted in a permanent detour from this normative revolution, or merely caused its temporary derailment. There is little doubt that the energies and attention given to the initiatives discussed above have been abandoned, especially in the United States, and replaced by a renewed foreign policy preoccupation with security and the dynamics of the war against global terror. In light of this shift, how should we interpret the overall impact of 9/11? Instead of seeking to build the structures of global governance, and strengthen further a global rule of law as a means of exerting constraints on sovereign states, the new emphasis is on claiming the authority to engage in whatever actions contribute to antiterrorist goals. This kind of claim to carry on violent conflict has two particularly disturbing aspects.

The first concern is that there has resulted the first borderless war in history. Both principal adversaries disavow respect for the territorial sovereignty of states. The Al Qaeda network declared a violent *jihad* against America, its cadres seem determined to launch attacks wherever such targets can be found, that is, anywhere in the world. The United States, in turn, claims the right to attack anywhere that it can locate an al Qaeda threat. This pattern of conflict is quite subversive from the perspective of international law, which evolved to deal with conflicts among territorial sovereigns. Of course, international law never enjoyed great success in relation to wartime situations, but it did have some role in moderating the scope of conflict by confining the zone of violent operations to the territorial domains of combatants.

The United States is militarily the most powerful country in human history. Since 9/11 its leadership portrays itself as the vehicle of good against this evil of anti-state terrorism. To destroy this evil, it is determined, as is the case with its Al Qaeda adversary, to suspend limits on the way force is used to achieve goals. Prisoners suspected of Al Qaeda connections are denied rights under the Geneva Conventions governing the standards of international humanitarian law. The White House issues orders to assassinate suspects in foreign countries as a permissible tactic. American investigative procedures have relied on relying on torture.[21]

There are additional reasons to be troubled. The antiterrorist banner is being waved, but the goals of American foreign policy were extravagant before September 11, and now seem to be pretending that the struggle against terrorism validates the project to exert control over virtually the entire planet. Such contentions can best be understood by reference to such other American strategic undertakings as the militarization of space, the realization that U.S. defense spending exceeds that of the next fifteen countries combined, and there have been Pentagon leaks disclosing an increased willingness to rely on nuclear weaponry in battlefield situations.

Under these circumstances can we, should we, search for new limits on the discretion to use force in world politics? This is a vital question, especially for Americans, which need to be addressed in the present world setting. I want to answer such a question rather subjectively, by offering some tentative thoughts about the reconstruction of limits, and how this might bear upon the wider agenda of humanitarian action. As a starting point, the only acceptable way to rediscover a framework of limits is to recognize that our own values and traditions as a free society based on constitutionalism depend upon nurturing a respect for law and for the opinions of others, including those situated beyond our borders, and a reluctance to embark upon warfare outside of the Western Hemisphere. This ethical outlook is part of the federalist idea and the republican vision that has guided our sense of ourselves as a country, despite notable departures from time to time, since the national point of origin in the American Revolution. To protect this heritage at this point, given the pressures of the mega-terrorist challenge and the ambitions of the geopoliticians in the White House and Pentagon, will require a high level of citizen vigilance. This vigilance must be provided by the American people, by interior states such as Kansas and Minnesota, by activism on college campuses, and by the religious community and organized labor. Even to contemplate such prospects may seem utopian at this point, given an aggressive nationalism that grips the country, reinforced by the disturbing passivity of Congress, the provocations of the Tea Party, and inappropriate cheerleading by the mainstream media.

At stake here also is the matter of fundamental national identity. Aside from this acceptance of the self-limiting character of the state is the traditional American claim to be a republic and not an empire. However, if you assess the plans put forth by the Pentagon or peruse recent issues of *Foreign Affairs*, it is assumed that America has become, whether intentionally or not, an empire. The issue that remains more uncertain in these interpretations is whether the United States is likely to be a benevolent empire or whether it will be its fate to be an irresponsible, and probably, self-destructive empire.[22] The question that has so far not been raised, at least in these discussions within the American establishment, is whether being an empire is itself subversive of the self-proclaimed constitutional identity of this country as a republic. To be a republic is to be sensitive to the fragility of power, including the acute dangers of its abuse. The main purpose of the constitutional structure, based on checks and balances, is to protect the society against the destructive effects and multiple dangers of unchecked power. This prospect threatens our liberties as citizens, but internationally, the menace of unchecked power involves ignoring the well-being and viewpoints of others who lack the means of resisting.

The second problematic aspect of the response to 9/11 was a missing part of U.S. foreign policy and political consciousness for many years, that is, diagnosing and responding to the legitimate grievances that exist throughout the world, which if ignored, give rise to severe resentment. This resentment is especially directed against those political actors that are perceived to be responsible for unacceptable conditions and possess the capabilities to fashion just solutions to outstanding conflicts. The United States, as the predominant actor throughout the world, is seen as having contributed to the suffering of peoples due to its relationship to some of these legitimate grievances. From the moment of the attacks, the American leadership has failed to connect anti-American sentiments, including those that give rise to political and religious extremism, and terrorist tactics with their real causes. Instead, avoiding the slightest willingness to allow self-criticism, the explanation of "why they hate us" is reduced to envy directed at our values and achievements.

These spiraling patterns of resentment pertain to the relations between the United States and the Islamic world, and especially the Arab Middle East. Of course, commentary is speculative. But it certainly seems much more likely that September 11 would not have happened if the Palestinian problems of self-determination had been solved years ago in a manner that was fair to both peoples. This conflict should have been dealt with long ago in a balanced way, not only for prudential reasons associated with regional stability, but as part of a more intrinsic commitment to a realization of the right of self-determination for the Palestinian people, who had been denied independence and statehood despite the dynamics of decolonization having swept across the world in recent decades.

Reviving the Normative Revolution: Temptations and Commitments

In effect, the construction of a humane framework for global governance, which was proceeding in a generally encouraging way in the 1990s, has been abandoned in this period after September 11. Can it be revived? Can global civil society renew its pressures that proved effective in the prior decade? What sorts of issues should take priority? Despite adverse trends, whatever integrity and courage are found, there remains the possibility of positive action with respect to the agenda of the normative revolution.

In conclusion, returning to the spirit of the normative revolution in the 1990s is not currently feasible. The continuing security consciousness, coupled with a prolonged economic recession, discourages use of energies and resources for humanitarian purposes. If this direct security threat is further diminished, a deeper security argument strongly supports the revival of the normative revolution, starting with fashioning equitable responses to legitimate grievances around the world. Without resuming the struggle to achieve humane global governance, the likelihood is that violent resistance will occur in forms that will jeopardize Western security in various ways. We need the moral and political imagination to realize that the security of the rich and powerful in a globalizing world depends over time on improving the circumstances and raising the hopes of the poor and weak. If September 11 has taught us anything, it should be that the weapons and tactics of the weak are capable of inflicting severe harm with significant adverse material and psychological consequences. To learn from such a traumatic experience means nurturing our ethical impulses as well as sharpening our swords!

The Academy and Humanitarian Action

Joseph A. O'Hare, S.J.

Humanitarian action is ordinarily understood to involve a response to the needs of individuals and communities afflicted by different kinds of calamities, both those that are natural, like earthquakes and typhoons, and those that are the result of human intervention, like wars and political repression. Some calamities, of course, represent a convergence of natural disasters and human mischief; famine, for example, can be the result both of climactic changes in a particular region and a flawed distribution system created by a world market dominated by a profit motive.

Humanitarian action can also be understood in a broader sense, namely the continuing attempts to achieve a more human world, one where wealth and opportunity are more evenly distributed among nations and among classes within nations. In this sense, humanitarian action is the enduring effort to create a world where a respect for human dignity and inalienable rights of the individual are the cornerstone of society.

At first glance, the world of the academy is more directly engaged in the second, broader meaning of humanitarian action. The expansion and communication of knowledge, which is the life of the academy, is more directly related to the continuing search for wisdom and a vision of the human than to the more episodic responses to the needs of victims of wars and famines. At the present moment, however, the possibilities of direct humanitarian action in support of the afflicted in different parts of the world are limited and threatened by a new kind of world conflict that is rooted in a clash of the fundamental values and traditions that have always engaged the energies of scholars and teachers. The possibilities of humanitarian actions, in the conventional sense of a response to a crisis but also in the broader sense of a continuing search for a more human world, are today linked together in an unusual and more immediate relationship.

In this chapter, I propose to first describe the specific character of the present world conflict that threatens the possibility of humanitarian action and the threat this conflict poses for the integrity of the academy or, more specifically, the freedom of the university. I will then argue that the dangers of the present moment underline the urgency of recognizing that the contemporary university must be an international institution, one that fosters authentic intercultural understanding and maintains an environment where interreligious dialogue can take place and religious traditions can be renewed. One important dimension of this conflict involves the inexorable process of globalization, which demands that contemporary education must be international in character, on every level in appropriate fashion.

The University and International Terrorism

The university, the most typical institution of academia, encourages differences, believing that the free competition of ideas is a necessary condition for the expansion of knowledge that can lead to a glimpse of the truth and the best available wisdom to guide our lives and our world. Given this inherent diversity, does the contemporary university offer a distinctive perspective on the possibilities of humanitarian action in a world where traditions and values can be locked in conflicts that can seem insoluble?

The dangers of the present moment arise from a network of international terrorists and terrorist organizations whose motivation and objectives are far more obscure than the causes that have, in the past, led nation-states into armed conflicts. International terrorism transcends national borders and political ideology. Its objective appears vague and shifting, its passion rooted in popular resentment rather than patriotic cause, its vision of the future vague and inarticulate. The amorphous character of international terrorism—the absence of any proposal for an alternative future coupled with its willingness to attack the innocent at random—only adds to the unsettling, because undefined, character of its threat to international society.

In such a climate of fear and uncertainty, legitimate concerns about national security can escalate into unnecessary restrictions on civil liberties and the repression of legitimate differences on how to meet the dangers of international terrorism. In the wake of the terrorist attack of September 11, the desire to retaliate overwhelmed the need to better understand the passions behind this murderous assault. Debate on university campuses over the Middle East crisis quickly became politicized, and the legitimacy of conflicting views on the Israeli-Palestinian conflict was challenged. In the rush of patriotic feeling, many were impatient with any call for an examination of the international posture of the United States as the sole remaining superpower in the world.

Yet, any attempt to contain and eventually eliminate the dangers of international terrorism must include a better understanding of its deep, involved roots. This search for understanding is the mission of the university. To fulfill this mission, however, the university must protect its autonomy and encourage the kind of academic freedom that is a condition of authentic discovery. Such freedom, which encourages the competition of ideas, is not a luxury that can be surrendered in a time of national danger, but a necessity if we are to understand the nature of the danger that surrounds us.

The Internationalization of Education

One source of the energy of international terrorism is resentment of the current division of wealth and power in international community. Such resentment can create coalitions of protest among groups with different agenda and ideologies. The demonstrations against the present economic order that have marred international meetings around the world have brought together a wide variety of groups and organizations; religious activists calling for the cancellation of the debts of poorer nations and anarchists seeking to undermine civil order, united only in a resistance to the inexorable but bewildering process of globalization, driven by the dynamics of world markets and information technology. In this world economy that transcends national boundaries, new wealth is created and whole societies can be transformed, but the distribution of this wealth is uneven and individuals and communities can be left behind and left out.

The very process of globalization seems to strip individuals and communities of their autonomy and self-determination, and provokes the fury of those who consider its cost, both economically and culturally, dehumanizing. These critics of globalization insist it has created a wider gulf between the rich and the poor, between nations and regions, and between classes within nations. Meanwhile, distinctive cultural traditions are being undermined by a homogeneous popular culture that comes with mass consumerism.

Resentment of the economic and cultural consequences of globalization is a common passion that connects a broad array of critics with different causes and agendas. The violent protests that have exploded at several international meetings have bewildered many, while legitimate questions concerning globalization have been obscured by the destructive behavior of radical groups. But the process of globalization, driven by the appeal of world markets and the revolution in information technology, cannot be reversed, nor should it be.

If the university is to contribute to a better understanding of both the challenges and the opportunities that globalization presents, then the university must be transformed into an international institution, recognizing that in our contemporary world, all education must be international in nature.

This does not mean that individual institutions must compromise their distinctive identities and missions. In the twenty-first century we live in one world, whether we like it or not, but it is a world of differences, and our challenge is not to diminish those differences or paper them over in the interests of some superficial unity. On the contrary, the challenge for the university as an institution is the same challenge that confronts all nations and institutions in this new millennium: How to make our differences a source of enrichment rather than division? How to better appreciate our own traditions and values by recognizing and respecting the traditions and values of others? How to redeem the promise of cultural and religious traditions of others? How to redeem the promise of cultural and religious traditions by a creative renewal of their deepest meanings? How to find in the renewal of such traditions a more human response to the opportunities made possible by the technological revolution? How to make it clear that modernization does not, in the end, mean Westernization?

The Development of Intercultural Understanding

The most obvious sign of the increasingly international character of higher education is the growth in exchange programs that brings students and scholars from other nations and cultures to our campuses here in the United States and encourages faculty and students from the United States to spend time at other institutions in other nations and cultures. But while the exchange of faculty and students is necessary, it is not enough. The university must encourage and support the development of authentic intercultural understanding.

The promotion of multiculturalism on American campuses can be an easy target for those critics who see it as a surrender of the defining values of Western civilization. It was with some chagrin that I learned some years ago of a campus debate here at Fordham that posed the question: multiculturalism versus the Jesuit educational tradition. We need only think of historic Jesuit experiments at inculturation, like those that led to the Chinese Rites controversy and the Paraguay Reductions, to realize that the Jesuit education over the past four and a half centuries has always been multicultural.

It is unfortunate that the debate about multiculturalism in American education has too often been mired in arguments about what texts should be included in college curricula in order to include underrepresented groups. It is a debate that has often degenerated into academic politics in its least appealing posture. To achieve the goals of an authentic intercultural sensibility, a program of immersion in another language and culture should be part of the required curriculum in any program of liberal studies. At present time, for example, the Beijing Center for Language and Culture offers a program for undergraduates at Jesuit colleges and universities in the United States that is far more demanding and far more rewarding in terms of an intercultural experience than prescribed readings, in translation, of a faculty member's favorite neglected author.

An understanding and appreciation of non-Western cultures should enrich our understanding of Western civilization and not diminish it. To achieve this end, however, the enduring goals of a liberal education have to be continually affirmed and realized. The study of other cultures should not lead to a collapse of community into separate national and ethnic enclaves but rather should lead to a deeper and richer appreciation of the common human values we share.

This process is assuredly not automatic. To be successful we cannot shy away from cultural critiques and ethical judgments. Accepting a bland moral relativism as the necessary corollary of multicultural appreciation will not guide the development of a more human world. At the same time, moral judgments that have no appreciation of different cultural sensibilities will remain irrelevant abstractions.

The Challenge of Interreligious Dialogue

The university has always been an institution where tradition is not only recovered and remembered but also renewed and transformed. In its classrooms, libraries, and laboratories, the wisdom of the past should confront each day the questions of tomorrow. In the life of the ideal university community, new questions are not feared and suppressed but welcomed and debated. In actual life, of course, university communities do not always resist the narrow politicization of activist and advocates that declare what is and is not acceptable thinking.

In the wake of the September 11 terrorist attack and the continuing violence in the Middle East, debate over the fundamental causes of the conflicts has often become polarized and the legitimacy of dissident scholars challenged because of their political views. If the university is to fulfill its historic role as a forum for competing views, we must insist on the conditions for civil debate: mutual respect and honest recognition of differences. Civility does not compromise moral commitment, although this is not obvious to campus activists who find demonstrations more satisfying than debates.

The need to balance passion and civility is particularly acute in the continuing conversation that should be interreligious dialogue. Perhaps the secular university is not the most congenial environment for such dialogue, since the recognition of the importance of religious experience and the legitimacy of intellectual inquiry into such experience can be absent from the prevailing ethos of the secular academy, the legacy of the children of the Enlightenment.

For the secularist, religion itself, with its absolutist claims, can appear to be the source of inevitable conflict, and certainly human history has demonstrated in many different ages that violence to the human spirit can be done in the name of religion. The terrorist attack on September 11 was not the only instance in history of the destructive purposes to which religious passion can lead. To protect the purity of the faith, heretics were tortured and beheaded in the name of Christendom. Closer to our own day, we have seen false messiahs inspire mass suicides by their followers.

Religious passion is a powerful flame that can inspire the radiant example of St. Therese of Lisieux and the heroic service to the poor by generations of missionaries. But religious passion, we recognize, can be turned to darker and more destructive purposes, as it surely was on September 11 when the terrorists committed the ultimate blasphemy of destroying the innocent in the name of the Almighty.

All religious traditions, if they are to be continually renewed, must be engaged in a dialogue with history. In the Catholic tradition, we speak of the development of doctrine, where the test of continuity is applied to new understandings of the received tradition. Every religious tradition, if the tradition is to be a living tradition, must deal with the tension between fundamentalism and modernity. There is no easy resolution of this tension; instead, it involves a continuing conversation, and the university offers a privileged forum for such a conversation. This has been the experience of Catholicism from the first development of the university as an institution born from "the heart of the church" (*Ex corde ecclesiae*) in the medieval universities of Europe.

This challenge of renewal confronts the powerful tradition of Islam. The dangers of Islamic fundamentalism can, in the end, only be resolved within Islam itself. The renewal of Islam, as a living religious tradition, must take place in the dialogue with history and modernity that must engage all religious traditions. The world of the university remains a privileged forum for this indispensable conversation and renewal. Those universities that are themselves animated by a living religious tradition would seem to be a particularly congenial home for such dialogue.

In our observance of the first anniversary of the September 11 terrorist attack at Fordham University, interreligious memorial services were held at each of our campuses. The readings for these services were drawn from the New Testament, Buddhist texts, and the Koran. Though obviously different in tone and accent, all of these readings converged on the primacy of human dignity as the test of any religious passion. Respect for those who differ from us in national identity or religious belief does not imply an indifference toward the truth. A healthy religious pluralism fosters the renewal of distinctive religious traditions and respect for the truth claims they make, even when one chooses to disagree with those claims. But the critical test of such claims is their relevance to the dignity of the human person. Does this religious vision recognize and enhance the human person or diminish and violate human dignity? While different cultures may manifest different expressions of what it means to be human, the assumptions of liberal education is that there is a common humanity we all share. To destroy the innocent on behalf of a religious cause is the ultimate blasphemy. Religious passion, then, becomes a vicious abstraction, demonic in origin rather than divine. Part of the legacy of September 11 is the painful reminder that religious faith can be betrayed by those who use it to justify violence. The search for understanding among differences, the mission of the university, is an essential guardian of religious integrity.

The fundamentalist instinct in all religious traditions, of course, can slide into a kind of anti-intellectualism that resists the kind of questioning of tradition that is part of the life of the university. The university, as an institution of inquiry rather than indoctrination, is suspect to the fundamentalist. The irony here is that without such inquiry religious tradition can become distorted, frozen into harmless irrelevancy or distorted into the more dangerous sense of absolute righteousness that can become absolute ruthlessness. Dare one suggest that the blasphemous attack of September 11 was an extreme instance of a religious tradition that had refused the essential dialogue with modernity that is the mission of the Catholic university and remains the best hope of a creative renewal of the deepest truths of the Islamic tradition?

Conclusion

The contemporary university should provide a context for humanitarian action in the broad sense of creating a more human world and enable individuals to respond to the need of the afflicted in the more narrow sense of humanitarian action by fostering an authentic intercultural understanding and encouraging the renewal of religious traditions, and particularly the Islamic tradition, through interreligious dialogue. In a world threatened by international terrorism, the university must resist restrictions on academic freedom that would inhibit the task of understanding the sources of the deep-seated, if inarticulate, resentment at the heart of such terrorist campaigns.

Government Responses to Foreign Policy Challenges

Peter Tarnoff

Different Paths to Common Goals

It is remarkable how much the preambles of constitutions have in common. Even when their authors come from different historical, religious, and cultural traditions, these documents extol the dignity of all citizens and defend the exercise of freedom and rights while proclaiming the unity of a people in a national politic. Founders of nations and their successors invariably appeal to universal sentiments common to all humankind. No doubt some of the constitution writers are sincere in evoking aspirations that elicit a general will to work for the common good. Other founders may be more cynical or manipulative, knowing full well that even a morally correct constitution does not always reflect the realities of governance.

In order to understand the true intentions of governments, we may want to distinguish between those that are value-oriented and results-oriented. Value-oriented regimes commit themselves to govern according to traditional—usually religious—texts or laws. The highest authorities in value-oriented states are clerics and the most venerated documents of state are scriptures. High religious authorities are empowered to interpret religious texts in ways that apply to everyday life including commerce, contracts, laws, and the definition and punishment of crime. In these societies, severe restrictions usually are imposed on the behavior of ordinary citizens and close ties with foreign powers are regarded with suspicion for fear of contamination or subversion.

Results-oriented governments aim to bring about tangible improvements in the well-being of society in areas such as health care, prosperity, education, public safety, national security, and infrastructure. When a government is results-oriented, its laws can be based on a body of traditional doctrine, but its constitutional foundation is consistently being interpreted and reinterpreted by secular, often elected, judiciaries and parliaments.

The U.S. government is, for the most part, results-oriented. Its constitution affirms the separation of church and state. A strong federal system and independent judiciary constrain the power of the central government. The two national political parties compete for public favor in terms of concrete deliverables. While public rhetoric, especially during electoral periods, embraces traditional values and moral principles, elections themselves usually are won or lost on the basis of policy prescriptions or records of achievement.

Can the same be said of American foreign policy? Is it also results-oriented, or is the propagation of an American value system becoming more central to U.S. objectives around the world?

In the immediate post–World War II period, American foreign policy was driven principally by the need to establish a network of coalitions under U.S. leadership that were prepared to defend—militarily, if necessary—the Western world against encroachments from the Communist bloc, led by the Soviet Union. During the forty-five years of the Cold War, there were superpower proxy wars in the developing world but no armed conflict between NATO and the Warsaw Pact. The two alliance adversaries made little effort to convert the other; both were principally concerned with controlling their own members and preserving their respective systems of governance and economic organization.

Suddenly, a quarter-century ago, the USSR collapsed and the Cold War ended.

An "end of history" was proclaimed by some and it looked to many Americans as if liberal democratic forms of governments and free market economies had triumphed over the Communist and totalitarian alternatives and that there would be a universal recognition that something close to a U.S. model had become the system of choice for most societies. In the absence of overarching military and ideological threats and a diminished need for the "sole remaining superpower" to tend to minding its alliances, there was more talk in Washington than before about a moral foreign policy and greater confidence that American values (often portrayed as "universal values") would be a central component of Washington's worldwide reach.

A Doctrinaire Foreign Policy

Doctrines and values are not new to American foreign policy. In the early nineteenth century, the Monroe Doctrine alerted Europeans that the United States "should consider any attempt on their part to extend their system to any portion of this hemisphere as dangerous to our peace and safety."

Shortly after World War II, the Truman Doctrine made clear that the United States would act to oppose any Soviet attempt to extend its influence into Greece and Turkey. Under President Jimmy Carter, human rights were placed high on the U.S. foreign policy agenda and, although Carter was denounced by balance-of-power realists for sacrificing American interests on the altar of idealism, his successor, Ronald Reagan, strengthened democracy-building efforts primarily to weaken the hold of the Communist regimes. The first President Bush announced the coming of a "new world order" that was understood to rely heavily on the American experience and influence.

President Clinton came to stand for what some of his aides described as a doctrine of "humanitarian interventionism," where the international community—assisted and sometimes led by the United States—intervenes, with force if necessary, to prevent or stop human slaughter.

The second Bush administration was more ambitious than its recent predecessors in proclaiming the need for a new doctrinal structure and the obligation to spread American political, economic, and moral values far and wide. It justified this redefinition of American interests and strategies on the basis of what is required to defend the United States against new enemies and new threats in the post–Cold War world.

The Bush II administration was, of course, heavily influenced by the need to retaliate following the attacks in New York and Washington, D.C. The new Bush Doctrine was published as the "National Security Strategy of the United States." The document makes clear that the United States intends to preserve and use its position as the dominant military power in today's world. Washington will decide what threatens the American way of life and, while there are passing references to international partners, it is clear that the United States is prepared (even eager) to act alone. It is not hard to see in the text the strength of the administration's unilateralist impulse that so concerned many foreign governments.

In the case of Iraq, the doctrinal and pragmatic strains of Bush administration thinking meet and fuse. President Bush repeatedly stated that the United States would act quickly, decisively, and alone (if necessary) to remove the threat that Saddam Hussein represented. He had been so clear and consistent that it is hard to imagine the President's being satisfied by anything less than a convincing cleansing of all weapons of mass destruction in Iraq and the ouster of Saddam as well. Most world leaders, including those in the Arab nations, would like nothing better than to rid Iraq of such weapons, and there was little support around the world for the murderous regime of Saddam Hussein. Yet, why then was there so much suspicion regarding Washington's demands when America's objective (Iraqi disarmament) was so widely shared?

For three reasons: The first is that many governments believed that American policy in Iraq was not based on a legitimate fear of Iraqi intentions or capabilities, but that Washington was using Iraq as a convenient excuse to assert America's paramount political power and military superiority and its willingness to use them. This skepticism was reinforced when it turned out that Iraq had no weapons of mass destruction. The second: Many Muslim leaders believed that the United States wanted to transform Iraq into a Western-style democracy. The third: The United States sought improved access to oil.

But back again to doctrine. Now that there was a clearly stated official Bush Doctrine, it became awkward for the administration to flexibly and creatively innovate new policies or react to new emergencies. But it did. The announcement by North Korea that it was pursuing a nuclear weapons program was a clear candidate for preemptive military attack by the United States. However, the Bush administration reacted cautiously and cooperatively to the North Korean program while defending itself against charges from the right that it was handling the challenge no differently from the way a Democratic administration would have reacted.

The United States forcibly installing democracy in Baghdad, and beyond, alarmed many in the Middle East who will not soon forget the crusader spirit of those American officials eager to assert that the United States has the right to remake Muslim societies. In the real world of international politics and diplomacy, imposing Western ways by force of arms following a military victory on countries determined to preserve their distinctive cultures and religions would have catastrophic consequences.

The Obama administration has generally adhered to the approach to foreign policy practiced by the predecessors of George W. Bush. It has stressed collegiality "whenever possible" and case-by-case decisions regarding the extent of U.S. involvement. And it has functioned at a time when the very nature of warfare and so-called soft nonmilitary pressures are rapidly changing.

Good vs. Evil: An Age of Absolutes

American presidents have called foreign adversaries "evil" before. Ronald Reagan labeled the Soviet Union an "evil empire," but he then went on to become a serious negotiating partner with Mikhail Gorbachev. The second President Bush described Iran, Iraq, and North Korea as constituting an "axis of evil," and he warned the rest of the world that countries have a choice: they can be either for or against the United States in the war on terror. But since World War II, the United States has worked harder at persuading and cultivating its political, military, and economic partners than at negotiating with its enemies. Presidents from Truman to Obama understood how much American security depended on having close friends and allies, even when there were differences of views to bridge and difficult compromises to swallow.

It is also true that diplomatic conditions have changed: America's new enemies are both more and less threatening: less threatening because, whatever their destructive power, they are unable to obliterate the planet (although some might do so if they could), but also more threatening because they do not seek to reach accommodations with us. They have no interest in summitry or state visits. In the Middle East, some have a political agenda: the destruction of the State of Israel and the overthrow of the Gulf monarchies, especially that of Saudi Arabia. They see the United States as the principal obstacle to their aims and have shown themselves ready to use terror to weaken and hurt us. In the case of the most fanatic extremists, no negotiation is possible, and the United States has no choice but to work with others to destroy them.

Does their suicidal fanaticism make all of the terrorists' demands evil? What happens when countries in the Middle East that we need for security cooperation and oil express some sympathy for the political agenda of the terrorists? The problem with labeling governments and groups as either good or evil and demanding (rhetorically, at least) that they be for us or against us is that it may play well in American politics but it outrages many important non-Americans whose cooperation is essential to us in the war on terror and who insist on making a distinction between the aims and the methods of terrorist states and organizations.

The overuse of "evil" to describe countries and governments also places an implicit obligation on the United States to dispose of such regimes. Although the United States can fight and win wars in many places at once, few in America want Washington to be the world's enforcer. Indeed, less talk of good versus evil and us versus them might allow the United States to recapture the moral high ground in the war on terror. The more insidious the threat, the more important it will be for the United States to be less absolutist in its approach. During the Cold War, the United States could have fought alone against the USSR. But there is no way that the United States can win the war on terror alone, even if America is statistically more powerful than ever before when compared to the rest of the world.

Shifting Fault Lines

Living as I do in an earthquake zone in California, I am extremely sensitive to the danger when fault lines start to shift, even to a small degree. I also know that it is hard to predict when and where these movements will occur and what will be the extent of the damage they are likely to cause. It is clear, however, that even the most democratic and well-intentioned governments behave uncharacteristically when they feel threatened or destabilized. For example, they can:

- relax their definition of what constitutes torture (e.g., waterboarding) and permit a degree of corporal punishment and nonphysical pressures (e.g., sleep deprivation, noise and light harassment, extreme and indefinite isolation, threats to family members, constant interrogation)
- resort to the extrajuridical and covert assassinations of suspected terrorists
- invoke a political form of "force majeure" as reason for selectively applying or ignoring the Geneva Conventions
- restrict immigration, especially from countries or cultures perceived to be strange or hostile. Anti-immigrant sentiment also leads to the formation of sometimes-powerful neofascist political movements in developed countries
- pay less attention to issues of discrimination against women and children
- amend domestic judicial practices so that terms of indictment and confinement are radically tightened. Punishments then become much more severe for crimes stemming from the new threats
- impose restrictions on the media that result in less information being made available to the general public. Invoking national security considerations is a frequent excuse for withholding information that might prompt citizens to oppose the policies of their governments.

It is reasonable, even necessary, for societies under threat to resort to extraordinary measures to defend themselves. But it is also essential that in open societies there be a continuing public and political debate about how much security can be gained by limiting how much freedom. Such a debate can be acrimonious but it becomes unhealthy only if stifled. As frustrating as it is to policymakers, the struggle between security and liberty is endless. Should conditions change, practices can be loosened or tightened. The tectonic plates of policy are always shifting and the number of independent variables at play in a crisis can be huge. Nevertheless, as long as governments are committed to the proposition that it is ultimately desirable for there to be more freedoms not less and more information not less, citizens can expect that liberties and openness will someday be restored. But beware of those— even in democracies—who seek to make emergency restrictions permanent, because the threat is potentially infinite. Their aim is to transform, not simply defend, society because they live in a world of absolutes, including the illusion of absolute security.

Because the very nature of post–Cold War threats is indefinite and universal, there are some who believe that it will be necessary to modify fundamentally the character of free societies in order to defeat them. We know wars that end with a V-E Day or V-J Day, and where we can see the battle lines changing in our daily newspapers. But there will never be a V-Terrorism Day.

Like foreign policy itself, the campaigns against the new global threats will be an endless process where success will be measured incrementally, never conclusively. In the long haul, however, it will be the free and open societies that are best able to sustain the efforts and sacrifices necessary to stay the course in the interminable wars against the new challenges of the twenty-first century.

All Alone or All Together

When confronted with complex and ever-shifting fault lines, governments incline either toward the unilateral or the multilateral. Smaller and more vulnerable countries—especially those firmly embedded in regional political or economic alliances—are prone to turn to their neighbors for help in times of crisis. Most Member States of the European Union act that way. Especially in matters of economic policy, the EU nations tend to stick together and face the rest of the world in a united fashion after setting common economic policies. However, EU solidarity is less firm in political and security matters. Since the United Kingdom and France are permanent members of the UN Security Council and most EU nations are also members of NATO, there are not yet common European diplomatic or security policies on most issues.

The unilateralist impulse is more prevalent in the case of major powers and those opaque and dangerous regimes sometimes identified as "rogue states." Major powers are the most inclined to act and stand alone. They have the wherewithal to operate with a high degree of autonomy and their domestic political climate favors policies of "national interest" over "international comity." China and the United States are prime examples of powerful countries that are readier than most to stand alone on matters of high policy and principle. In the case of what might be called "outcast regimes," their very isolation and opaqueness create a shield that makes it hard for outsiders to have a clear view of their intentions and capabilities. North Korea is such a case in point.

The world and the cause of peace would be better served if international organization and agreements were effectively respected by all nations. In principle, most countries claim that they favor a rule of international law and order that prevents conflict and humanitarian chaos.

But nations differ over whether a threat to international peace and stability exists and, if it does, how international players should react. The discussions in the UN Security Council over how to disarm Saddam tended to overshadow international concerns about the scope and nature of the threat itself. Since the United States and others invaded Iraq, the multilateral approach to solving international problems has suffered a blow unless it makes the major powers more circumspect about using their armed forces to achieve political aims.

In principle, the new global threats of the twenty-first century are mostly multilateral in nature. They include environmental degradation, international crime, proliferation of weapons of mass destruction, ethnic and religious conflicts, disease, extreme poverty, and violations of human and civil rights. These threats generally know no borders and governments are not usually the sole entities with influence and resources. In fact, governments are coming to understand that nongovernmental organs (business, labor, the media, academia, religious groups, and private voluntary organizations) are increasingly important components of international affairs.

Today's multilateral diplomacy extends vertically to nonstate entities and horizontally to like-minded governments and international organizations. Effective international coalitions are no longer limited to ministers and generals. Nonstate players from business, academia, labor, private voluntary organizations, and the media are represented at the diplomatic negotiating table whether or not they are physically present. International diplomacy is now played like multidimensional chess.

Sanctions and Fence-Mending

When countries clash over what they consider to be important issues of policy or principle, there is always a risk that they will resort to military force. However, most governments at least pay lip service to the proposition that they will use force only as a last resort and many leaders actually do their best to resolve disputes peacefully. Moreover, there has emerged in recent decades a long menu of ways that governments and international organizations can bring nonmilitary pressure to bear on adversaries or outlaw states:

Economic Sanctions

Multilateral: Usually imposed by the UN Security Council. Generally regarded as the most effective because the most widely observed. Can be lifted once offending country meets certain conditions but requires a confirming vote by the UN Security Council to do so.

Unilateral: Country-to-country. May have political/moral effect, but porous economically because most countries are not bound to restrict trade or investment with targeted regime. If sanctioning country has sufficient power in International Financial Institutions (IFIs), it can block IFI loans and grants as well.

Extraterritorial: Sanctioning country applies economic penalties to third countries trading with targeted country. Hotly contested politically and legally by countries unwilling to accept jurisdiction of sanctioning country over their sovereign trading practices.

Coalition of the Willing: Although generally referring to military groupings, there can be coalitions of sanction imposing governments operating without formal UN Security Council approval. The imposition of economic sanctions can, however, be a broad and blunt weapon. Unless they are targeted on the offending country's leadership, sanctions can cause serious suffering among the civilian population. If the pain from sanctions on the innocents is prolonged and serious, states—especially in the region—will circumvent them. The United States has imposed sanctions more than any other country in recent years, but because most American sanctions are bilateral, they have had only marginal economic effects.

Moral/Political Sanctions—Multilateral or Unilateral

This form of sanction is often applied in the area of human rights. The UN Human Rights Commission meets annually to pronounce itself on alleged human rights violators around the world. Charges and countercharges are debated in Geneva before the violations are put to a vote by the Commission. In addition, and uniquely, the United States publishes annually a human rights report describing and condemning what it considers to be human rights violations around the world.

Shunning

A more discrete form of official displeasure occurs when a country decides to have no or limited diplomatic representation in another capital. Shunning can be augmented by ordering its diplomats to avoid all contact and dialogue with representatives of the foreign power.

Sanctions are nonmilitary methods of pressure and punishment, but the diplomatic arsenal also contains devices to promote reconciliation and dispute resolution. They include:

Mediation/Arbitration

Ideally, such interventions occur before international disputes turn violent. Successful conflict prevention is better than settlement negotiations but resolving conflict that has already erupted is sometimes the only way that peace can be restored. International organization negotiators (usually, but not always, with the UN) abound but there are skilled national mediators as well. For decades, the United States has played a unique role in the Middle East peace process and now, more recently, in the Balkans and the EU is reinforcing its dispute resolution capacities. Regional organizations should play greater roles in settling disputes, although the disputing parties must also be convinced that there are positive consequences for them to settle. This means that the developed countries and the IFIs have to be prepared to provide financial rewards for good political behavior.

Constructive Engagement

This is a diplomatic way to describe "good cop, bad cop" routine for dealing with a recalcitrant state. It involves at least one outside government maintaining contact with the regime that is under pressure to change or to cease and desist. Constructive engagement works best when the "good cop" coordinates its initiatives with the international community pressing for change. Often times neighbors are good in this role although it helps to have a major power also involved so that the "target" country believes that any eventual political and economic rewards it gains in return for compliance will have broad international support.

How Democracies Should Make Foreign Policy

When governments are confronted with cataclysmic threats or emergencies, traditions, values, and humanitarian actions can be incinerated by the intense heat of the moment. Especially in democracies where public pressure on governments is greatest, political leaders often feel that they have to act first and ask (moral) questions afterwards. In the United States it is commonly accepted that the president's first responsibility is to come to the defense of the country. Voices calling for measured and appropriate responses consistent with a nation's traditions and values rarely hold sway in the command centers and cabinet rooms of beleaguered governments. There are, however, ways that elements of morality and humanism can be inserted into the decision-making process.

The first way is to have the public be as well informed as possible about exceptional measures that a government believes it must undertake. Ultimately, it is the public and its elected representatives that should have the final say when it comes to deciding how drastic and how durable these measures must be. But without fairly full disclosure, the public will be kept in the dark and domestic discontent will grow.

The second way is to improve the legislative oversight of foreign policy. For the first two hundred years of our nation, it was generally accepted that foreign policy was the purview of the executive branch. Only rarely were presidents and secretaries of state subjected to the degree of scrutiny that administrations received on domestic issues. Then came the Vietnam War and television news. Trust in government was further eroded by Watergate, and serious oversight of foreign affairs by the Congress began. As a result, American foreign policy may be less coherent and well managed than before. But foreign policy is also more transparent than before and it turned out to be no harder than domestic policy for the American people to understand.

The third way is to broaden the uniquely American practice of having high officials shuttle between private careers and public service. Government careerists find our system arbitrary and inefficient and it often is. But a government dominated by career politicians and civil servants runs the risk of isolation and excess. Moreover, having men and women who were successful in nongovernmental careers appointed to high diplomatic office increases the chances that decisions will better reflect the attitudes of society at large and that policies will be made by people who are used to being held accountable for their actions because they come from professions where rapid merit-based advancement and abrupt dismissals can occur.

The fourth way is for citizens to understand that values are as essential to their security as military might and economic strength. A country true to a legacy of humanism is easier to defend and harder to attack. Its population will rally to the defense of the homeland. Its government will have standing in calling for international aid and support. Its enemies will know that world opinion will turn against them. Such a country is not guaranteed to be invulnerable but it will be much safer if it makes every effort to adhere to practices and conventions accepted by most of humanity as genuinely beneficial to all.

In modern democratic societies, the pressures for demanding high levels of accountability, freedom, and openness come from the bottom up not the top down. Governments under threat will always seek greater control and autonomy and it is hard to strike a perfect balance between a government's ability to manage a crisis and a free people's need to know, judge, and change what a government is doing. Still, if the balance of power tilts too strongly and indefinitely in government's favor, the new global challenges that it is trying to manage will be hard to overcome.

Disasters and the Media

Jeremy Toye

For the media, a disaster is not a tragedy. It is a challenge, an opportunity. A challenge for the traditional media to find out what is happening, how to get there, what is at stake, who is to blame. For the nontraditional media, the tweeters, Facebook friends, and bloggers, it is how to get the message out, who to include, when to retweet someone else's tweet. And for all of them, there is the chance to inform, to activate, or to enrage, for a vast audience always turns to the media whenever a disaster strikes.

Those are some of the challenges, but there are opportunities too. It is not necessarily wrong, nor even cynical, for a decent journalist to see a disaster as an opportunity to get a good story. Journalists wept at the site of the Twin Towers falling. But they and their employers had a job to do, and in a disaster, no matter whether it is "natural" or "man-made," it gets harder but potentially more rewarding. And most media outlets will claim that they are there to serve noble ideals, that challenging authority and revealing the facts will lead to change for the better.

For the owners of commercial media, there is not only an opportunity to show expertise and concern for suffering but also a chance to revive flagging circulations and audiences.[1] In that large slice of the world where the state controls the media, it is a chance to show that government can move fast and help—unless, of course, it is the regime itself which is to blame for the disaster. For those among the millions of social media users who want to go beyond their circle of friends and what they had for breakfast, disasters spell a chance to get help, to rally support, or to let their compassion or concern show through.

The media have traditionally been reactive to disaster. It has happened, so now let us surf the feelings of revulsion and compassion and maybe someone will do something about it. But the explosion of digital connectivity via instant satellite links, social media, and above all the cell phone is leading some to question whether the media should do something more about disasters before they happen: to educate, teach, and inform people in areas vulnerable to drought, famine, or flood; to build, plant, save water, stock grain, or practice first aid. While more traditional media may argue that their role is to present the facts and let others decide, social media opens the door for communities of all stripes to take charge of their destiny.

It is left to the readers, listeners, and viewers who turn to the media, particularly in times of disaster, to distinguish reality from rumor, fact from fiction, promotion from propaganda. In the middle of all this cacophony sits a wide variety of enterprises lumped together as "the Media" (often friends, sometimes foes) and the "aid professionals," whose role is not only to find out what is going on in what they may call a disaster-related scenario, but also to do something about it.

Media and Disasters

Disasters have always been part of the media's staple diet, but in early times the dish was eaten cold. After the eruption of Vesuvius in A.D. 79, before anyone had time to react, the elegant city of Pompeii was preserved in ash.[2] By the time of Abraham Lincoln's assassination in 1865, the invention and rapid expansion of the telegraph system meant the news spread across the United States in minutes.[3] Two world wars tested first print, then broadcast journalism (and the extent that censorship would be tolerated), while advocates for change used media to move into the public glare. The suffragettes battling for votes for women, who chained themselves to London railings, calculated well that their photos would be used around the world.[4]

The Ethiopian famine of 1983–84[5] was a milestone in putting a remote human disaster into the living rooms of what used to be called the first world. But even in the world's first TV war in Vietnam,[6] instant communication to the public, and therefore instant reaction, was rare because of limited technology and high expense. And there was still time for judicious editing along the way: The most gruesome scenes could be cut, prompting accusations of media manipulation and official sanitization.

CNN coverage of the bombing of Baghdad bridged the technology gap to show the Iraqi capital as it was bombed. Later, mobile telephony, web-cams, and YouTube matched technology with portability and minimal price. The death of protester Neda Agha-Soltan,[7] broadcast from a cell phone camera in an Iranian demonstration attacked by government forces, took the process to a point where the traditional media, in the sense of providing a link between event and audience, were almost redundant.

The events of the Arab Spring of 2011 showed that not only could you use the new media to inform the uninformed and marshal support, you could also tell your fellow demonstrators what was going on just a few meters away. And since there is a dark side to almost everything, security forces could monitor those same calls and sift through YouTube videos for the faces they could identify. A sinister side of social media was demonstrated in the UK riots in 2011,[8] when rioters with no political agenda could use encrypted messaging to give news on which shops were ripe for looting. BlackBerrys, so long seen as the smart tool for the wheelers and dealers of the commercial world, found a new, unwelcome market among gangs of youths who knew open SMS messages would be monitored by police. Huge numbers of passive security cameras recorded images of looters blithely trying on shoes.

Like a knife or an ax, media in the wrong hands can be a fearful weapon. The videotapes of Osama bin Laden fueled al Qaeda's campaigns and inspired its followers to further violence. As in the filming of journalist Daniel Pearl's murder in Karachi in 2002, instant communication was another weapon to be used to support a campaign.[9] Pearl's death was also a reminder that dozens of journalists have been killed in conflicts such as Iraq, Afghanistan, and Syria.[10]

No wonder, then, that much of the monitoring of social media and instant communications is being done by representatives of the more traditional media. Twitter feeds, recalling for wire-agency veterans like me the brief Snaps and Bulletins used to alert media outlets to breaking news, could keep a single journalist in touch with a dozen places at once. Backed by two-way satellite communications and an array of gear, the BBC's man in Beirut, Jim Muir, could keep track of a host of Syrian cities under attack by the forces of a government that refused entry to anyone identified as a journalist.

While journalists on the frontline donned flak jackets to ride with rebel forces into Tripoli, others were scouring the airwaves in case Libyan leader Muammar Gaddafi should suddenly send an SMS message that he needed, say, sticking plasters. When he was found, his summary execution on screen[11] caused genuine shock, even in a world becoming inured to the blood and gore of battle. The execution was carried out by individuals in a remote place, but a cell phone camera made it a public event.

Natural disasters seem to happen most where access is least: an earthquake in the mountains of Pakistan; a tsunami from a quake deep below the Indian Ocean; drought and famine in one of Africa's most forbidding spots, Somalia. Yet even when a disaster happens in a country as sophisticated and accessible as Japan, and affects an industry as modern as nuclear power, the media are often hard pressed to get there. That being said, the single-minded determination of a journalist seeking out a story means that relief agencies often find that the media are alongside and even ahead of them.

No matter how reliable the firsthand source, or how venerated the wire services, every media outlet worth its salt wants its own staffer's byline, voice, or face to tell the story. And that costs money. Cut-price airfares suddenly fade away as affected airports close, helicopter hire soars like the machines themselves, and even the cost of a taxi will multiply if the driver thinks he might not be able to get back.

But for a while, some parts of the media seemed to have money to burn. The second half of the twentieth century saw a major expansion in the money spent gathering news of all kinds, especially disasters, and much of it was driven by television. *The Guardian* editor C.P. Scott could famously predict that "no good" would come of television,[12] but one of his rivals[13] in the UK's first commercial network could equally famously boast that he had been issued "a license to print money." The rival U.S. networks of NBC, CBS, and ABC could outbid each other in their coverage, each fronted by a household name, while CNN in unfashionable Atlanta endeavored to unseat them. The era of twenty-four-hour news channels had arrived, concentrating on breaking news, whatever its actual significance. On quiet news days, they would play the same video or audio clip again and again. On the disaster days, they would swing into action, using prearranged links to a welter of broadcasters whose own styles have moved inexorably from studio sets to street scenes.

In the twenty-first century, mobile telephony has opened whole continents to information access like never before. African villages that may still have only one communal TV set now have smart phones. African populations have made an enormous leap across a technology spectrum that had offered them nothing before.[14] Contrast this with a few years ago when the headmistress of a large secondary school in Swaziland told me that her pupils had no idea where their World Food Programme (WFP) aid came from—"and neither do I."

With a little help, that headmistress could now show her pupils where the food comes from, tapping into smart phone links on YouTube, or running Skype chats with the people who might help them grow better crops themselves. Such access might encourage the donors to ask their "beneficiaries" what is required before they supply, and also combat the stultifying fatalism that leaves so many children just as stunted as their lack of vitamins. Media campaigns, such as *The Guardian*'s regular reports from the Ugandan village of Katine,[15] help that process, but real change may come when means of communication sit firmly in the hands of the villagers themselves. And that day is not far off, as cell phones spread like wildfire across the world.

For many, information overload led directly to compassion fatigue. A new drought in East Africa—or is it West Africa? (In fact, in 2011, it was both.) Urgent pleas for donations from a familiar group of agencies were met by an unusually slow response from Western governments battling budget cuts and fighting to maintain levels of aid pledged in rosier times. Members of the public gave generously, but there were legitimate questions about how many more times they would be asked to save the starving child. Proponents of development rather than emergency handouts trotted out the cliché that if you give a man a fish, he will eat for a day, if you teach a man to fish, you will feed him for life, to which a weary aid official responded: "Yes, but the lake's dried up."[16] Templated stories gave the idea that disaster was recurrent, predictable, and followed patterns: from rubble to tented cities to cholera outbreaks to stories written on the first anniversary that so often begin with a child's name: "Muhammad lost half his family . . . ."

With global financial turmoil gripping both the developed and developing worlds since 2008, the media could not escape a cold blast of reality. Famous titles disappeared from the newsstands as rising costs and falling audiences swamped them.[17] Equally famous names such as the BBC found financial support waning, forcing news teams from different divisions to work together to keep down costs. Advertising revenue, in particular for television and print, dropped away.[18] (Insurance costs alone could scupper the chances of sending a news team to cover an event that may or may not turn into a major disaster.)

In some cases, the use of social media mirrored the agendas of the more familiar news outlets: delirious flattery for the latest music sensation; rage at a rape case; fervent support or ferocious condemnation of politicians like President Obama, who used the network brilliantly to help his election, and perhaps came to rue its impact on his ratings. At other times, the social network made its own agenda. A thirty-minute video that attracted more than 70 million online viewers in a week is a case in point. A small charity had a committed filmmaker produce a video on their work and on one of their targets—Joseph Kony.[19]

So it is no wonder that many branches of traditional media turn to cell phone screens, blogs, and onsite video channels to supplement and even substitute their own coverage. In one sense, they have been doing this for years: the international wire agencies[20] were the Twitters of their day, with largely anonymous correspondents filing reports from every capital and major city as wholesalers to the world's media retailers. They too have had to change their approach, providing elements of their coverage without charge on innumerable websites while charging premium rates for their very best material—most of it related to financial and commercial markets.

But disasters have a habit of echoing right through those trading floors, as carefully analyzed scenarios are turned upside down by events on the coast of Japan or in Haiti.

Disasters and Stakeholders

While the traders hit their keys in response to the latest disasters, a disparate set of groups spring into action. These are the "stakeholders," in the parlance of the aid world, who are thrown together whenever a disaster strikes:

> the government departments whose job it is to safeguard a nation's health, safety, security, and general well-being;
>
> the official international agencies, such as the United Nations (UN) humanitarian family, with global mandates to serve the vulnerable and dispossessed, backed by national and international funding; agencies such as USAID and Europe's ECHO;
>
> the myriad nongovernmental organizations (NGOs), ranging from the Red Cross/Crescent Society and Bill Gates's Global Fund, to religious charities, to a couple of Texas carpenters building one home at a time for tsunami victims, all responding to the natural wave of sympathy and support that a disaster brings;
>
> communities, national, regional or local, that may be drawn from the victims of a disaster or from others threatened by it, or from generous people far away.

Almost all of them, in an emergency, will find themselves seeking the oxygen of publicity—or being sought out by a demanding media when they are already overwhelmed. How these groups use, and might better use, the media is a key factor in whether they emerge in the aftermath of disaster honored or ignored.

Stakeholders, Disasters, and the Media

Alistair Cooke, once the doyen of foreign correspondents with his weekly broadcast "Letter from America," remarked that the only way to judge a journalist was by the quality of his sources. Anyone in media hoping to present her readers, listeners, or viewers with a portrait of what is happening in the world of aid would make little headway without sources within the community of stakeholders. Some sources would be known to many, such as a minister or an agency head. Other sources may never show their faces in public—the "Deep Throat" of Watergate, the "usually informed" or "reliable" sources where trust lies more with the believing journalist than with the potentially opportunistic whistleblower.

How the potential sources among stakeholders interact with the media may not directly affect the work they do or should do. But how their supporters and critics see them, and how their supporters react when asked for help or reject hindrance, can be influenced by how the stakeholders are presented in the media.

Governments, Disasters, and the Media

When disaster strikes—either on a national or regional scale, or closer to home, say, within a government agency itself—is the time when a government's relationship to the media is put to the test. It may have to face international media if the crisis attracts global attention, but it is often at local and national levels that a good relationship with the local press pays off best.

Until the onset of social media, some governments could bask in the comfort of an entirely state-controlled media. They had little to fear from the Soviet-era *Pravda*, President Mubarak's fawning *Egyptian Gazette*, or the broadcasts of Radio Peking under Mao Zedong. While a more open press has flourished in many countries since the fall of the Berlin Wall, radio and television, both with a wider reach, have remained a principal tool of dictators everywhere.

The products of such systems are invariably dull, pedantic, and so far removed from reality that even a disaster can be buried alive. Editorial staff who work under the yoke of malicious state control lose their perspective in their constant search for the ultrapositive. For the rest of the world, a lively, driven media may actually get read, heard, or seen—but it means their governments have to work harder to get a sympathetic hearing.

One of the first acts of any new government is to appoint an information minister. For journalists, alas, they rarely live up to their title.[21] The government spokesman (occasionally a woman, but more often than not, a man) usually has more to say, and, if they are truly professional, will always be ready to say it. But a journalist who relied on speaking only to spokespersons of any hue would have a lackluster career, because the spokepeople must invariably be "on message" and, if threatened, must guard the gates of government against assault.

Given half a chance, the spokesperson will attempt a more sophisticated role, that of "spin-doctor." Turning a nightmare catastrophe into a glorious triumph by becoming a spin-doctor is much resented by journalists, but there will always be those officials that cannot resist trying to put a positive spin on a clearly negative story. Another more mundane role of the spokesperson is equally important: They are a route to the top. Most journalists want to speak to the organ grinder, not the monkey, and they work hard to get the most senior voice they can. A friendly word with a spokesperson often works. This cozy relationship between the media and their principal sources may not look much like the bombast coming out of a dictator in front of his cowering head of broadcasting, but the aim is the same—to keep the message sweet.

In disasters beyond the control of government, events themselves will take precedence over the words of even the most powerful leader. But sooner or later the spotlight turns on who needs to fix the roads, drain the fields, house the homeless and open the airports. Invariably it is government that finds itself in the limelight. For journalists, the questions are easy: Why was help too slow or too rushed; why has so little or so much been spent; why wasn't this fixed last time; what's to stop it from happening again?

Counterintuitively, the sooner those questions get posed, the easier they will be to answer. A good government mouthpiece should be out there immediately saying what is known so far. At that stage, few journalists will have their own information to challenge what is being said. But if the government waits "until the situation becomes clearer," chances are it will have become muddier. The spokesperson may now have some beautiful charts to show what has been done, but the enterprising journalist has been there, seen a different picture, and has the quotes and photos to challenge the official line.

It is at this point that officialdom starts to stonewall and denials multiply, not only of facts but also of obvious conclusions.[22] Some spokespersons are very proud of being able to handle any question, no matter how tough. The trouble is they can look like a boxer who builds a great defensive shield but fails to land the punch that wins the bout. Some spokespersons defend so well that they rarely get around to saying anything positive about the organization that pays them so well.

Some are masters, however: The U.S. ambassador to the UN under George W. Bush, John Bolton, once declined to answer a tough question. When it was asked again in a different form, he said, "Go ahead, it will be interesting to see how many times you pose that question before you give up." It was Bolton, the archetypal neocon, who also said that you could chop ten floors off the top of the United Nations building in New York and "it wouldn't make a bit of difference."[23]

The UN, Disasters, and the Media

Lose ten floors off the UN HQ and a journalist might miss a couple of useful sources, but it is more likely to have a greater impact on the ground. When the UN Offices in Baghdad were bombed in 2003 it robbed the UN of sixty staff including its highly respected Iraq chief Sergio Vieira de Mello. Furthermore, it robbed journalists covering the conflict in Baghdad of the expertise, experience, and data gathering that makes the UN much sought after by the media.

In times of disasters, journalists can rely on the UN for more than just quotes—for access, for vital statistics to back up their own anecdotal evidence, for protection if the story gets too hot. That is not to say that the UN is universally popular among journalists who often like to see themselves as much more in touch with events on the ground. It is quite easy to paint a picture of the UN as overpaid suits operating behind heavily protected walls, breezing around town in gleaming white Land Cruisers and ready to cut and run at the slightest hint of trouble.

What is undeniable is that the UN's hierarchical system of checking and rechecking can mean that its reports and responses take days to appear. It can also lead to heavy self-censorship to avoid upsetting the Member States who in the end own the UN—and some of whom themselves see the UN as the enemy within.

UNICEF is widely judged by its sister agencies in the UN to be the most adept at news management. "They don't move without thinking about the media," grumbled a UN veteran who knows his agency has fewer media professionals worldwide than UNICEF has in one office. Another agency organizing a huge convoy into Iraq seethed when UNICEF turned up with a handful of trucks emblazoned with its name—and stole all the media thunder.

But one other reason why UNICEF is so well known—in spite of having an acronym whose original meaning is often forgotten[24]—is that it has National Committees. These organizations, independent of the agency itself and of each other, run much of the publicity and fundraising at the local level in many developed countries. Other agencies rely on their top executive to get their message across. Josette Sheeran came from a media background to head the WFP, and frankly, her glamorous appearance did no harm either.[25] UNICEF chief Carol Bellamy[26] may have been a tough taskmaster, but she could turn on the gritty charm for the media whenever required.

Increasingly, UN agencies are looking to social media to go beyond their own circles to the public at large. Punchy blogs stripped of the UN's love for acronyms and words like "psychosocial" are posted within minutes of an event, as are emailed invitations to support a named child with a small donation.[27] Yet for many senior UN staff, releasing the genie from the social network bottle means losing control, and increased risk of stepping on the toes of their masters.

Some of those toes belong to the funding agencies, the donors whose decisions can make the difference between life and death in a disaster. For the UN and most other aid agencies, funding only flows in when a disaster strikes, the result of urgent appeals that make up so much of the early media coverage. But once funds start to arrive, the UN teams on the ground are in the eye of the storm, and part of that storm is whipped up by another set of initials, the NGOs.

NGOs, Disasters, and the Media

One UN agency counts more than 1,100 NGOs as its partners. Though the term NGO might not be on everyone's lips, the individual names are among the world's best-known "brands"— the Red Cross and Red Crescent, World Vision, Oxfam, Save the Children, Greenpeace, *Médecins Sans Frontières* (MSF). And they are so well known because above all they know how to use the media.

The suffering child with huge eyes and a swollen belly is an enduring symbol of innumerable campaigns. Though glossy or homespun posters, charity workers shaking tins on street corners, and subsidized advertising play their part, it is the extent of media coverage that marks the successes from the also-rans. Public relations lore suggests that an unpaid article written by a real journalist is worth many times more than paid advertising space. The one-minute video promotions shown between TV bulletins may be fully sponsored, but an interview embedded in the bulletin itself will have a greater impact.

In disasters, television leads the way—and some of its material is made by the NGOs themselves. The high quality of even the smallest cameras, complete with realistic shaky images, means that broadcasters can show aid workers as they move in. NGO bloggers and tweeters have much more freedom than their UN counterparts not only to describe what they are doing, but also to pin down those they feel should do more. MSF is renowned for calling everyone to task, lambasting all and sundry. The impact can be twofold—to prompt the slow-footed into action, and to raise funds from members of the public who admire their forthright manner— which in turn won MSF a Nobel Peace Prize.

As with the UN, NGOs are not universally popular. Their heavy guns sent into an emergency can shoulder aside their local colleagues and sour the work done in building good relations on the ground. Their solutions, worked out around a desk in a distant capital, might not gel with local communities who resist change. In their home countries, NGOs are frequently questioned about how much of the funds they collect actually go to their beneficiaries and how much is spent on administration or travel.

And in all the turmoil of a disaster, the media are there looking over their shoulders. Once behind a lens, a news photographer will stop at little to get the shot—and if there is a crowd, they will jostle along with their text counterparts. Like the UN, NGOs spend many hours training their staff to accept media as a necessity rather than a mere nuisance or an actual hindrance.

Some of the larger agencies try to ensure media coverage by taking selected journalists in with them. The journalists might insist on paying their way, and though they will be grateful for the access, the best of them will still keep their professional distance, and the wise trip organizer will keep a watchful eye in case the whole thing goes wrong.

Courting publicity for any cause can backfire. An aid worker in West Africa complained bitterly that a campaign to help people deliberately mutilated by rebel forces had turned sour when insistent photographers made them "into a freak-show," prompting revulsion rather than sympathy.[28] The maker of the Kony video mentioned earlier won notoriety himself when he was filmed running naked and in distress near his home.[29]

Providing access is only one of the ways an agile NGO can improve its media coverage. High-quality data-gathering pays off if boiled down to easily assimilated facts. Introductions to the main players or even something as simple as offering recorded samples of local music to a radio reporter yields dividends. Willingness to answer questions while providing graphic details on the importance and success of their work is the hallmark of an excellent NGO spokesperson—and they will be sought out wherever they land.

The Public, Disasters, and the Media

Journalists love to recount their adventures in getting to the scene of a disaster against insuperable odds. But even the most agile reporter cannot beat the victim of a catastrophe who pulls out a mobile phone, snaps a surprisingly high-quality shot, and sends it off around the world (even if in fact it was only meant for a faraway member of the family). Communities of such people have begun to exercise their advantages of local presence and knowledge to campaign on their own behalf.

Some communities use the NGO route, though it can be difficult to sort the genuine from the grifters.[30] Social media work well at the other end of the pipeline, too. Email campaigns based on the old principle of chain letters can raise large amounts of cash in very few days—though they too need careful scrutiny for scams and spams.

As the instant access of social media spreads to every corner of the planet, the possibilities of community-inspired media getting ahead of a disaster are increasing. Rather than wait for a drought to hit, a well-organized community can launch a targeted appeal for money to buy grain, or sponsor wells, or agricultural extension work to identify more resilient crops. This puts powerful mitigating tools in the hands of those most affected.

Disasters and the Big Picture

Earthquakes, drought, floods, and fire have been with us since time began, and media of all types know about handling them. But what of the big-ticket items that worry so much of the world's thinkers and planners: climate change, environmental damage, deepening poverty, crippling disease, and the demand for universal education? If the media are adept at handling instant disasters, they are perhaps less assured in how to deal with these ongoing challenges. And while the media struggle, voices in the wings insist that they can do much more than report passively what they see and hear.

All media, from the self-important "Thunderer" (as the *Times of London* once styled itself) to the humblest blogger, thrive on change. But they are also addicted to speed, and no matter how big the looming disaster of climate change, no matter how destructive rising poverty to the future of the global village, actual change can be very hard to spot and track day by day. Add a third motivator, which is controversy, and much of the media will struggle—to use an old print-era phrase—to "hold the front page!"

For example, it is well established that human-made climate change will have a catastrophic impact, but perhaps not for years to come. Polar ice melt will swamp whole island nations but is just an almost imperceptible drip-drip every day. The media might report the first findings and the most dramatic, but struggle to find the vital new "angle" they need on a regular basis to avoid the unforgivable journalistic sin of running the same story twice. That the vast majority of the world's experts agree that human-made climate change is a huge threat and must be checked makes matters worse: Where is the opportunity for the "on the one hand, on the other hand" adversarial style of most established media?

No small wonder, then, that to the fury of the conventionally wise, the mavericks that decry climate change as "media hysteria" themselves become the ones who find journalists beating a path to their door.[31] Mix in the fact that media love a rogue more than a saint, and "good causes" have a hill to climb. There is also a risk that well-meaning campaigners will "cry wolf," overstating their case in the interests of people who are genuinely suffering.

Concerns about life-threatening health risks fare better in the media. Bulletins from the World Health Organization about bird or swine flu are given huge publicity, which in turn drives governments to act fast.[32] Most journalists try hard to be careful with stories on the latest miracle cure for cancer, but it can be tough to separate hyperbole from reality when a highly respected agency or a world-famous actor is warning that an entire region is about to suffer the worst disaster it has ever faced.

Human-made disasters, principally wars, have an easier route to the front page. This time the old cliché that the first victim of war is truth is difficult to avoid for the media and their sources alike. Like soldiers sending letters home from the front, almost all media will respect a degree of censorship in wartime—unless they are reporting for the other side, but then that tends to be called spying.

On the inside pages and in the TV and radio documentaries, there is a chance to take a more nuanced view of the long-term impact of a slow- burning threat, and many responsible media outlets do just that.[33] Plus, media outlets can hardly be blamed if the public prefers the celebrity scandal, the reality TV show or, enormously important for most media, the sport. So, can the media be more proactive in saving the planet, and can they ever be seen, as some would like, as "a Force for Good"?

Media: A Force for Good, Neutral, or a Necessary Evil?

Whenever media are in the dock—as they were after journalists at the Murdoch-owned *News of the World* in Britain were found to have hacked into the phones of a large number of its targets—the charges are familiar. The media are intrusive, abusive, disrespectful, money-grabbing, salacious—and everyone knows that because they all read, see, and hear the media.

When a media house does a clear public service—the *Washington Post*'s exposure of Watergate, the *Sunday Times*'s campaign on behalf of disfigured victims of the thalidomide drug—its achievement is honored by jealous peers and grudgingly respected by the public. But since the media can only be judged by their latest story, the glory fades fast. Some media identify with carefully selected good causes, especially at festive times such as Christmas in Western countries.

Campaigners[34] argue that the media can do much more to educate and advise their audiences on critical issues affecting their lives. In the case of disasters, members of the public could be advised to stock certain types of food during periods threatened by drought, to erect flood defenses, to build stronger quakeproof houses, to boil drinking water, or to sleep under malaria-proof bed nets.

Along with every other communicator, the media cannot just say useful things. They must also say interesting things. Unlike a boss who can oblige a subordinate to read her demand to cut down on paperclips, the media cannot oblige anyone to look or listen to what they write or say. Journalists constantly look for new angles on old stories, but the burden also rests on their sources to make their material interesting, and not just important.

So, can media ever be neutral, a disinterested but by no means uninterested recorder of whatever happens? The unsung heroes (to this entirely biased writer) are the local, national, and international news agencies, the "wire services" who feed a constant flow of as-it-happens reports to almost all the world's established media, who then choose what they will use.

The blunt instrument of media can certainly be evil in the wrong hands. The radio stations in Rwanda that goaded and screamed the murdering gangs into genocide were using the same basic medium that Aung San Suu Kyi in Burma used to address her followers after years of government-imposed silence.[35] The walls of the Schindler's Factory museum in Poland display chilling Nazi newssheets alongside schoolgirl letters describing the devastating effects on their wartime lives.[36]

To get the most good out of media, campaigners for any cause must make what they say as persuasive and interesting as possible. Fortunately, there are some well-tried tools that help do the job.

Tools for Disasters

The dedicated media campaigner can tap into a range of tools that have long been used successfully to attract and maintain media attention, but first a word about preparation. "I have no idea what this interview is about" is an awful admission. A campaigner should use any encounter with the media as an opportunity to get across what is happening, what is being done and what is needed. Translating everything into the language of the café from that of the office is a vital step. Only then will the maximum benefit come.

The humble press release remains a staple of almost all aid agency media campaigns. It should be brief, tightly edited and contain all the salient facts, backed up by a powerful quote or two, and supplied with useful contact details. Thousands upon thousands hit the media every hour, and sadly most end up "spiked," in the bin.

A news release can be reworked as a series of tweets, a usable set of Q&As, or an op-ed piece penned by the most senior person available. But for maximum impact, a human being is required. And an interview, broadcast live, is still one of the best ways of getting the messages across. While it is more comfortable to chat with a reporter on the phone or (rare in these hectic times) over a beer or lunch, the journalist involved remains at liberty to select whatever elements he wants. A live interview reduces that risk dramatically, and a well-prepared and practiced interviewee will win out almost every time over even the most aggressive interrogator.

Once a journalist is "hooked," a field trip to a disaster area is a popular means of promoting a cause. Careful planning is essential, as is monitoring of results, as such trips are rarely cheap in financial terms and sometimes very expensive in terms of reputation.

Perhaps most risky of all is a poorly planned news conference, because if one journalist is a threat, a group of journalists is a radioactive hazard. Our advice at MediaTrain is to explore every aspect of media relations before resorting to a press conference, and then have it very firmly handled by a seasoned press officer who is not afraid to be a policeman for the day.

Whatever tools are used, they all need regular polishing. Practice interview techniques in front of a mirror, write a new report in the alternative style of an op-ed piece, sit in on a press conference with the journalist's best-loved tool, a notebook. Many worry that too much practice can make messages sound overrehearsed and stilted: In this author's experience, the vast majority of people facing the media are far away from reaching that point in their media-facing lives.

Disasters and the Media: A Never-Ending Story

Whether a disaster is instant, such as an earthquake, or ongoing, such as climate change, the basic human urges to know what is going on, and to listen to a frightening story, will remain.

Whether the media transmit information to the inside of your eyeball, or boil it all down to an entirely arbitrary 140 characters, or blast it out of rows of loudspeakers no one can ignore, the awful, the terrible, the catastrophic will always be with us.

Though the media may never want to be a force for good (and sometimes want to be deliberately evil), there are going to be well-meaning people who, with skill, speed, and ingenuity, can make the media a critical part of their toolbox. In turn, that may help prevent, predict or mitigate an impending disaster. Whatever happens, the media, in one form or another, will always be there to report it.

Humanitarian Civil-Military Coordination

Looking Beyond the "Latest and Greatest"

Christopher Holshek

There is a tendency, in a world of increasingly ephemeral attention spans, to pay greater attention to the "latest and greatest" developments to generalize about current topics. Behavioral psychologists and economists call this the "availability heuristic." The well-publicized tensions between nongovernmental organizations (NGOs) and particularly the U.S. military at various times would suggest that civil-military coordination in humanitarian crises has been perpetually poor. However, when the span of these relations is examined both horizontally across the globe and vertically through time, a more assuring picture comes into view. By and large, the humanitarian civil-military relationship has had more stories of success than failure, suggesting it is not doomed from the start.

Even amidst the most contentious moments in the humanitarian civil-military relationship, in 2005, the U.S. Institute of Peace noted that "interaction between humanitarians and militaries had deepened over the last decade to include formalized exchanges, coordination, and institutional development of centers and institutes. Indeed, an emergent consensus on coherence—coordination of intervention and humanitarian action—was emerging by the turn of the millennium."[1] Nonetheless, the difficulties experienced in post-9/11 international interventions such as in Afghanistan and Iraq evinced serious ongoing challenges. An overview of how these relations have evolved would not only provide some perspective, but point to some ways ahead.

After the Cold War, the relationship between the military and civilian organizations providing relief services in the wake of natural or man-made disasters or conflicts was maturing. While the 1990s were by no means a halcyon era, demand for the services of both civilian and military providers of humanitarian services grew exponentially. During that time, some clear trends with impact on this relationship emerged. A report by The Challenges Project noted:

> One obvious change in peace operations over the last decade has been an increase in the numbers and disciplines of contributors: international and national, gov-

ernmental and nongovernmental, and military and non-military. The inability, however, of this broad, diverse and complex set of layers to conceive, plan and work together in managing a crisis and implementing a peace plan, despite the massive commitment of financial and human resources, is a major challenge in crisis management and modern peace operations today. On some occasions, civil and military elements have worked together constructively and harmoniously, but on others the inability to achieve an appropriate level of cooperation has seriously weakened the overall effectiveness of the mission. The reasons are many and, although experience varies, the all-too-frequent instances of inability to cooperate willingly, to coordinate effectively and efficiently and to pursue common objectives collectively and professionally are sometimes referred to as the "Civil-Military Cooperation Issue (CIMIC) issue."[2]

Beyond the mere proliferation of players, however, civilian relief organizations grew increasingly more capable of taking on a greater role—indeed, the lead—in humanitarian assistance operations. The United Nations has steadily improved since the initial implementation of the 2001 *Report of the Panel on United Nations Peace Operations*, better known as the "Brahimi Report," in the wake of the peacekeeping disasters of the 1990s. Better resourced, more professionally staffed, and more operationally adept, the UN, NGOs, and (as of late) regional organizations and even private industry have been taking on roles and tasks that the military had been performing, more or less, by default since before the Second World War.

With its own maturation, the "humanitarian community" eventually developed a universal set of principles and guidelines for the conduct of humanitarian assistance—what the military calls "doctrine"—beginning with the *Code of Conduct for the International Red Cross and Red Crescent Movement and Non-Governmental Organisations (NGOs) in Disaster Relief* in 1994 as well as the first humanitarian civil-military guidelines: UNHCR's *UNHCR and the Military—A Field Guide*, now in its second edition. By the middle of the first decade of the new century, the maturation of the UN's Office for the Coordinator of Humanitarian Assistance (OCHA), which has become an authority on humanitarian civil-military coordination, resulted in additional guidelines, the most important of these being *The Use of Foreign Military and Civil Defense Assets in Disaster Relief*, better known as the "Oslo Guidelines." This is the preeminent document codifying what is known as "humanitarian space" defined by the principles of humanity, neutrality and impartiality—for many humanitarian organizations a catechism if not a doctrine.[3]

They have also developed their own coordinating structures, first in conjunction with UN lead agencies such as UNHCR, and then with the adoption of the

UN's Inter-Agency Standing Committee (IASC) "cluster" approach in 2005. In many cases, the relationship between these lead organizations or consortia and many of the especially smaller NGOs are contractual or subcontractual in the sense of market specialization in relief or predevelopment services.

This growth in civilian capability and sophistication has been good news, but it has also led to the corresponding need for the military to better understand and coordinate with civilian activities, as these actors demand a greater say, not so much in the international political decision-making process, but in related operational decisions on the ground. This has complicated matters for the military.

Even more significant, however, NGOs now appear in many more forms, including the local or indigenous NGO, which tends to take over the brunt of relief activity, either supplanting international civilian relief groups or as competing organizations, as the situation develops. In addition, many (especially indigenous) NGOs, are sponsored by (or affiliated with) political and religious organizations, thus blurring the distinction between a humanitarian NGO and the plethora of like but different "civil society organizations." The humanitarian space, in turn, has experienced its own version of "mission creep," in which development organizations, advocacy or activist groups, and some other private assistance organizations have cloaked themselves in the humanitarian principles. Beyond making it much more difficult not only to define what an NGO is, this has made if vastly more complex and difficult for the military to determine by what rule sets these organizations should indeed play. (This is why it is instructive to "follow the money"—i.e., investigate the donor sources of an NGO in order to determine its real aims and interests.) And what of those NGOs, more established and having a record of adhering to the principles that should afford them their special status, that choose to collaborate with, albeit for practical reasons, less impartial and neutral organizations, or obtain funding from government agencies? Has their own impartiality and neutrality in this process been compromised? These questions have further exacerbated the challenge of civil-military coordination.

As for the military, Karen Guttieri, in "Civil-Military Relations in Peacebuilding," notes:

Just as we must ask *which civilians* form the civil-military relationship, it also matters *which military forces* are involved. Some militaries bring international political baggage. Accepting troop contributors from interested regional actors or major powers may increase the odds of military effectiveness at the expense of political impartiality. Secondly, militaries have different orientations toward society. Some have been segregated from society and oriented toward defense against uniformed adversaries on a defined battlefield.... Other militaries have more recent experience with counter insurgencies and other internal control functions.[4]

In spite of all these developments, the military remains a relatively dominant player. Beyond leadership, planning and training, the military enjoys comparative advantages in organization, intelligence, operations, logistics, medical services, engineering, etc., along with large amounts of funding. Parallel to the rising competence of civilian organizations has been the military's growing ability for civil-military synchronization, often at the hands of specialists. In the United States, it is called civil affairs (CA); in NATO, civil-military cooperation (CIMIC); and, in the UN, civil-military coordination (CM-Coord for civilian humanitarians, UN-CIMIC for peacekeeping forces).

Depending on national policies, the civil-military relationship, and doctrinal culture, civil-military operations could mean different things. CA, for example, grew out of the U.S. Army's experiences with military government dating back to the 1830s. Now, its "full-spectrum" capabilities support U.S. global strategy, concerned lately with antiterrorism and counterinsurgency. NATO CIMIC, looking to coordinate numerous national approaches, was formed by post Cold War adventures in the Balkans and other "out-of-area" operations, emphasizing support of the military mission within a specific political mandate. The UN concept, which is newest, is less about command and control and more about coordination. This diversity of civil-military approaches has likewise complicated matters for civilian organizations trying to work with the military.

Furthermore, the "complexity of interdependence between civilian-military is not simply because both communities are engaged in all functional categories of peace operations, but due to other complicating factors"[5]:

The plethora of civil and military organizations in number, type, and status, as well as their activities in a given mission area;

The relative impact of progress or failure in one activity on another (among them, security operations on humanitarian assistance actions);

Changes in the roles and capabilities among players at various times;

Obstacles, misunderstandings, and dilemmas (discussed below) impacting civil-military cooperation and coordination, some derived from fundamental differences in corporate culture and others from circumstances;

> The ability and willingness of each community to appropriate resources, personnel, money and technology to civil-military coordination.

However, an additional complication came into greater play following 9/11; namely, the simultaneity of conflict and peace operations. Again, the Challenges Project noted:

> In the 1990s . . . peacekeeping followed a sequence: if conflict prevention failed then one moved on to various means of peacemaking; once there was an agreement to pursue a peaceful solution then traditional methods of peacekeeping could be applied; and finally, once peace had taken hold, peace-building could begin. . . . The reality of today's operations, however, is that there is essentially no such tidy sequence. Conflict prevention, diplomatic peacemaking, peace enforcement actions, classic peacekeeping, peace-building and nation-building (development) are often all taking place simultaneously. In addition, humanitarian assistance operations have been required in addressing the consequence of these recent conflicts.[6]

More than any other complicating factor, it was the commingling of conflict and peace operations that caused the greatest rub between NGOs and U.S. forces in Iraq and Afghanistan. The major difference is that, prior to 9/11, relief workers had been used to being much more in "postconflict" situations and thus relatively permissive environments for humanitarian assistance. Working under more hostile conditions was more the exception than the rule. Following 9/11, the reverse happened. In short, peace operations, to include humanitarian assistance, have become a considerably more dangerous business for the military and civilians alike.

In response to methodologies used by U.S. forces, many NGOs issued strong protests, fearing these methods compromised the neutrality of NGOs and, in blurring the ostensible distinctions between combatants and noncombatants, endangered NGO personnel working with or in proximity to military forces attempting to "win hearts and minds" through humanitarian actions and in attempts to "coordinate" civil-military humanitarian responses. Some, such as U.S. Special Forces troops, operated in civilian clothing in order to better blend in.

Already by December 2002, NGOs began to articulate what were to become enduring concerns about these methodologies as employed in Afghanistan. While NGOs "welcomed the shift in Coalition focus to the establishment of a more secure environment in which reconstruction can take place," they also contended that "using military structures to provide humanitarian assistance and reconstruction support will both prematurely deflect attention from Afghanistan's deteriorating security situation and also engage the military in a range of activities for which others are better suited." Namely, they were concerned that "(1) long-term impact will be sacrificed for short-term political and military dividends, (2) communities that oppose the current government may get different levels of aid than those who support the government, (3) communities in conflict areas may receive different levels of aid than those in areas considered stable and (4) the military will aim to use NGOs as "force multipliers" to achieve political or security-related ends."[7]

The NGOs also posited that "(1) military expenditures on assistance activity could go much further in the hands of assistance professionals, and (2) because those expenditures will be counted as a contribution to the assistance on Afghanistan rather than as an internal expenditure of the military, this commitment will substitute for, rather than supplement, the commitments that the donors have already made to help rebuild Afghanistan." Then came the crux argument, as detailed in a local coordinating agency report:

> Local populations on the ground often cannot or will not distinguish between soldiers and civilian aid workers engaged in humanitarian and reconstruction activities. Military participation in assistance may significantly enhance antagonism towards humanitarian professionals and the risks that those the military chooses to disengage from its reconstruction efforts, NGOs will be required to take over and will be perceived as agents of the larger political and military strategy as a result. While military-led assistance may be short term, the impact on community perceptions of civilian humanitarians may be lasting.[8]

In addition to having the military focus exclusively on security missions, the NGOs recommended that the military "should not engage in assistance work except in those rare circumstances where emergency needs exist and civilian assistance workers are unable to meet those needs due to a lack of logistical capacity or levels of insecurity on the ground," and if it does engage in such activities, that they should fall under civilian leadership, be documented through a "transparent accountability mechanism," and be held accountable to a "code of conduct agreed upon between the military and representatives of the civilian assistance community." This led, in great part, to the Oslo Guidelines of 2006–2007.

The Pentagon's response to this was, having already ordered soldiers back into uniforms in the spring of 2002, to create Provisional Reconstruction Teams (PRTs) to create more "whole-of-government" U.S. military and civilian interagency responses for stability and reconstruction in outlying areas in Afghanistan, including military CA personnel and civilian representatives from governmental agencies, mainly the U.S. Agency for International Development (USAID), but not NGOs. More familiar coordinating mechanisms such as civil-military operations centers (CMOCs) were also employed. Despite all this, many NGOs maintained their objection to the military conduct of humanitarian assistance per se. In July 2004, following the murder of five of its aid workers, *Médecins Sans Frontières* (MSF) announced its withdrawal from Afghanistan under protest, marking the nadir of the humanitarian civil-military relationship.

Yet, the dilemma remains that, while civil-military coordination is essential to the success of either community, civilian interaction with the military risks compromised humanitarian space. In finding a way through the thicket of civil-military issues in humanitarian assistance operations in general and under semi- or nonpermissive conditions in particular, it is helpful to reorient through examination of these essential characteristics of the two communities.

Regardless of the level of progress in civil-military coordination over the years, there are essential differences in the *modus operandi* of military and civilian organizations. While the military normally focuses on reaching clearly defined objectives through linear operational (planning and execution) progressions with given timelines under a unified command and control structure, civilian organizations are concerned with a process of fulfilling changeable political or social interests through a fluctuating sequence of dialogue, bargaining, risk-taking, and consensus-building.[9]

British Army Major General Timothy Cross, in an earlier publication in this Series, provides an excellent detailed analysis of the differences between military and civilian organizations in humanitarian assistance fundamental to corporate cultures:

Any operational development has a number of "lines of operation"; the military line is alongside the political, diplomatic, legal, economic, media, and humanitarian lines. To be effective, military commanders must face up to the challenges of shattered societies as well as direct military threats. They need to remain focused on their primary imperative, that of establishing a secure environment to enable the other lines to be developed, but balancing the various frictions is not easy . . . taken to an extreme the military can be too "task" orientated, becoming over-controlling, autocratic, and critical; the individual is held to be subservient to the greater good. State focused, with legitimacy coming from the State, the military are, by definition, political servants and are neither neutral, impartial or independent. Too often we can forget individual needs and close our minds to others' views; often our head rules our heart.[10]

Cross lists the strengths of NGOs as: being principled in humanitarianism, which is the basis for their legitimacy; knowledgeable, in having served in many countries and skilled in their work; committed to the longer-term, which is often the nature of such operations; networked with other organizations and locals, much more adept at "relationship-building"; linked to the media and thus able to command a moral imperative for humanitarian intervention; and enhancing the role of women. Their weaknesses, however, often include low material resources, the inability to respond quickly to changing conditions, overemphasis on single issues and a view of other organizations, military and civilian, often as competitors. Cross notes:

> The NGOs exhibit softer, more manageable cultural traits than the military; traits that make them, generally, less confrontational and, generally, fairly effective in multicultural environments. There is rooted in their souls, a "bloody line" divide . . . put there in their early years and which many struggle to cross in their search for moral and ethical virtues and a "what I stand for" doctrine. Nonetheless, taken to extremes, they can be self-indulgent, too focused on their particular human issue and, living within a "rights-based" culture, they can be resentful of control, morally arrogant, and blind to the dark side of individual human nature; often their heart rules their head.[11]

These differences between military and civilian organizations are also reflected along the "security-development nexus," suggesting they are more fundamental when seen across the whole spectrum of peace and conflict. As Fouzieh Melanie Alamir has noted:

> By nature, security and development actors are ascribed to different roles and mandates in peace-building processes. . . . Different roles yield different self-conceptions and organizational cultures. While the military is entitled with the mandate and capacities to use force, development policy relies on mutual acceptance and cooperation. Consequently, this results in opposed self-conceptions: being an instrument of power on the one hand, and a provider of aid/supporter on the other. The point of reference of the military is the nation state; its ultimate legitimacy (in democratic societies) is the political will of the legitimate authorities, based on national interests. The point of reference for development actors, however, is ambivalent and differs among donor nations. . . . Military actors conduct operations, development actors implement programs and projects. This is not only a difference in terminology, but also in approaches, procedures, and time horizons.[12]

The considerable differences between the nature and *modus operandi* of military and civilian organizations cannot be eliminated: The gap can never be closed. It can, however, be considerably narrowed through mutual acceptance and a careful balance between humanitarian space and civil-military coordination. Instead of focusing on differences, the impetus for better civil-military coordination in humanitarian assistance can be well understood by thinking of such differences as comparative advantages, which can be managed to achieve a workable degree of complementarity (rather than compatibility):

> Although civilian organizations have taken the lead in crisis responding and "nation-building," the military maintains certain comparative advantages which complement the operational shortcomings of much of the civilian peace operations community. . . . Beyond its primary role of securing the peace operations environment, the military can play a vital role in . . . the success of the civilian peace operation community. This is particularly true in the early phases when civilian organizations are not as well-deployed and resourced in the field as the military, yet at the very time when certain actions, taken or not taken, can have long-lasting impact on the legitimacy and effectiveness of the international presence. This, paradoxically, is in the direct interests of the military and sending states in order to minimize the military's role—i.e., in supporting the "exit strategy" and reaching the "end state."[13]

Particularly in the post-9/11 world, military and civilian players are more codependent than ever before, driven by two overarching strategic imperatives: the constraints of a transforming environment for peace and security; and the restraints of diminishing resources in the face of higher costs, risks, and demand for intervention. In other words: we all have to do more, together, with less.

The roots of both confrontation and cooperation in civil-military relations in humanitarian assistance extend well before 9/11; if anything, the more dangerous and complex environments in Afghanistan and Iraq have demonstrated to experienced soldiers, diplomats, and aid workers an even greater need to find more practical means to work together and bridge their more principled differences.

Thus, while it is important for the military to understand and respect the principles under which NGOs operate, it is likewise important for NGOs to understand that their involvement has an unavoidable political context. If anything, because of the emerging realities explained earlier, NGOs are now more politically relevant—or at least perceived to be—than ever. Thus, while NGOs and other civil society organizations should never abandon humanitarian space, which sets them apart from other intervening entities, they must also temper their principles with a certain degree of pragmatism, in order not to defeat their own purposes. One author reflected that:

> In any case, inasmuch as [the] military community needs to better understand and accommodate the ways of the civilian community whose success in peace operations is essentially a prerequisite, civilian organizations and their practitioners in peace operations—the majority of whom have no military experience—must likewise be prepared to work with the military, operating from its side of the Clausewitzian continuum, this time between politics and peace. Nevertheless, "the natural reluctance of governmental and nongovernmental agencies to be seen as working with the military in complex emergencies has diminished in recent years, and NGOs in particular are finding that collaboration can benefit all parties."[14]

Even before 9/11, terrorists, insurgents, criminal organizations, and many other informal power structures against the international interventions that can be called "spoilers," particularly in areas where culture and religion shape the dialogue, often have little to no interest in NGOs improving life for indigenous populations—unless they can take credit for it or at least have it perceived that way. If the spoilers cannot co-opt or gain advantage from the presence and activities of NGOs, they will do everything or anything necessary to frustrate them—from intimidation tactics to kidnapping or even killing them. Because the spoilers are often most interested in the status quo or status quo ante, they resent the presence and activities of relief and development organizations that help people to move toward and become more oriented on the future, regardless of their association with the military or any other government organizations. Moreover, NGOs and other "change agents" come with information and perspectives (such as the role of women and public education) that resent competing ideas to the orthodoxy of many spoiler groups, helping to connect these hitherto disconnected societies to the world outside.

It was no accident, for example, following the bombing of the UN compound in Baghdad in August 2003, that many relief workers were killed, kidnapped, or otherwise dissuaded from continuing to be a force for positive change in that country. In military terms, this was a deliberate campaign to attack the "operational center of gravity"—the presence, willingness, and ability of these change agents to transition local dependence on the military and other "occupiers" to more sovereign political and economic control, a key feature of the "exit strategy." In short, by attacking NGOs and other civilian relief and development groups—again, often regardless of their relationship with the military—the spoilers are attacking the military and the political cachet it represents and at least the perception of legitimacy so central to their operations. The presence of NGOs and other change agents helps to legitimize this process of change—the more an international intervention looks like the whole-of-world (let alone the whole-of-society or whole-of-government) has come to help a distraught population, the more legitimacy it has. This essential impact of the presence of NGOs has been one of the main reasons why the military sometimes—and incorrectly—terms NGOs as "force multipliers." The error is not so much in recognizing the reality of this legitimizing factor, but in particular U.S. forces forgetting that good civil-military operations are essentially an application of the civil-military relationship in democratic societies.[15]

The military, however, is not alone in its clumsiness. In a rejoinder to the MSF arguments for quitting Afghanistan, a *Wall Street Journal* journalist noted:

> It's a different world out there, and unless they want to get out of the aid business altogether, they'll have to come to terms with it. . . . The new generation of terrorists does not spare unarmed humanitarians. They do not leave clinics, schools and other benign civilian projects untouched: They destroy them especially because they want civilians to suffer and reconstruction to fail. Fear and backwardness are a kingdom they can rule; healthy, secure and prosperous populations have no use for them. This means that humanitarian aid workers are not neutral in the eyes of the terrorists; rather, because they work to make things better, they represent a threat. . . . Whoever supports progress, stability and the well-being of civil society is the enemy. In this deeply regrettable new situation, security, development and aid are parts of an inseparable whole.[16]

The question, therefore, should not be whether there should be civil-military coordination in humanitarian assistance, even in the least permissive of operational environments, but how. Fortunately, much has already been developed on the ways and means that military and civilian organizations can cooperate—and more needs to be written. Nonetheless, any discussion of humanitarian civil-military coordination should include an exploration of the following areas:

Security. While security is primarily the military's job, it is not exclusively their concern. That is because security has become "more than globalized; it has also become more humanized, civilianized and democratized."[17] "Human security," which is predicated on the security of the individual and the community, has gained ascendancy over "national security," which is state-centric. On one hand, the delivery of a secure environment, which is primarily a military responsibility, may have a much wider application for the military than either community is at first willing to admit, especially in less permissive environments. Unfortunately, the military often falls into the trap of security becoming an end in itself, rather than as an enabler to the broader goal of peace. On the other hand, relief organizations not only have an increasing stake in the security situation, but also a greater impact on stabilization, which the military now sees as essential to security.

Often, immediately following a conflict or crisis, there is a vacuum of governance in essential public services (among them security), which intervening military forces have no other choice but to fill (or the spoilers will) until competent and legitimate civilian authorities are in place. The rule of law, repair or development of essential political, economic, and communications and transportation infrastructure, and so on, are necessary to initiating a virtuous cycle of security and relief and recovery in that critical period. Freedom of movement, for example, is as important to security operations as to humanitarian assistance. At least early on, the military will need to be involved more directly and robustly in humanitarian assistance, providing it themselves, securing civilian relief supplies, convoy escorts, clearing mines, and unexploded ordnance, and so on. In any case, any military humanitarian involvement should be done with a view to creating a lodgement for humanitarian space, then looking to "civilianize" and "localize"—that is, turn it over to international or, ultimately, local civilian authorities for service delivery.

In this respect, the military should actually look at how it can be a "multiplier" to civilian relief capability and efforts. In this respect, the role of the military should be seen as "enablers," because the success of the change agent is a prerequisite to the success of the military. This is in keeping both with the quest for an "exit strategy" and the longer-term intent to empower locals. Understanding this enabler-change agent relationship in terms of the applied democratic civil-military relationship is the crux to resolving the security-relief conundrum and maintaining the delicate balance between military and civilian interveners.

Security, for example, has both physical and psychological dimensions, as well as humanitarian, economic, political, social, and cultural elements. While the military may rely on more physical means to provide security, civilian organizations such as the ICRC depend on their transparency and neutrality to be able to work among all sides. The Red Cross or Red Crescent on their vehicles may have greater protective value than the armor plating of a 70-ton tank. Who can contribute what to a safe and secure environment must be clearly understood and respected by all players in the intervention, regardless of mission and operating principles.

Information. Information transparency is the engine of civil-military coordination, in both directions. While NGOs often have knowledge of the local culture and community, socio-psychological conditions, and humanitarian needs, the military is privy to information on the security situation and threats to safety, mines, infrastructure assessments, weather, topography, and so forth. Information management and database sharing, from the Afghanistan Information Management Service or AIMS (www.aims.org.af) to OCHA's One Response (http://oneresponse.info) to humanitarian clustering, used with great effect in the response to the Haitian earthquake, have made great strides in humanitarian coordination over the past few years.

Still, there is much progress to be made, particularly considering every organization's tendency to work with its own systems and information sets, the "information-is-power" psychology that pervades many organizations seen to be in competition with others, and the military's sensitivity to information and thus operation security and the habit of classifying information that may not require classification. Because of the sensitivity of certain information, such as regarding spoilers, mines, and other critical elements NGOs may encounter, civilian organizations need to understand that providing the military such information, especially on a voluntary basis, may serve their interest in helping the military create a more secure environment. The military in turn must view civilian organizations only as sources of information—not intelligence. Despite the clear value of civilian organizations as sources of operationally exigent information, particularly in what the military calls "human intelligence" (more important to stability, antiterrorist, and counter-insurgency operations), both communities must establish, in advance, clear rules of engagement on the collection, dissemination, and attribution of such information—the more discreet and indirect, the better.

Coordination. Beyond virtual means of civil-military information exchange, specific physical coordination nodes, often built by the military, are necessary to facilitate the most efficient and effective use of humanitarian assistance resources, to the benefit of the affected population. This not only avoids the issue of duplicity and underlap, but it also helps to minimize the military's direct involvement in humanitarian assistance, helps collectively prioritize projects, takes advantage of shared information in support of decision making, and most importantly, enables civilian organizations to more quickly take the lead in humanitarian assistance, mainly because it provides an overhead capability many (especially smaller) civilian relief organizations lack in terms of resources and management expertise to put together. It also often helps mitigate a common problem in humanitarian assistance areas, which can simply be called "assessment fatigue."

From the point of view of the recipients of aid, there is nothing more frustrating than watching countless organizations, civilian and military, show up to assess—rather than address—their needs before aid finally arrives. In this respect, there is no quicker way to delegitimize even the most well-intentioned relief efforts, and not just for a few. Whatever these coordination nodes are called is secondary. The deployment of liaisons to help deconflict civil-military issues in the planning and preparation phases, as well as to provide the civilian relief community the opportunity to exercise its advocacy in reminding the military of its humanitarian obligations, for example, is targeting.[18] Beyond that, it suggests the idea of civil-military preventative actions—before the outbreak of a crisis.

Among these actions could be capacity-building among regional organizations and local governments. The most important thing is that the civilian organizations take control of the coordination effort—the sooner, the better. In addition, both organizations need to be disciplined about personnel designated to play a liaison role. For the military, this should be civil-military specialists (CA, CIMIC, etc.); for relief organizations, it should be designated liaison personnel, preferably with a background in working with the military (e.g., CMCoord), to represent one or many organizations. This not only minimizes confusion, but also protects both communities from under- and overcommitment. As with security and information, clear lines of coordination, through commonly agreed civil-military rules of engagement, are even more important in hostile or semipermissive environments, and as any business person knows, always with an eye to the market.

Logistics. Next to security and information, this is the most practical—and most benign—area of civil-military cooperation. In fact, ideally, the majority of issues between military and civilian relief organizations are and should be logistical. Better shared resourcing not only enables more effective civilian-led relief, but also minimizes the resources the military has to draw from its core security operation—mitigating "mission creep." Nonetheless, the military may need to realize the quickest and most effective way to get civilian relief activities up and running effectively is to provide an initial surge of logistical support effort. Logistical information-sharing tools have vastly improved the ability of military and civilian organizations to work together. And logistical support and especially logistical information-sharing is perhaps the most discreet way the military can enable the success of change agents like NGOs in a low-key, less visible manner with less risk of compromising (at least the perception) of humanitarian space. Notable examples include AIMS, One Response, or the Humanitarian Logistics Software developed by the International Federation of Red Cross and Red Crescent Societies. In addition, logisticians—or logistically versed operators—from both communities should be key members of the civil-military planning and coordination cast.

Training and Education. As mentioned before, one of the greatest comparative advantages the military maintains is in professional development, due to the tremendous value many militaries place not just in training and education but also in lesson-learning. In the U.S. Army, for example, an officer can spend as much as 40 percent of his or her career going to school. Unlike most civilian relief organizations, the military can and must afford the overhead. While training and education should be seen as an "allowable expense" by both civilian executive and donor boards, the military (and other government agencies), again in the role as an "enabler," as a matter or programmed budgeting, should open the doors of many of its institutions to civilians. This is enlightened self-interest, not just in improving the capacity of these organizations to more quickly espouse roles the military (and other government agencies) would ultimately rather have civilian relief (and development) organizations take on.

Moreover, their presence—prior to operations—has a co-educational value, for operators and not just executives. Such steady state relationship-building helps improve cross-institutional understanding, deconstructs often long-held stereotypes, and ultimately improves civil-military and interagency coordination. It reduces the learning curve while operators focus on the problem at hand and critical time is going by, in addition to feeling out implementation partners. It also enables selective collaboration on training and capacity-building of regional and local organizations and leverages localization by allowing local players to more quickly become stakeholders in the peace process and thus mitigate the threats of spoilers.

Civilian institutions, however, are themselves offering more and more high-quality training in many areas of peace operations such as those created by OCHA and the Peace Operations Training Institute (www.poti.org). Some are, in fact, collaborations between civil and military providers. There are too many to list here, but many are listed with the International Association of Peacekeeping Training Centers, or IAPTC (http://www.iaptc.org). Both civilian and military organizations should redouble efforts to host information seminars and problem-solving oriented workshops to allow executives and especially operators to come together and inform each other on their views of civil-military coordination and respective principles and procedures, as well as capabilities and limitations, in order to mitigate obstacles, misunderstandings, and dilemmas—before the intervention takes place and precious time and credibility is lost on both sides. This is an application of the insight that what you do in the "steady state" builds the strategic and operational capital upon which players draw during crisis response operations or in the field in general, with corresponding levels of success or failure. That is because peace operations, including humanitarian assistance, are more than a knowledge-based enterprise; they are essentially about building relationships. For that reason, beyond training and education, it should never be forgotten:

> We can promulgate all the information and education in the world, but the face-to-face coordination of two to eight people is irreducible. This NGO/military relationship is about people. The ones controlling the operation in theater are the most important linchpins in the entire endeavor. Good people matter—they must be selected carefully.[19]

What is remarkable about especially the development of civilian (or collaborative) references, guidelines, and tools on humanitarian civil-military coordination, is a tacit recognition of more than the inevitability of such, but more important its value—by both sides. With all the talk about "paradigm shifts" in the civil-military relationship in humanitarian actions over the past few years, the basis of the civil-military imperative in these situations, years before the situations in Afghanistan and Iraq made them center stage, has long been recognized:

> Operating to the principle of altruistic self-interest allows each community to more properly assume its comparative advantage. Each community has something unique to offer. NGOs bring humanitarian expertise, a familiarity with the affected area, and sustained commitment. The military brings in infrastructure that provides communication, logistics, and security. In its most simple form, the equation works like this: the military's infrastructure leverages the NGOs into collaboration, which the NGOs provide the military with their ticket home. In other words, NGOs are willing to participate in collaboration and eventual coordination because of the need for a comprehensive effort, not to mention that the military will sometimes move their relief supplies and personnel for free. The military, on the other hand, needs to transition to civilian agencies in order to withdraw quickly—something to which both sides agree.[20]

While the challenges to civil-military coordination in humanitarian assistance are greater than ever, due to the more complex, difficult, and dangerous operational environments facing both military and civilian organizations, the risks and rewards, likewise, at a higher level, are increasingly intertwined between these two communities, who have become more co-dependent than ever to achieve respective and collective success. If the interventions in Afghanistan and Iraq have demonstrated the limits of civil-military coordination in humanitarian assistance in non- or semi-permissive environments, the widespread international and multilateral efforts to provide assistance to the victims of the tsunamis and earthquakes are reaffirming its potential. Much has been achieved and much has yet to be achieved. They key will be continuing to improve understanding the relationship between these communities of actors and the political, social, and other human equities they represent. This is where civil-military coordination writ large should be seen as an application of the societal civil-military relationship.

Above all, the civil-military coordination in humanitarian assistance should be about managing expectations, within and between these organizations and with the affected population itself. The nirvana of complete integration and unity of effort is just that, but it is also not necessary. Often, it is about mutual understanding of the principles and missions that define their presence and operations, looking for common aims and interests. Even if you agree to disagree, it may, as a minimum, be about getting together in order to stay out of each other's way. Coordination on the practical issues of security, information management and information sharing, coordination mechanisms and methods, and logistical matters should be the greater area of concentration, and will help balance out the thornier issues of philosophical or even political differences. As in business, the customer (i.e., the recipient of humanitarian assistance) should be king, and therefore have the greatest common priority. One thing is clear—failure in civil-military coordination means not just the failure of one or the other, but the failure of all and the suffering of many.

PART V

Operational

In this section, four humanitarian specialists with extensive operational experience consider some of the specialized approaches that are essential in providing a comprehensive and efficient response to a complex emergency. There are accepted methods for rapid health assessments that will guide the early days in a disaster, helping to bring the most appropriate assistance in the shortest time to those in greatest need. Team building is an indispensable requirement for both immediate and sustained response.

The techniques to achieve effective collaboration under trying circumstances are presented here. The development of educational programs and an appreciation of the contributions that indigenous people make in disaster risk management are other topics that were selected from many other valid options.

Evidence-Based Health Assessment Process in Complex Emergencies

Frederick M. Burkle Jr., M.D.

Disaster assessment is defined as the "survey of a real or potential disaster to estimate the actual or expected damages and to make recommendations for preparedness, mitigation and relief action."[1] In natural disasters, such as rapid onset earthquakes and cyclones, the health consequences are usually the direct results of injury or death. Often, however, the greatest toll on humans comes from the unappreciated long-term secondary effects as seen with slow moving droughts and massive flooding.

Zwi has defined complex emergencies as "situations in which the capacity to sustain livelihood and life are threatened primarily by political factors and, in particular, by high levels of violence."[2] The most common complex emergencies of the past two decades have involved famine and forced migration. Since the 1980s, few famines have occurred that were not human-induced, and many famines catalyzed the onset of complex emergencies.

The most severe consequences of population displacement have occurred during the acute phase, when relief efforts have not yet begun or are in the early stages.[3] Refugees (populations that cross internationally recognized borders) and internally displaced populations have experienced high mortality rates during the period immediately following their migration. Internally displaced populations, in contrast to refugees, do not enjoy the immediate protections under international law that are afforded to refugees by the UNHCR (United Nations High Commissioner for Refugees). They must fend for themselves without the benefit of basic health-care services, food, water or sanitation that make up the protective infrastructure of refugee camps. Therefore, in complex emergencies, the health consequences are both directly and indirectly related to the conflict itself (Table 22.1).[4]

Historically, response activities in both natural and human-generated disasters have often been ineffective, both because of the poor quality of the information available as well as the manner in which an assessment was conducted. Disaster assessment and assistance activities are often hampered by organizational

Table 22.1. Direct and indirect effects of complex emergencies

Direct Effects	Indirect Effects
Injuries/Illnesses	Population displacement: internally displaced and/or refugees
Deaths	Disruption of food
Human rights abuses	Destroyed health facilities
International Humanitarian Law violations and abuses	Destroyed public health infrastructure
Psychological stresses	
Disabilities	

problems that ultimately diminish the effect of these efforts on the population they intended to help.[5] Unfortunately, lack of personnel, medical records, and financial resources often hinder the assessment of the health situation in a complex emergency by conventional epidemiological methods practiced in traditional development programs. Epidemiological methods established for situations of restricted resources employ a simpler method of statistical analysis to be performed. The technique offered by these epidemiological methods became known as a "rapid assessment."[6] The outcome of an appropriately organized and directed assessment is an efficient and effective response. During the decade of the 1990s, both health and nutritional assessments in complex emergencies gained a reputation for quality. With critical advances in indicator identification, epidemiological analysis, data retrieval technologies, and in education and training of relief personnel, health and nutritional assessments have continued to improve as an art and science.

The immediate priorities of assistance in complex emergencies are the protection of the affected populations and the reduction of mortality and morbidity.[7] The effective response to complex emergencies requires timely, accurate public health information and data.[8] The rationale for an assessment is to provide objective information for planning, prioritizing needs, implementing health programs, evaluating the relief process, and identifying health issues needing further investigation.[9]

The humanitarian community (international organizations, nongovernmental organizations, private governmental organizations, and peacekeeping militaries) has a professional obligation to base the assistance on the best evidence available.[10] This assumption is the cornerstone of the concept of evidence-based healthcare. The need and demand for health care in complex emergencies are increasing at a rate determined, in part, by the rate at which public health infrastructure is destroyed and the moral integrity of governance disappears. Initially, healthcare needs may be greater than the rate at which resources are being made available.[11] Use of an evidence-based approach makes it possible for decision makers (policy, operational, and field levels) to differentiate the needs of the population, the resources available, and the costs of any decision. An evidence-based approach helps to differentiate between what is supported by evidence and that made on unsubstantiated assertion. Health assessments today are expected to be reliable and valid; and as such, are inextricably linked to the analysis of specific performance and outcome indicators, region- and disaster-specific epidemiological studies, and measures of effectiveness.[12]

The assessment tool used can vary depending on the phase of the disaster event: prevention, preparedness, response, recovery, rehabilitation and reconstruction. There is much written concerning the assessment process in each phase of natural and human-generated disasters. This chapter concentrates on the rapid health assessment of a complex emergency where disaster managers and decision makers require immediate and accurate data necessary to rationally allocate available resources according to the emergency needs of the humanitarian organization.

Rapid Assessment Process

All health and nonhealth interventions in support of public health in complex emergencies are determined by rapid assessments, focused surveys and surveillance. Poor surveillance design, at all three levels, will lead to a predictable resurgence of disease and public health disruption. If survey indicators and surveillance methodologies are incomplete or inaccurate, the ability to monitor the sensitive relationships between health, nutrition and environmental indicators, endemic disease, injury prevention (e.g., landmine injuries), and gender and age specific vulnerabilities will be lacking. Evaluation and monitoring programs based on these three levels are the essential management tools for all health and nutrition-related programs in complex emergencies. The important role of epidemiological surveillance in infectious disease control in a long-term refugee camp is illustrated in the applications of simple epidemiological methods in camps on the Thai-Burmese border. Here, agency collaboration organized a Health Information Office to facilitate the collection of demographic and vital statistics data, administration of a disease surveillance system, regular monitoring of hospital and outpatient discharge diagnoses, and investigation of disease outbreaks.[13] This was the forefront of Health Information Systems (HIS), that are now an essential component of all refugee camp protocols. How rapidly and how accurate an assessment and an HIS can be implemented is often used as a measure of efficiency and effectiveness of camp management.

The objectives of a rapid assessment in the emergency phase of a complex emergency are to:[14]

determine the magnitude of the emergency

identify existing and potential public health problems

measure present and potential impact, especially health and nutritional needs

assess resources needed, including availability and capacity of a local response

determine and plan an appropriate external response

set up the basis for a health system

The initial or rapid assessment comprises both situation assessment (a definition of the problem and an assessment or measurement of its extent) and needs assessment (a systematic procedure for determining the nature and extent of problems experienced by a specified population, that affect their health either directly or indirectly). This is performed in the early, critical stage of a disaster to determine the type of relief needed for immediate response. It must identify the impact on a society, its infrastructure, the most vulnerable population groups, and the ability to cope. A rapid assessment requires data and interpretation of data.

Therefore, data critical to interpretation of the needs of a population affected by a complex emergency begins with background data on the political, social and economic status of the country (and also the region where refugees might migrate), the size and demographics of the population, and vital health information.

Facts and figures are "indispensable tools" for health personnel.[15] A simple graph of daily mortality rates can work miracles by catalyzing the mobilization of human and material resources, focusing the attention of decision makers, and guiding and refining the assistance program that is being put into place. The five areas that are most useful are: mortality; incidence of the most important diseases; nutritional status; "activities data" such as immunizations performed; and the "vital sectors," namely food, water, sanitation, shelter, and fuel. All assessment tools have been minor variations on this original theme. An effective way of presenting information is graphically, so that everyone can see the trends over time.[16]

Data collection commences before the field assessment and originates from existing country profiles, maps, census data, previous demographic and health surveys, early warning system tools, and previous or ongoing in-country assessments.[17]

endemic diseases

mortality rates

morbidity-incidence rates

nutritional status

sources of health care

impact of disruption of health services

More detailed assessments, in the form of surveys and surveillance, will follow as the emergency develops and needs evolve. Assessment never stops.[18]

Initial assessments serve to provide a structural cornerstone for a more robust survey and surveillance system. There is often an overlap of the rapid assessment and the process implemented by the more organized survey teams. Field surveys are intermittent focused assessments that collect population-based health, nutritional and environmental data found to be of concern or potential concern during the rapid assessment phase. To increase the power of a survey, it is combined with statistical analysis. To increase the validity of a survey and affirm or deny the suspicions drawn from the initial assessment, surveys are repeated after a certain time has elapsed or after some intervention (e.g., vitamin A) has been completed.

In addition, surveys are performed to gather baseline data on endemic diseases, locally and regionally, and serve as the foundation for an ongoing surveillance system. The quality of the survey instruments used and the population studied increases as one moves from the rapid assessment to the more sophisticated surveillance system. In the survey and surveillance phases, the evaluation process screens and monitors all children within the camp and at the time of entry and registration.

Data and Information Sought

Assessments must be sensitive and specific enough to identify the most vulnerable groups and to appropriately target them with assistance. In complex emergencies, indicators are used as assessment, monitoring, and evaluation tools to inform practical decision-making in the field. Indicators are defined as quantitative or qualitative criteria used to correlate or predict the value or measure of a program, system, or organization.[19]

In the acute emergency phase, based on best practice, only the most essential indicators should be selected.

Rapid Assessment Indicators

Population size and demographics: this data is necessary for determining the denominator for indicator rates (e.g., infant mortality rates), to determine who and how many people are entitled to material assistance, and to facilitate legal identity and protection of those at risk. The age and gender structure (age and sex-specific rates) of the population is also necessary to identify the vulnerable groups and to target necessary assistance programs (e.g., immunizations). In a refugee camp setting this data is obtained early on from the camp registration system, convenience and cluster sampling of the camp population, aerial photographs and global positioning system (GPS) assisted population estimates.[20] Humanitarian assistance is slowly moving to an urban setting where the majority of the world's poor now reside.[21] In an urban setting, household surveys, records of beneficiary of aid, and city and country records (if recent) can be used.[22]

Vital health information: The goal is to confirm or deny the above background data against actual field data. The indicator data required from the field is summarized in Table 22.2.[23]

These rates are essential for the recording of disease, trend analysis, a comparison of populations at risk, and to develop a baseline for future surveillance. A public health emergency may be defined as a situation where the daily crude mortality rate (CMR) is significantly higher than the baseline level in the affected population. A threshold of one death per 10,000 people per day is commonly used to define an emergency in a developing country.[24] In Africa, the CMR has been as high as

Table 22.2. Vital health data

Crude mortality rate (CMR): this is the most specific indicator of a population's health. It is recorded as total deaths/10,000 population/day. In the post-emergency phase this reverts to total deaths/1,000 population/month

Under age 5 mortality rate (U5MR): measured as total deaths < 5 years/10,000/day

Cause specific mortality rates: Specifies proportion of deaths according to cause, e.g., trauma

Case fatality rates (CFR): proportion of individuals with a specific disease that die within a specified time, e.g., CFR for children with malnutrition that die from measles

Age and sex-specific mortality rates: incidence rates collected during survey phase

SPHERE PROJECT MINIMUM STANDARDS in HEALTH SERVICES add:

Sex and age-specific breakdown (at least < 5 years and > 5 years)

Average family and household size

Age and sex-specific incidence rates of major problems and diseases

60–80 times the baseline rates.[25] Unaccompanied orphans, not easily recognized in densely populated refugee groups, lack care and protection usually afforded by adult supervision. As such, it is not unusual for them to experience CMRs over 200 times the baseline. CMR benchmarks are illustrated by Table 22.3.[26]

A concerted effort must be done during the assessment process to identify these vulnerable populations. The most common causes of death among refugees and internally displaced persons are diarrheal diseases, measles, acute respiratory infections, and malaria.[27] Most people become refugees only after their health and security has been severely compromised, and during their flight the health status deteriorates even more. Except in retrospective assessments, those that died prior to reaching the camps are usually never recorded. In addition, mortality rates, particularly among those under age five (U5MR) and infants, increase when the rate of newly arriving refugees is higher.[28]

Protein energy malnutrition (PEM) has three components: malnutrition, micronutrient deficiency diseases (especially vitamin A, C and B_1), and secondary infections. PEM is often used instead of kwashiorkor or marasmus to define the state of illness. Indeed, many cases are mixed (marasmus-kwashiorkor) in their presentation and difficult to clinically distinguish. Nutritional assessments are performed by population convenience samples, screening new arrivals at the refugee camps, and through cluster sample surveys (Table 22.4). The malnutrition rate of children under age 5 years is next to crude mortality rates as the most specific indicator of a population's health.[29] It also determines the urgency for food ration delivery and requirements for supplementary feedings and therapeutic feeding centers. Some interventions are now so routine that they no longer require an assessment before implementation in the acute phase of complex emergencies. Most demonstrable is the use of vitamin A and measles vaccines in refugee populations in developing countries.

Studies from the early 1990s in complex emergencies have shown that vitamin A will reduce mortality and morbidity in malnourished children, especially those with

Table 22.3. Crude mortality rate benchmarks

Normal rate in developing countries	< 0.5/10,000/day
Serious condition	> 1.0/10,000/day
Emergency condition	> 2.0/10,000/day
Severe famine or disaster	> 5.0/10,000/day
Effective relief effort	< 1.0/10,000/day

Table 22.4. Nutritional assessment

Goal: Prevalence of acute protein energy malnutrition (PEM)
Prevalence of micronutrient deficiencies (especially vitamin A, C, B_1)

Data retrieval: Rapid Screening: Mid-upper arm circumference (MUAC)
Survey and Surveillance phase data: Weight-for-height, Z-scores
Clinical evidence of micronutrient deficiencies

Levels of acute malnutrition: Minor, moderate, serious (presence of edema/Kwashiorkor)

Prevalence of malnutrition: > 10% of < age = population = SERIOUS STATUS
> 20% of < age = population (with edema/Kwashiorkor) = CRITICAL STATUS

measles (active, susceptible and exposed) and other respiratory illnesses. Indeed, vitamin A supplementation reduces all-cause mortality in children.[30] By the time measles becomes identified in a population in a dense camp environment, the mortality and morbidity rate may already be out of control. Based on this evidence it has become protocol to provide all children between 1 and 6 years of age, at the time of registration into the camp, both measles vaccine and vitamin A.

This being the case, the initial assessment will focus on identifying the population in need of services and on ensuring continuing monitoring through program outcome surveys and surveillance. Relief programs emphasize a primary health care (PHC) approach, focusing on oral rehydration, feeding centers, immunization, promoting involvement by the refugee community in the provision of health services, and stressing effective coordination of programs and information sharing among the nongovernmental organizations that deal directly with the recipients of care.[31]

As the nutritional assessment moves from the rapid assessment phase through to the surveillance phase, the evaluation methodologies used become more sophisticated. For example, in the rapid assessment phase the MUAC studies performed through convenience or cluster sampling provides the decision makers information to determine whether a serious malnutrition problem exists, but not necessarily the full extent (i.e., micronutrient status, age and gender specifics, etc.). By moving to more exact weight-for-height and Z-score monitoring in the survey and surveillance phases, the evaluation process screens and monitors all children within the camp and at the time of entry and registration.

Environmental health assessments: disruptions in basic water, sanitation, shelter and fuel indicators are indicative of public health infrastructure loss and most commonly contribute to rising acute respiratory illnesses (e.g., pneumonia, tuberculosis), and gastrointestinal diseases (e.g., dysentery, cholera, common pathogen diarrhea). In large refugee camps the mortality may increase as the population of the camps exceeds the environmental resources available.[32] In the last decade, environmental health assessments have become increasingly a critical means of defining the causes of the mortality and morbidity seen in complex emergencies (Table 22.5).[33]

Epidemiological-Based Definition of Complex Emergencies

The core evidence (knowledge) base for war and public health management comes from these assessments, surveys and surveillance studies that, with other more advanced epidemiological research, provide a working definition and description of the phases of complex emergencies. Burkholder and Toole first described complex emergencies in developing countries as having acute, late, and post-emergency phases, each of which is characterized by predictable patterns of health indicators and expected public health responses.[34] If these patterns are addressed with appropriate management responses, a decline in mortality and morbidity, and a shortening of the duration of each epidemiological phase will occur.

In this developing country model, the acute phase is characterized by high mortality rates for infants and those under the age of 5 years from severe malnutrition and outbreaks of communicable disease. Epidemiological indicator studies in the acute phase in developed countries (e.g., Yugoslavia, Chechnya) appear to be characterized more by violent trauma from advanced weaponry and untreated chronic disease (e.g., diabetes, high blood pressure and stroke), increased incidence of communicable diseases and malnutrition in the elderly, and in neonatal health problems.[35]

Table 22.5. Environmental health assessment indicators

Water	Sanitation services	Shelter	Fuel
Quantity: 15-20 liters/person/day Quality of supply Sources of water and accessibility	Types of facilities: e.g., latrines, defecation fields, etc. Recommended pit latrines/family: *minimum*: 1 pit latrine/20 people *serious*: < 1 pit latrine /50 people	Types of structures: e.g., tents, plastic sheeting, etc. % households without water resistant shelter % households without any form of shelter Recommended area: 3.5m2/person	Types of fuel, access, and security Recommended: 5 KG of wood/family/day

Measures of Effectiveness

With an increased understanding of the knowledge base and consequences of these internal conflicts resulting in complex emergencies, the humanitarian community has moved to attempt to define whether the interventions to provide relief and assistance have actually been beneficial or not. A theme of many recent humanitarian evaluations has been that the effectiveness of the relief process has been lacking.[36] In part, this has been attributed to a lack of clearly stated program objectives and monitoring information used in both the overall program and the sector and project components.

To answer this problem, the humanitarian community is mandated to use clear and explicit statements of objectives starting with the initial assessment phase. This mandate has encouraged that assessments be redefined over three levels of management and response: strategic (or policy), operational and field levels all using goals based on indicators most relevant to the individual level. For example, "strategic frameworks" should be established to set system (country and region) wide objectives by the international community. Second, "country (operational response) strategies" should be clearly articulated by the donor organizations, and "logical framework analyses" (LogFrame) are valuable as a way of articulating the goal, purpose, outputs and indicators for humanitarian projects in the field. Some donor organizations have made LogFrame use mandatory.[37]

Outcome or performance measures of effectiveness (MOEs), developed primarily from analysis research, use quantitative or qualitative criteria (indicators) to correlate or predict the value or measure of a system or organization, and to make decisions or judgments on performance. MOEs criteria should strive to follow these desiderata (Table 22.6).[38]

MOEs have been used in complex emergencies to correlate a variety of diverse but interrelated humanitarian, security, economic, and infrastructure indicators, and to determine whether effectiveness or success of assistance goals exists within the overall relief program. MOEs can be used with medical and public health indicators to determine trend analyses in various sectors, compare geographic sectors and programs, and identify areas where additional program scrutiny or security is needed.

Medical and public health MOEs rely on data that are already collected in the initial assessments and surveys. For example, a crude mortality rate is a MOE that is an indicator of improving or deteriorating health status and is used to show impact of the overall mission. As a security MOE, the measured number (fraction) of the security assumed by the security guards at the distribution centers by the host nation indicates the ability of the host nation to conduct the security mission

Table 22.6. Desired qualities of MOE criteria

Appropriate	Mission-related	Consistently measureable	Cost-effective	Sensitive	Timely
MOEs should be appropriate to the objective of the stated mission	MOEs should be related to the mission	Those measuring MOEs should be able to assign a value	MOEs should be reasonable	Must be sensitive to the goals and objectives of the mission	MOEs should be responsive to changes
1) to help the decision makers understand the status of the situation in different geographic areas	1) the mission is clearly understood by all participants	1) quantitative values (i.e., indicators)	1) so as not to levy too high a burden on limited resources	1) must change as progress toward meeting the mission objectives change	1) must be sensitive in time to what the participants are trying to measure
2) to present information to higher authorities	2) focus on assessing the effectiveness of the mission and not on the accomplishment of the supporting tasks	2) qualitative descriptors (i.e., criteria)		2) not be greatly influenced by other (external) factors	3) must be timely enough for participants to act
3) to support authorities in making better decisions	3) cover all aspects of the mission and expand as the mission expands			3) be measured in sufficient detail that changes will be apparent	

themselves, and functions as a transition indicator (measures capability of host nation to assume responsibility).[39] In a complex emergency, there are always MOEs (at a minimum) that address security, infrastructure, medical/public health and agricultural and economic factors.[40] Additional MOEs may address more directly the human rights issues (improvements) as a measure of success in aid relief.

Characteristics of Complex Emergencies That Result in Assessment Bias

Decision makers require data rapidly in order to clarify rumors and make reasonable judgments on response management. Early on, there is much pressure to act. Complex emergencies result in a rapidly changing situation in the field, in and out migration of the population at risk, and a higher vulnerability to disease and injury. The rapid assessment is time dependent, suffers from limited data resources, data quality, and occurs within an unstable or disrupted infrastructure that is insecure and intolerant of scrutiny. There may be pressure to interpret data to reflect a certain political or media agenda (e.g., intervention versus nonintervention).[41]

Several examples are illustrative of the need for well designed and measured assessments. In the early stages of the Somalia debacle, many countries were eager to obtain data that would justify a larger intervention. Media reports described a rural area where there were few if any children under the age of four left alive. The report suggested that the children had died from the violent conflict that raged throughout the country. The report immediately became a rally point for intervention and began to drive the logistical efforts for relief. Several months later an assessment team visited the area. They confirmed that there were few children under age four alive, but that the reasons for this were more likely due to prolonged infertility from secondary amenorrhea of malnourished women of childbearing age, and lack of adult males who were either killed or long absent and fighting in another area of the country. Childhood deaths from violence of trauma were not above the expected norm.

Similarly, the peacekeeping forces were eager to show success in the humanitarian mission, transfer duties to other organizations, and redeploy their troops. The singular indicator they were following was the infant mortality rate that had skyrocketed with the onset of fighting throughout the country. They used as an objective the baseline infant mortality rate present before the conflict escalated. When this objective was reached, mission success was unilaterally declared and plans were put in place to begin redeployment. Concurrently, the UN Secretariat spoke to the humanitarian community on the status of the relief effort and communicated that there was a tenuous and alarming situation with infants, in that half were still considered ill and half remained malnourished. In both examples the data were interpreted to support a particular self-interest and decision.

Many early studies were "often hastily planned rapid assessments, executed under less than ideal circumstances, and too often did not culminate in a formal report."[42] Of twenty-three assessments studied in Somalia between 1991 and 1993, all revealed extensive methodological differences. Target populations and sampling strategies varied widely. Of sixteen that assessed mortality, only eight assessed cause of death. None of the studies provided confidence intervals around the point estimates of the rates. Use of units of measurement and inclusion of denominators in rate calculations were inconsistent. Concerns were that some studies may have influenced policy and program management decisions, but even here, these effects "may have been limited by failure to adequately document results and by differences in objectives, design, parameters measured, methods of measurement, definitions, and analysis methods."[43]

Because there is no clear population denominator, it has been said that complex emergency assessments consist of numerators searching for an accurate denominator. With denominator estimation, data accuracy may be uncertain ("dirty").[44] Unfortunately, incomplete assessments or unscrupulous interpretation of assessment data has led to misuse of scarce resources and incorrect analysis of the etiology of observed mortality and morbidity.

Given the context of shifting populations and unstable political conditions, population size is especially difficult to assess.[45] Hansch stresses that current methods are inadequate for dealing with large-area emergencies, especially where populations are unregistered, uncounted, migratory and likely to be mobile in response to aid.[46] In these situations relief agencies must employ improved sampling strategies and population tracking and unique demographic retrieval techniques, such as advanced satellite and GPS/GIS methods.[47]

In conflict areas where there is little or no data available, collected or analyzed, proxy or surrogate data collections have been employed. Cross-border assessments of North Korean migrants seeking assistance in China have provided the most accurate view of the nutritional status within the country. This data is limited to one province and may not reflect conditions elsewhere.[48] Although there will never be complete accuracy in the rapid assessment phase, the assessment must emphasize uniformity in analysis and appropriate restraint on descriptive judgments to act.[49]

Summary and Future Directions

Rapid assessment is the first step in designing and developing a surveillance system in complex emergencies. The data interpretations of the rapid health assessment will launch the initial phase of assistance, and is expected to result in a decline in mortality and morbidity. To be accurate and timely, initial assessments and the follow-on surveys and surveillance protocols must be:

1. evidence-based;
2. incorporate valid indicators;
3. derive verification from epidemiological studies;
4. build a data foundation by which one measures relief effectiveness.

By this process, initial assessments build the foundation by which the humanitarian community gains the knowledge and understanding of causes and consequences of the particular complex emergency and how it compares and contrasts to others.

The process of assessment of complex emergencies has advanced considerably and standards now exist for the process and the indicators. The humanitarian community has learned a great deal but much needs to be done. Spiegel emphasizes that to ensure an evidence-based assessment environment, more research is needed, especially in a grading system for existing indicators (type and levels which lead to improved health outcomes) that address the different phases of complex emergencies and the level of development of the country in which the conflict occurs. This would provide "credibility and a strong foundation" for decision makers and future research. He specifically sees indicators as being evaluated in four areas:[50]

1. type of indicators;
2. manner in which they are implemented and interpreted;
3. standardization within and between different NGOs and settings;
4. their effects on program implementation.

Experience this past decade, the 1990s, has shown that complex emergencies are longer lasting, more complex, more dangerous, and more widespread than previously thought. This information, to a great degree, came through a variety of assessment and monitoring events, both political (e.g., economic, social) and medical. The violence perpetrated against the civilian population in complex emergencies has caused unprecedented mortality and morbidity as well as the destruction of vital public health lifelines. Societies have ceased to function, govern or protect their citizens. Arguably, complex emergencies are appropriately referred to as catastrophic public health and human rights emergencies that often require the total rehabilitation and reconstruction of the entire country. Assessments have been critical in painting this epidemiological picture for decision makers.

Unfortunately, attempts to intervene in a complex emergency by the humanitarian community are often severely restricted by a claim of sovereignty by the country in conflict. With health indicators deteriorating, healthcare providers frequently become "peace builders" by negotiating and mediating ceasefires to immunize and feed children and other vulnerable groups. The assessment data are used in these negotiations as a public health argument and as an educational tool for the warring factions to realize the extent of the destruction caused by the continued warring.

Teamwork in Emergency Humanitarian Relief Situations

Pamela Lupton-Bowers

The Importance of Teamwork in an Emergency Operation

Effective team functioning in disasters is often underestimated until it can no longer be ignored. The importance of teamwork to the success of a mission cannot be overemphasized. In the urgency of a disaster or a sudden public health threat everyone's energy and focus is given to the technical components. WatSan engineers plan how best to provide life-supporting water to affected communities; logisticians organize how to reach them; health experts collect data, assess risk and set out options of how governments and the humanitarian community ought to respond. Only later in the after action reports are people cognizant of the often debilitating dysfunction of the multidisciplinary, multi-stakeholder, multicultural, and multilingual teams involved in the response.

Humanitarian professionals know the frustration of working in a dysfunctional team that fails to:

Consult broadly when collecting necessary information or problem solving.

Share information with all affected stakeholders.

Include stakeholders adequately in initial analysis.

Invite all essential partners in to the decision making process.

Respect local partners and affected communities in their interactions and early assessments.

Recognize and handle obvious power struggles and potential conflict within the multidisciplinary team and among involved partner organizations.

Handle inappropriate behavior as soon as it starts.

Invest in setting up processes for ongoing information sharing and decision making.

Set standards about the working culture of the team and the quality of interactions and products, both internally and externally.

The vast majority of humanitarian workers are deployed with little or no preparation for the tensions and complexities of working in a multicultural team, in an emergency situation, and often in unsafe and unpleasant living conditions. Too often lip service is observed in the agendas of leadership development programs where priority is awarded to technical topics. The result is painfully inadequate for changing behaviors and developing skills. Yet those same behaviors and skills are consistently identified in evaluation reports as those that could have made the difference between the success and failure of an operation.

Fortunately, some people "get it." The global polio eradication initiative coordinated by WHO emphasizes quality teamwork and team leadership critical to overcoming the final hurdles in those countries most challenged by eradication. Recognized internally and reinforced by independent review, team leadership training has been organized for operations in Nigeria, Pakistan, Afghanistan, Chad, and Congo. The purpose of the training is to improve accountability through more personal responsibility to achieve objectives, to encourage working more collaboratively to tackle entrenched problems, to identify more creative solutions, and to provide leaders with the basic skills of managing performance, and of understanding that building and leading the team is real work.

During a training program in Southeast Asia to prepare a group of medical experts for deployment in teams in risk assessment of acute public health outbreaks, the leader's debriefing conclusion was this: "It really struck me how important teamwork is to the success of the mission when I witnessed what should have been the strongest group technically come out with the wrong assessment decision." The team was not working well together. One person arrived late to the workshop and missed the team building session. Typical of character, he dismissed it as unimportant relevant to the rest of the technical sessions. He soon imposed himself as the de facto leader—he was Anglophone, Western, male, and quite tall, especially compared to his Asian counterparts. The rest of the group initially acceded to his leadership; however, cracks were forming. There was dissent—some obvious, most passive. Some team members did not support the decision but did not assertively express their difference sufficiently. Fortunately we had invested in a tutor support process similar to the one modeled by the International Diploma in Humanitarian Assistance (IDHA)—more on this later—and we were able to address some of these issues so as to divert more serious emotional scars.

Unfortunately, these behaviors are not limited to training programs; the same thing happens in real field teams. The result is exhausting, demoralizing and unacceptable, especially when one considers the potential impact on people's health.

The Benefit of Good Teamwork

When teams work well together things are in synch, ideas flow; people are clear about what has to be done; they communicate openly with one another; they are comfortable with decisions, and they work in complementary harmony. An atmosphere of fairness and inclusivity reigns, and team members respect and support one another. There is a sense of personal as well as team fulfillment, and, most importantly, teams are effective. The combination of knowledge and ability can result in superior outcomes.

The complexities of a humanitarian response today demand more than ever a multidisciplinary approach.

Effective behaviors of high performing teams (HPTs) include:

Improved communication: They gather and share information as an essential part of their work.

Achieved results: HPTs focus on deliverables and outputs, recognizing that success depends on the knowledge and skills found in more than one person or one discipline.

More creative and more efficient problem solving: HPTs that combine multiple perspectives have the skills and tools to create more innovative solutions.

Higher quality decisions: Good leadership and appropriate process combine to assure shared decision making.

Increased quality in product and services: HPTs understand what people expect of them, control the quality of outputs, and have the interpersonal skills to manage relationships.

Lean processes: HPTs are not hampered by unnecessary internal bureaucracy; they identify obstacles and redesign processes to remove them, speeding up responses.

Motivated members with a thirst for learning: HPTs allow people with different kinds of knowledge, opinions and approaches to work together. They learn together and grow together. Participation in such cross-functional teams strengthens and develops individuals and can contribute to the sustainability and strengthening of organizations and partnerships.

Despite the clear added value of powerful teamwork to humanitarian work, organizations rarely invest in building HPTs. Some refer to the limited contracts as excuses for their decisions, while others assume that the group dynamics involved will occur naturally without conscious effort to establish or maintain them.

"We don't have time to deal with that. We are there to do a job, everyone knows what they have to do and they just get on with it." So said a health coordinator in Brazzaville in 1999, following an upsurge of violence in Congo. It could just have easily have been said yesterday. In their defense, emergency response team members are typically motivated by a clear commitment and drive to respond to the often overwhelming humanitarian imperative.

In the first hours and days of an emergency response, time is of the essence; the operational priority is saving lives, ensuring protection and sustenance, reducing the vulnerability of the victims, or of risk in the case of public health outbreaks. It is an understandable focus but it is short-lived. Emergency management may be condoned for immediate reaction, but far too often in humanitarian assistance operations "emergency management" becomes the accepted modus operandi. It also ignores the fact that the relief team is not a hermetically sealed unit able to operate in isolation. The members must operate with other actors including multiple, sometimes competing, agencies, and the local communities.

Investing time and resources in ensuring strong team performance in emergency missions has real advantages to the work.

1. The overall success of the operation: A well-prepared team with strong common values and beliefs, robust structure processes, and fair management style will influence action on the ground.
2. Improved relationships and image with beneficiaries and local communities: Humanitarian workers can operate more effectively and more safely in communities where they have established trust and transparency. More and more emergencies involve a new profile of the beneficiary. Articulate communities of people accustomed to power themselves, respond to relief personnel who provide prompt and effective services in a fair, respectful, and compassionate manner. They reject the traditional and essentially patronizing dynamic of the agency-beneficiary relationship that legitimizes an authoritative approach.
3. Improved potential for creating opportunities for capacity building: One of the great challenges of the relief operation is to exploit opportunities to share knowledge and capacity wherever possible and no matter how minimal. Fieldworkers who can listen, who are able to cooperate and collaborate as well as coordinate, will be those who are most effective in transferring know-how and building the capacities of the local communities and individuals.
4. Well being of their own staff and the strengthening of their organizations: Good team and interpersonal relations contribute to raising people's coping abilities

with stress. Stress is a common factor in the humanitarian world. Regardless of the presence or absence of conflict, the human tragedy associated with all disasters, the absence of family, friends and the traditional support network, added to unfamiliar climate and conditions all contribute to increased anxiety and stress for any humanitarian worker. However, when humanitarian workers benefit from good leadership support, collaborative efforts on the part of colleagues, respect and recognition for his/her contribution then the stress of the mission can be considerably reduced.

More and more relief workers are reporting that while they are competent in their functional expertise, they are unprepared for, and overwhelmed by, the ambiguous and confusing situations on the ground, which they complain get in the way of doing the job. An example would be the reaction of a senior manager who had been thrust into a "crisis" situation. He explained that he had not had time to properly meet with his team in the five months since he had been appointed. This was an HQ-based team working in the same building! One of the critical issues he wanted to deal with in a hastily arranged retreat was internal strife and conflict, as well as criticism levied at the team from their operational partners. In the words of Tao, "that which we haven't time for, we have not prioritized."

The IDHA Investment in Teamwork

The authors of Fordham University's flagship course, the International Diploma in Humanitarian Assistance (IDHA), understood the value of effective teamwork to the success of emergency missions. For this very reason the course is designed to emulate, to the degree that an academic program can, the operational conditions emergency teams find themselves having to cope with: being thrust into a group of incredibly diverse individuals with whom they have to live and work, and on whom the success of the mission depends. In IDHA programs students are selected into the most diverse "syndicates" possible and must study and perform as a team, only succeeding if the team succeeds.

However, unlike many organizations, the IDHA recognizes that the syndicates have an increased likelihood of succeeding if they are prepared for the challenge and supported in their development as a team. The first days are dedicated to helping the group bond and establishing a consensus of a culture. In addition, each syndicate group is allocated a tutor who will assist the team throughout the course. The tutor's role is to observe the team's working culture and dynamics, providing insights and support as they struggle with increasingly difficult assignments and personal study demands.

The tutor support is a big investment to the program, but one that has proven itself over and over in the forty-odd month-long courses, which have more than 2,000 graduates from 133 nations. IDHA rationalizes its investment on the following realities:

The demand for a higher caliber humanitarian worker. Large-scale complex situations requiring international response are dependent more and more on relief workers who are highly educated, skilled, and experienced. Gone is the belief that a technical relief worker need simply to follow clearly defined standard operating procedures to be able to function successfully in a predefined disaster situation. The whole playing field has less clear parameters, which demands more flexibility to deal with the ambiguity in which they work.

More complex environment. Modern disasters are less routine, and more expanding and emerging. There is a greater variety of vulnerable populations, extending over all cross-sections of society. Stakeholders can include warlords, local and international media, military, and armed guards as well as local communities, churches, and agencies. This complex scenario demands a more sophisticated response.

Longevity and permanence of complex emergencies. Both are increasingly distinctive features of relief operations, and agencies are seeking new models of operation that can cope with the crisis within emergency and that include principles of "operationality in turbulence." A number of situations provide vivid examples, among them long-term disasters such as Palestine, Sudan, and Somalia. Often what starts as an emergency response evolves into long-term relief as reconstruction is hampered by the magnitude of the disaster, and frequently followed by periods of renewed crisis as a result of the community disturbances and violence.

Sustainability and continuity of their own staff and organization. The humanitarian relief field suffers a high turnover of staff. On one hand, this is not surprising, since many relief workers approach the work as temporary or occasional. However, it poses threats to organizations if they lack professional career relief workers able to strategically manage their projects and to be able to build on institutional memory and learning. Poor team leadership and interpersonal relations contribute to this drain of talent. The stress created by the dysfunctional working environment can have a serious impact on the health of their staff. This has been documented in research in the general work environment.

Human Resources (HR) studies report that it is exacerbated many fold in the conditions the humanitarian relief workers find themselves in. There is also the warrior's code of "it's part of the job, we can handle it." This contributes to a pattern of denial, which, combined with a lack of access to professional debriefing, leads to accumulative stress syndrome, causing serious and long-term effects on the humanitarian worker. The consequences of inappropriate management and poor interpersonal relations with supervisors and colleagues are a major contributing factor to this stress. In debriefing sessions psychologists report that a significant number of humanitarian workers leaving the profession cite unsatisfactory relations with managers or colleagues as a major reason. Said one first-time Danish relief worker returning from a posting in Macedonia in 2000:

> I went straight out to Macedonia. I didn't have time for a briefing, I didn't see my manager for several weeks. I went out as a driver and ended up coordinating a team. I had no experience for that. I had no support. I don't think I did a good job. I am completely burned out. I don't think I'll be going back.

Building the Team

The IDHA program models its approach on the emergency relief situation. Groups of strangers are placed together within the first hours of arriving. They are organized into syndicate groups and expected to operate immediately as productive "teams." The majority of them do; a few of them do not. What is it that binds them? What helps to build the team? What prevents them and causes their failure? These are questions that are explored within the first day of the IDHA program, because when team formation is hampered the entire outcome of the team can be jeopardized.

A major contributing factor to the function—or dysfunction—of a team is the underlying values and beliefs that motivate the individual to engage in humanitarian work. This influences decision making and relationships with colleagues and especially with host communities and victims. The driving factors that lead people to seek humanitarian relief work vary considerably. Some people are driven by fundamental humanitarian values and a need to "do good," others by religious beliefs, but many are driven by less altruistic values, the excitement, the risk, the exotic locations, or simply the desire to get away from day-to-day life back home.

We can neither assume nor rely on an agreed moral basis for modern humanitarianism. For many the concept of "deserving poor" no longer holds true, and many aid workers suffer from that deception in an increasingly politicized world. Impartiality, long considered an essential of humanitarianism, was questioned during the Rwanda operations, in Bosnia, and during the Arab Spring and associated civil uprisings. Within the paradox of motives and context is a real need to establish a common sense of identity and purpose.

Through a series of personal reflections and group discussions I facilitate a team through a process that allows them to do just that. It is achieved by inviting members to share their own experiences of good (and bad) teamwork, to build a model that everyone buys into. The bottom line is when a team has a common purpose, it can establish a common identity and work more effectively toward a commonly agreed goal.

The Three-Component Model for Effective Teamwork

A simple model for establishing effective teamwork would include the *what* (that is, the team objectives), the *who* (internal and external relations—the human dimensions, in short), and the *how* (organizational procedures) of a situation. All three of these components have to be aligned to assure success.

A misperception is that a group of people thrust together to respond to the urgency of a humanitarian disaster will naturally pull together and work together immediately and consistently. Unfortunately, this is rarely the case. Interpersonal dynamics create daunting challenges that some teams just cannot overcome.

Mastering team effectiveness means mastering complex relationships and learning agendas. Team members are usually confident about their own subject matter excellence, but the emergency demands much more of them in terms of the cultural, political, and organizational challenges that are an inextricable part of the complex fabric of the disaster environment. There are several paradoxes to building strong teams. Here are some of them:

Team members have to learn to work together; however, they cannot really be taught. To be truly successful, the team must design its own model.

People generally identify strong leadership as a successful factor to great teamwork and then bristle against it when it does not allow them inclusivity and contribution.

Managers have a right and obligation to lead, but when they assert this right by virtue of position they are at their weakest.

What: Common Goals and Objectives

The "what" gives the team its purpose and legitimacy. It describes what the team has to do, and more importantly what they must achieve.

The common goal has to be agreed and accepted by all. It should be in line with the organizational mission and agreed with other stakeholders and partners. This is not always as easy as it sounds. In today's complex environment more and more partners are involved in any response and they expect to be included in decision making that affects them. Partners are no longer accepting that lead agencies, despite their mandates, make decisions on behalf of all concerned. This reality demands more frequent and more skilled coordination and collaboration.

Experts and specialists bridle against what they see as interference and slowing up of responses. Clearly this perception is delusional. While lead agencies may have made decisions unilaterally in the past, they were not easily acknowledged by partners; precious time was lost, and impact reduced by the passive or active resistance to those decisions. It makes much more sense to include partners in the early information gathering and sharing, and in the initial decision making so that all concerned operate from the same sheet of music. This type of collaboration demands a more sophisticated management relationship and communication competence than many team leaders currently display.

Individual objectives develop out of the agreed, common goal. Personal objectives should be allocated fairly and according to specific technical abilities, skills, and competencies of each of the members. They will usually be based on a person's terms of reference, but these alone are rarely sufficiently detailed enough to capture the specific objectives expected of personnel or provide an adequate basis to be able to hold them accountable for their results. They should also take into consideration, where possible, individual style and preferences. They should equally consider the conclusions of recent research in motivation, which reveals much about how and why people work.

Many emergency response team leaders claim they do not have time for all of this while responding to an urgency. I would challenge that thinking and say, "You don't have the time not to." Emergency response teams often travel together, wait in airports together. I have briefed teams in capital cities as we wait for transport to the final destination. I have also provided briefs to team leaders to conduct in the vehicles en route. The time you invest at the outset clarifying overtly expectations in terms of contributions and quality standards will save precious time later on.

Who: People

The mantra here is "Know your people." There is nothing to replace your knowledge of your team. The leader and the team need to know and respect individual differences, cultures, and preferred work styles. You do not have to be a psychologist, but you do have to understand that people have different thinking and problem solving styles.

Team members are typically selected because of their specific skill set, and in many cases their contribution to the team's task is clear-cut, but a leader must be aware of, and put to use, team members' general potential and preferential work. There are many general activities that need to be accomplished in a team, above and beyond the individual technical contributions. It is important for the team to know who are the accomplished negotiators, report writers, counselors, organizers, budget handlers, and so on.

A medical team demonstrating a purely logical approach to identifying an unknown virus causing public health dangers may ignore the complex relationship-building and communication required to ensure accurate and trustworthy information from an affected community. A reconstruction team trying to get access to a village of victims after years of mistrust with the local religious leaders may fail to consider new and innovative approaches because they are so entrenched in the way things have always been. A leader used to working from his "gut" and ready to take risks may ignore facts and data that might suggest a more analyzed and considered response. And most emergency response teams ignore the value of establishing systems and investing in sustainable procedures, which often contributes to the lack of a seamless transition to on-the-ground NGOs or communities, and to an effective exit strategy.

To be thoroughly effective, the team must think through all these issues despite their primary mandate. To ignore them is to risk ignoring an essential part of the picture. When the team members understand one another's preferred thinking, deciding, learning and communication styles the working culture is improved and the team can be more efficient and effective. Mutual understanding and respect empowers each member to achieve within their respective roles, and as representatives of the team.

Motivation

Another critical component effecting the functioning of the team is motivation. One could assume that all members of the team are primed to be fully motivated in any emergency response situation. Yes and no. Yes, in that they may set off in that frame of mind; however, circumstances can very soon change the drive. Emergency health professionals, logisticians, lab technicians as well as security personnel have all described the demoralizing and demotivating impact of inappropriate and uncaring behavior from colleagues and team leaders.

In a wide study undertaken by the Saratoga Institute on 20,000 exit interviews exploring why people leave their jobs, 85 percent of managers believed that people left for better jobs and higher salaries, while 80 percent of people reported leaving because of dysfunctional teams or poor bosses. In debriefing during the African Great Lakes disaster, 90 percent of Red Cross delegates reported their reason for leaving or not extending contracts as related to internal issues with the team or the person's manager. Examples or behaviors contributing to poor morale and defection include:

Inadequate welcome or induction into the team

Unclear or no objectives set

Uninspiring work

Seemingly disconnected work with no obvious added value to the team task

Work that does not reflect the skill set or ability

No direct contact with the leader—being ignored

Not being consulted about decisions in the team

Receiving no feedback on performance—formal or informal

Being reprimanded in front of others

Disrespectful language or attitude (both verbal and nonverbal)

These driving principles lead to several clear key points about the motivation of individuals:

People like targets. Without something to aim for, work is just a job. The targets should be agreed with the team member themselves to encourage autonomy and ownership. Whereas long-term goals are essential for the team, individual targets should be relatively short-term (particularly in emergency response), or else they are too far off to be real.

People like to feel good. When people feel good about themselves they work better. People feel good when they succeed, that is: meet their targets, and are praised by people they respect. It is easier to raise people's standards by raising their targets and praising achievement than by criticizing them for their faults.

People like to work to their strengths. People tend to be more effective and successful when they are involved in work that matches their preferences. When people's work emphasizes more of their weaknesses than their dominant preferences (or auxiliary preferences) then they are more likely to become disillusioned

People are different. Different people want different things out of their life and work. Check out the psychological contract (what they intrinsically believe is their relationship with the organization) if you can; it may not be what you think it is.

As a team leader, this leaves you with a set of paradoxes:

Do not tell people what to aim for; it is better if they work out their goals for themselves.	Do emphasize that they must work out some precise goals against which they can measure success or progress.
Do not shout at people who make mistakes; it will paradoxically make them try less hard.	Do insist that they learn from their mistakes and they set new goals for next time; forgive the sinner but condemn the sin.
Do not assume that everyone is like you; they may be driven by other reasons.	
Do not give only negative feedback; it will diminish either a person's self-concept or his or her view of you.	Do encourage people to be explicit about their psychological contract, what they expect to give and get from their work.
Do not make promises for good work; it creates only dependent pigeons, and you will get locked into never-ending promises	Do take opportunities to praise good work; give feedforward[1] about what you'd like to see more of.
	Do make sure that people know when their work is good; create obvious signs of success/ progress that people can read for themselves.

Last but not least in this section, I challenge you to ask, "Who is the team?" When I work with a team in the field, I ask them who they work with on a day-to-day basis. When I first joined the International Federation of Red Cross and Red Crescent Societies Secretariat I challenged the target audience of the heads of delegation workshops, since they did not include headquarters (HQ) managers. In every organization there has been tension between HQ and the field.

How: Process

Processes describe "how" the team will operate, and how each member will contribute and participate. Processes need to include agreed procedures for:

Participation—How the team members will communicate with one another, with the team leader, with other teams and with external partners; how they will share information, status updates and changing intelligence; how they will provide feedback to line managers, to external agencies as well as to one another. There may be a mix of informal and formal mechanisms. Both are essential; both need to be respected.

Decision making—There are different methods of decision making, some are more appropriate than others. A key factor in the effective working of mature teams of professionals is that they have input into decisions. This is referred to as participative decision making. It does not mean that everyone gets to make the decision, but that everyone's opinion is heard before the decision is made. Although many technical thinkers frequently found in medicine, science, finance, and logistics are comfortable when decisions can be based on factual evidence, the ambiguity of a major disaster does not often lend itself to numerical or logical sequencing. A lot of decisions have to be made under pressure of time and limited information. A lot of decisions are made on experience and gut reaction. A good team leader will be comfortable with a variety of decision-making methods: sometimes relying on "the expert" in the team, sometimes on a majority agreement, sometimes able to rely on the evidence or data, but sometimes just going with his or her gut. At times any decision is the right decision.

Contribution and performance—The team should agree on levels of quality that they all aspire to meet. It is also helpful to make explicit, and to agree on the values and competencies that describe the way the team will operate. How will it deal with strong and weak personalities? How to ensure the team has whole brain thinking and that all quadrants have been explored. How will it handle conflict if it emerges?

Progress—How will achievement be monitored and evaluated? How will your progress be measured? Again, be cautious of recognizing all achievements. Quite often in emergency response some of the more critical work is unseen. A lot of the backup work is unrecognized. I remember standing on the tarmac of the airport at Dar es Salaam unable to board a flight for Kasulu, where I was to do some leadership training for local relief workers in the refugee camp because there was no cash to buy the fuel for the plane. A finance person in Geneva had not completed a necessary procedure for the request to the Humanitarian Aid and Civil Protection department of the European Commission (ECHO), formerly known as the European Community Humanitarian Aid Office. When people are so disenfranchised and disengaged from a mission that they are unaware of the consequences of their work, the person in the field will suffer.

Celebrate—Last but certainly not least, the team must pay attention to informal relationships: how it celebrates success, how it commiserates, how it maintains the energy and enthusiasm, how it deals with stress.

There are more questions than answers. There are no absolute answers as to how a team should operate. Of course, certain omissions will negatively effect team performance: lack of targets, lack of systems and appropriate filing and reporting, and so forth. But many of the answers will depend on the task to be achieved, the length of time of the mission, the composition of the team, the predominant culture of the team, the location it finds itself, even the availability and tolerance for alcohol.

Feedback

We have made reference to providing feedback, or preferably "feedforward." One might assume that once standard operating behaviors have been established, team members will moderate their behavior to match the agreed culture. The capability of a person to change, the behavioral flexibility, involves both the motivation and the ability to adapt. Inextricably linked with success in teamwork is the assumption that individuals are agreeable to change and that change involves learning new skill sand adopting them. The extent to which members are able to give and take timely, honest and constructive feedback will depend on having clear operating behaviors, and an atmosphere that encourages discussion and sharing of expectations.

Feedback: The IDHA Model

The following factors contributed to the success:

1. Ongoing: It was a regular and natural part of the working day.
2. Specific: Team members were encouraged and helped to give detailed examples about what happened and the impact it had. It was not enough to say "Good job." People were encouraged to explain why they felt it was a good job, so that it was clear what the person was to continue doing.
3. Immediate: So that the person relates the comments directly to the behavior or incident that occurred that day.
4. Present- and future-based: We wanted to dissociate with being reprimanded. Members were taught to objectively describe behavior and then to provide feed forward of what they would like the person to do in the future.
5. Helpful and constructive: The intention of the comments was to help the person improve the behavior, so that they were able to perform better, more effectively, more efficiently or more diplomatically the next time.
6. All-way: All members of the team including the team leader were open to feedback.
7. Work-related: Comments were directed at the behavior and not at the person. Participants were encouraged to describe what the person did or said, rather than make statements about what the person is.

8. Given privately: Although all team related comments were handled in the team meeting where facilitators had personal interjections with the most difficult situations, individuals were taken aside and given the opportunity to reflect or respond and to save face. People are generally less likely to accept feedback if they feel threatened, challenged, or humiliated.

A word of caution about feedback in emergency situation: People are often in a highly charged emotional state in the early phases of an emergency. They may be sleep-deprived and stressed. In such situations, feedback—even feedforward—may be misconstrued and unwelcome. Another reason for establishing standard operating behaviors or agreeing to common language to describe behaviors is that personal insult can be reduced when discussion is being compared to standards already accepted.

The Team Leader

The difference between leader and manager has been the subject of discussion and exploration for many years. It is important to keep in mind Bennison's[2] distinction between leadership, which is more about setting a new direction or vision for a group to follow, and management being more about controls and directing people/resources in a group according to principles or values that have previously been established—either by a group or by the organization it represents.

In emergency response situations the role is more about managing to agreed goals within accepted mandates, taking a shorter-term view and complying to standards. There is no doubt that to achieve this task leadership must be demonstrated and role modeled. Great leaders demonstrate this by:

Creating and communicating the vision

Acting as powerful role models

Aligning people towards a common goal

Bringing out the best in people

Acting as change agents

Staying calm in crisis and challenge

Today's workforce is the best-educated and most qualified in history. Managers can no longer expect them to leave their brains at the door when they come to work. Sadly, managers from many authoritarian cultures and others representing cross cultures behave as if this is the case, in their belief that they alone are qualified to interpret information, resolve issues and make decisions. Such beliefs and practices create quite a challenge to promoting facilitative approaches to team leadership.

Good leadership is about giving a sense of real purpose to the team. It starts with self-awareness—the first step to what is now referred to as Emotional Intelligence. According to the widely recognized work of Daniel Goleman,[3] Emotional Intelligence is a combination of self-awareness, self-management, social awareness, and relationship management. It is also about being proactive and thinking ahead—this requires innovation, creativity and future planning, and being comfortable with ambiguity and paradox. Good leadership is not about being liked but about being effective. It is not about the status, position, fancy 4×4 vehicle, or other perks. It is about doing the right thing and doing it well.

Trust: A Critical Factor in Establishing High-Performing Teams

From project managers to emergency health responders, a critical factor identified as contributing to or destroying a team is trust. It appears as the superglue that holds teams and organizations together. Without it there is dysfunction and suboptimal performance.

In numerous exercises conducted around the world and in numerous organizations, the following list emerges:

What creates trust	What destroys trust
Giving credit to others	Pushing to be understood
Listening to understand	Breaking promises
Keeping promises	Being unkind and discourteous
Being kind and courteous	Being disloyal
Being loyal to the absent	Being prideful and arrogant
Being available and open	Blaming others
Offering apologies	Lying and double standards
Keeping commitments	Rejecting feedback
Being open to feedback	Personal attacks and criticism
Being emotionally stable	Taking credit for others' work

Summary

Society in general is demanding more of humanitarian action, whether it is the Gates Foundation demanding measurable results or cooperating partners demanding more involvement with lead agencies. Today's situations demand a more cooperative and inclusive approach, and workers involved in them need to employ effective cross-functional, cross-disciplinary, and multicultural teamwork. An inherent assumption of this approach must be that the competencies of individual relief workers and particularly team leaders must include skills in facilitating these processes. Among some disaster relief workers there is still a reluctance, even embarrassment, on the part of humanitarian agencies to give credit to this kind of training and preparation. But, the consequences for not doing so are serious and may be fatal to the program, those who need assistance, and to the humanitarian workers themselves. There are a number of advantages to getting this right.

1. The improved functioning of teams: Just as an organization's values and beliefs influence the actions and ethics of its people, so too does the structure, processes, and management style. By extension, both will influence the functioning of its teams on the ground and the overall perceived success of the organization.
2. Community relations: Not only can humanitarian workers not operate in communities where they have not established trust and transparency, but their lives are also sometimes at risk.
3. A new profile of beneficiaries: "Articulate communities of people used to power themselves" describes relief personnel who provide prompt and effective services in a fair, respectful and compassionate manner. They reject the traditional and essentially patronizing dynamic of the agency-beneficiary relationship that often legitimizes an authoritative approach.
4. Capacity building: Good team and interpersonal relations contribute to raising people's coping abilities with stress. Stress is a common factor in the humanitarian world. Regardless of the presence or absence of conflict, the human tragedy associated with all disasters, the absence of family, friends and the traditional support network, added to unfamiliar climate and conditions all contribute to increased anxiety and stress for any humanitarian worker. However, when humanitarian workers benefit from good leadership support, collaborative efforts on the part of colleagues, respect and recognition for his/her contribution, then the stress of the mission can be considerably reduced. As one aid worker said, "In Abidjan when the violence was at its worst, the team spirit and relationship with our colleagues in other agencies was so good that we were able to handle the worst situations with a sense of humor and without being totally stressed. It would have been impossible to have survived without."

Education as a Survival Strategy

Sixty Years of Schooling for Palestinian Refugees

Sam Rose

In times of war, still photography retains a singular ability to transfix and disturb. From the carefully crafted and sometimes dissembled compositions by the legendary annalists of the American Civil War to the "trophy shots" of torture and abuse of Iraqi detainees in Abu Ghraib, war photography can chronicle the horrors of conflict and the vulnerability of its victims with breathtaking power and emotion.

Among the most arresting images from the military operation (Operation Cast Lead) that Israel waged in Gaza in December 2008–January 2009, are a series that illustrates both sides of the artistry of the photojournalist. They tell the story of the shelling of a UN school in the northern town of Beit Lahiya by the Israeli Army on the last day of the war.[1] In the initial photograph, an Israeli ordnance round can be seen exploding above the school, while another lands in the playground, trailing a plume of white smoke. In the next, scores of miniature fireballs rain down on a UN compound. Subsequent pictures convey the panic and heroics of those under bombardment—civilians flee toward the camera while paramedics dart in the opposite direction. They disappear into a blanket of dense white smoke, which has now engulfed much of the schoolyard and buildings, where almost two thousand Palestinians had been sheltering. Soon, the medics are also in flight, as firefighters struggle to douse the flames.

Suddenly, the mood and pace (and most likely the photographer) changes, and we are taken through several more stylized compositions portraying the aftermath of the attack. Women and children return to the blackened classrooms where they had been sheltering before the bombardment; aid workers and local residents sift through the remains.

We now know that the ordnance used by the Israeli Army that day was filled with felt wedges steeped in white phosphorus, a fiercely incendiary and highly toxic chemical. Although permitted under international law under certain circumstances, it is prohibited wherever there is "a concentration of civilians,"[2] a description that Human Rights Watch has concluded applied on that day in Gaza. We also know that two children, aged five and seven, who were inside the school were killed, and thirteen persons were injured.

The Beit Lahiya Elementary School sustained extensive damages. It is operated by the UN Relief and Works Agency (UNRWA), which provides basic services to around one million Palestine refugees in Gaza, approximately two-thirds of the total population, and another 3.5 million in the West Bank, Jordan, Syria, and Lebanon. Thirty-six of the organization's schools were damaged during IDF Operation Cast Lead; forty-five were turned into temporary shelters, hosting more than fifty thousand displaced civilians.

This is not the first time that UNRWA installations have been damaged or destroyed during military operations. The organization's entire compound in Nahr el Bared camp in Lebanon, which housed five schools and several other UN and NGO facilities, was leveled by the Lebanese Army in the siege of summer 2007. Ninety of UNRWA's one hundred schools in Gaza were damaged or looted during the 1967 Arab-Israel war. The almost serial nature of such incidents and the repeated breaches of the immunity and inviolability of UN assets that they imply should in no way reduce our shock and duty to protest in the strongest possible terms.

IDF Operation Cast Lead ended on January 17, 2009. A week later, on January 24, following makeshift repairs, UNRWA reopened the Beit Lahiya school. Teaching resumed at all UNRWA's schools in Gaza that day, for close to 200,000 refugee pupils. This was arguably the most significant step taken by UNRWA in the immediate aftermath of the war. As well as creating space for children and parents to come to terms with their trauma, it helped to provide structure and stability for those young people whose lives had been shattered by war, reinforcing a return to "normality," insofar as such a word has meaning in Gaza. It also held significant symbolic value, emphasizing UNRWA's intent to reorient itself rapidly toward longer-term development goals and its commitment to supporting the Palestine refugees of Gaza during the recovery process.

The Early History of UNRWA's Education Programs

Behind the incident described above lies the story of one of the largest education systems in the Middle East and one of the most important in contemporary Palestinian society.

While long-term crises and sudden shocks in the past decade have forced UNRWA to direct an increasing share of its resources to emergency relief, over the course of its sixty-year history the organization's primary role has been to provide social services—mainly education and health—to an ever-growing population of refugees. Each day of the academic year, 500,000 children aged between five and fourteen pass through the doors of almost 700 UNRWA schools in Jordan, Lebanon, Syria, the West Bank, and the Gaza Strip, at an annual cost of US$328 million.[3] Since operations began, UNRWA has educated three generations of refugees, or around four million children.

It is in the sphere of education that UNRWA has made by far its most significant contribution to Palestinian human development. However, this was not the original intention of the UN when it began to seek funds for Palestine refugees following the 1948 Arab-Israeli conflict. In what was thought would be a temporary emergency operation, no provision was made for education by the UN's Disaster Relief Project for the victims of the war, which began work in July 1948, or in the first budget of its successor, UN Relief for Palestine Refugees (UNRPR).[4] The few schools there were in the refugee camps that had sprung up across the region had been set up by voluntary organizations, including the Quakers in Gaza and the Red Cross Society in the West Bank, and were supported by UNESCO.[5] They survived on sales of used materials, special appeals and grants from other UN organizations.[6]

When UNRWA assumed responsibility for the education of Palestine refugees in the middle of 1950, it took over sixty-one schools from the UNRPR, with 730 teachers and 33,600 pupils, representing just over a quarter of all school aged refugee children at that time.[7] A director was assigned from UNESCO to lead the agency's education programs, in an arrangement that continues to this day. However, the share of education in the organization's first budgets was negligible: between 1950 and 1955, it accounted for only 5 percent of total expenditures.[8] While understandable given the context—more than 700,000 refugees had recently been uprooted from their homes and livelihoods—it also reflected the prevailing approach of the major powers to the Palestine refugee "problem."

Unable to repatriate the refugees as per the terms of UN General Assembly Resolution 194 (III) of December 11, 1948, the international community instead sought their regional resettlement and "reintegration." This was to be achieved through public works projects that would (1) help displaced communities to become self-sufficient; (2) strengthen the economies of the host countries; and (3) allow UNRWA to delete large numbers from its ration rolls in fairly short order.[9] Projects developed to meet these goals ranged from local construction works, for example, of shelters, roads and camps, to regional initiatives of a scope and ambition that have not been seen since in more than sixty years of peace-building efforts for Palestinians and Israelis.[10]

UNRWA had already begun increasing its expenditures on education, partly to support the goal of economic rehabilitation, but also given the longer-term character the refugee crisis was gradually assuming. Another consideration may have been a rebuke from UNESCO's Executive Board to the effect that the UN would be in breach of the Universal Declaration of Human Rights if it failed to make further investments in educating Palestine refugee children.[11]

Although food parcels still accounted for the majority of UNRWA's budgets, there were major leaps in allocations to education during the first half of the 1950s. By the middle of the decade, its accounted for almost one-fifth of total expenditures. Almost 100,000 pupils were being taught in 264 UNRWA schools by 2,700 teachers, with subsidies provided to house another 55,000 refugee children at government or private schools.

Most teaching had moved out of tents and into specially constructed premises or rented buildings. UNRWA schools were the first permanent structures in many camps and became a symbol of an increasingly education-centered approach to refugee assistance. UNRWA was also operating two vocational training centers in Qalandia and Gaza and had links with regional organizations and host governments to secure placements and employment contracts for its graduates at the end of their courses. Course materials were developed with regional market needs—and UNRWA-funded large-scale development projects—in mind, supported by specialist UN agencies. University scholarship and teacher-training programs were also offered, albeit on a very small scale, while tens of thousands of adult refugees benefited from adult literacy courses.

As the 1950s progressed, skepticism about the feasibility of the much-trumped reintegration and resettlement schemes continued to grow. The failure to resolve the Arab-Israeli conflict as per the terms of Resolution 194, the intransigence of Israel and host authorities, and the paucity of donor funding for development plans were all contributing factors. Perhaps most importantly, the refugees refused to be part of what they considered to be a conspiracy to liquidate them and deny them their internationally recognized rights.

The Suez crisis of 1956 signaled the abrupt end of the era of regional refugee-development schemes. After this time and the final acceptance that there could be no resolution of the Palestine refugee problem absent political accommodation, UNRWA began to reorient itself away from relief toward education. The seeds of this strategic transformation had been planted in the five-year education plan of 1955–1959 and were given full voice in the watershed annual report of 1960.[12] In that report, UNRWA's fourth director, John Davis, announced a three-year plan for "well planned and promptly executed programmes for improving general education and expanding specialized types of training" that would harvest the "latent productive talents" of refugee youth that had so far been laid to waste.[13]

Proposals included the formalization of a three-year, lower preparatory cycle; increasing the number of vocational trainees from 500 to between 2,000 and 2,500 through the construction of six new training centers and the establishment of a joint vocational and teacher-training school for girls and a separate men's teacher training center; doubling the number of university scholarships awarded by UNRWA each year, from 90 to 180 per year; and institutionalizing UNRWA's loans and grants programs, designed to help refugees become self-sufficient.[14]

These initiatives, which placed UNRWA at the vanguard of regional education policy, laid the foundations for a series of remarkable successes. They established UNRWA as a significant educational force, far ahead of the curve in the Middle East and North Africa region, and endowing refugees with an "educational advantage" over their non-refugee peers, which persisted for many decades.[15] To this day, literacy rates of Palestinian refugees are higher than for the Middle East and North Africa region as a whole, particularly among females.[16] UNRWA's initiatives were often groundbreaking, especially in girls' education and vocational training, where graduates were highly sought after and an UNRWA qualification effectively guaranteed employment. The organization had a reputation for innovation, dynamism, and vision in its approach and commitment to education, a commitment that was shared by the refugees.

Beginning in 1961, the share of the budget spent on education began to increase significantly, and by 1970 it had become UNRWA's largest program. Five years later, education accounted for more than half of all program expenditures.[17]

The Successes of UNRWA's Education Program

The successes of the program can be attributed to a number of factors. Some were circumstantial, others a result of direct choices and support by UNRWA, refugees and host authorities. Considered as a whole, they provide compelling evidence of the opportunities for development and progress that can emerge from crisis and tragedy.

The First Decade

Even before the Palestinian exodus or nakba of 1948, education levels among Arabs in mandate Palestine were relatively good by regional standards, despite Palestinians' primarily agrarian backgrounds. This was partly the result of investments by the British in the last years of the mandate period. It also reflected a growing desire for learning among village communities at that time, with many contributing labor to build their own schools and the government providing the teachers.[18] Nevertheless, overall attainment levels were quite low, and enrollment was far from universal. Most schools were based in towns, limiting access for rural population and girls in particular, who fell victim to cultural barriers regarding unaccompanied travel.[19] Estimates of illiteracy among Palestinians at that time range from between 60 and 70 percent, with around half of all children—and four in five girls—not receiving any kind of education.[20]

The *nakba* removed many of the barriers to physical and cultural access, particularly for rural Palestinians, who formed the overwhelming majority of the residents of the refugee camps. The network of schools established by voluntary organizations offered a platform that UNRWA could capitalize on and support with resources and technical expertise. Within months, many thousands of Palestinians now had educational establishments within walking distance. Enrollments by girls increased with each year, as cultural norms which had conspired against progress in normal circumstances were rapidly overcome at a time of crisis.

If UNRWA's attitude to education in the 1950s could be seen as somewhat ambivalent, the same charge could not be leveled at the refugees. As early as 1951 refugee communities were urging UNRWA to devote more of its resources to education,[21] and while often skeptical of its overall intentions and those of its power-brokers, they viewed education as an apolitical form of rehabilitation, which did not compromise their right of return. UNRWA's commitment to education from 1960 onward was also framed explicitly in these terms.[22]

For the first generation of Palestine refugees, education was both a short-term and long-term coping strategy. As a result of the *nakba*, a predominantly peasant society had lost access to its land and needed to secure alternative and reliable means of livelihood. Education and training were viewed as well suited to their needs and capacities; the human capital that they generated could not be destroyed or taken away.[23] However sepia-tinged this analysis may appear, there is no doubt that study offered a route out of poverty, and as such, investment in education—particularly higher education—was embraced as a "family project"[24] by many households. Some researchers have further suggested that refugees' desire to better themselves partly reflected a sense of inferiority next to Israelis. Bridging the gap thus became part of the national struggle, one in which education partially replaced the homeland as a focus for Palestinian efforts.[25] There were also more mundane considerations: Children who had previously worked in the fields no longer had the opportunity to do so and needed alternative ways to occupy their time.

The 1960s and Beyond: The Impact of the Davis Reforms

Davis's plan yielded almost immediate results. It fostered the growth of what could be described as a virtuous circle for education similar to those seen in many Western European states following the Second World War, and which acted as a vital engine for economic growth in the postwar period.

The institutionalization of a third year of preparatory education, formalizing the lower secondary cycle in UNRWA schools and with it nine years of compulsory education, was critical. This enabled refugee students to graduate to upper secondary and also tertiary education, which was often provided free of charge by the host authorities and Eastern Bloc countries.[26] By the end of the 1960s, the ratio of Palestinian university students to total Palestinian population was considerably higher than for the Arab region as a whole and comparable to many developed countries. The fact that most of these students came from families who would have been fortunate to have access to even basic education a generation earlier makes this achievement even more impressive. As was the case with primary education, girls in particular benefited, and host country data show major leaps in refugee females' participation in higher education from this point.

The expansion of UNRWA's education and training programs enabled refugees to tap into the professional opportunities offered by the opening up of regional markets, particularly in the Gulf. Oil-rich governments were making massive investments at that time, including in schools and hospitals, and UNRWA was quick to pinpoint these states as potential employers for graduates. Market surveys and systematic analysis of labor market needs across the Middle East, played an important role, continually informing the content of training courses at the new vocational colleges.[27] UNRWA's own employment placement centers, originally set up to facilitate refugee resettlement, provided further support. Investment in education quickly became self-reinforcing, as remissions from graduates of UNRWA schools and colleges working in the Gulf funded the education of future generations of Palestinians from the camps. Importantly, such remissions also helped to support the Palestinian national movement.

Likewise, the development of public institutions and infrastructure in Arab host countries and UNRWA's own expanding education and health programs ensured a ready stream of work for qualified job seekers, particularly for women, for whom teaching and medical jobs were well suited and culturally accepted, and for graduates of UNRWA technical colleges, who built much of the furniture used in agency schools.

Although partly driven by the failure of attempts to ensure refugee repatriation, UNRWA's reorientation towards education services in the 1960s had a transformative effect. It allowed the organization to transcend the temporary nature of its mandate and focus on longer-term human development goals. For the refugees, whose role in shaping UNRWA's priorities should not be underestimated, this move effected a qualitative change in their human capital and living levels.

The Challenges

Achievements in education have come despite chronic underfunding and repeated national and regional emergencies over the past sixty years. The cumulative effect of these has been a dramatic narrowing of refugees' educational advantage and opportunities in recent decades, at a time when new labor force entrants face ever-growing competition for employment in an increasingly global job market.

Funding Shortfalls

UNRWA's dependency on voluntary financial contributions was identified as a major structural shortcoming as early as 1951, in the UNRWA Director's Interim Report of that year, which covered the first five months of operations:

> The Agency's financial situation has never been a happy one . . . At no time in its brief career has the Agency been able to see its financial position assured for more than a few weeks ahead. A large and complex program cannot be adequately planned and administered efficiently when it depends on the receipt of voluntary contributions in unknown amounts, to be delivered at unknown times.

Financial shortfalls had an immediate impact on UNRWA's education programs, consistently limiting capacity to invest in the human and capital resources needed to accommodate a rapidly growing student population. From the early 1950s UNRWA was forced to operate schools on a "double-shift" basis, with one group of students studying in the morning and a second in the afternoon. Although the planned elimination of such a system became a mantra of Annual Reports, with each passing year the proportion of double-shifted schools grew, and some schools in Lebanon were eventually forced to operate a third shift. By 2004, more than three-quarters of UNRWA's schools operated two shifts each day.[28] As a result, school days have had to be shortened to accommodate the second shift, resulting in fewer hours available for learning, use of specialized facilities and extracurricular activities.

Construction plans to reduce class sizes and teacher-pupil ratios and replace rented premises, many of which dated back to the early 1950s and were increasingly ill suited to the demands of modern learning, were prepared and updated but were routinely under-resourced. At times, the funding crisis became so grave that programs were threatened. In the late 1970s, the provision of university scholarships was frozen, while spiraling inflation over the course of that decade led the Commissioner-General to propose the closure of all preparatory schools in 1979. A year later, UNRWA was considering shutting down all its schools for financial reasons.[29]

A Deteriorating External Environment

UNRWA's inability to upgrade and develop its educational resources, facilities, and systems undoubtedly contributed to the eventual narrowing of the educational advantage of Palestine refugees over their Arab peers. Other external factors, which had helped to create such an enabling environment for education throughout the 1960s and 1970s, also began to recede. By the early 1980s, the demand for professional expatriate labor in the Gulf, which had fed the drive for education and whose remittances had supported the education of future generations, was down. The Gulf States were becoming increasingly reliant on their own nationals to fill teaching and other public sector roles, a professional cadre and system whose development owed no small debt to Palestinian migrant workers. At the same time, massive investment in education systems by other Arab States, designed to absorb their rapidly growing, increasingly urban-dwelling, young populations, paid dividends for host-country nationals and led to greater competition for jobs. The same pattern was repeated in the West Bank and Gaza after the establishment of the Palestinian Authority in 1994: donors made significant investments in systems and structures that had been heavily neglected by Israel in the years since 1967. Even so, the Gulf States remained an important source of employment for professional Palestinians until the end of the first Gulf War in 1991, when an estimated 300,000 Palestinians were expelled from Kuwait. Particularly for those in the occupied Palestinian territory and Lebanon, there were few domestic alternatives to these professional employment opportunities.

For Palestinians in the occupied Palestinian territory, the Israeli labor market offered a major alternative source of employment. Following the 1967 war, Israel had immediately sought to integrate the Palestinian economy into its own. It incorporated the surplus of low-skilled Palestinian labor—mainly male—into Israeli construction, service, and industrial sectors in jobs that were unattractive to its own workers. Access to relatively well paid job opportunities in Israel from 1967 onward also influenced the attitude of young Palestinian males in Gaza and West Bank to higher education, further reducing the educational dividend for Palestinians.[30]

Perpetual Emergencies

Perhaps most devastating, though, have been the repeated crises across UNRWA's fields, which have forced the closure of schools and led to the suspension of classes and the diversion of funding and attention to more immediate, life-saving concerns. In the Gaza Strip and West Bank particularly, these emergencies have become the norm in recent years. Often political or complex in nature, crises have had both immediate and long-term, irrevocable impacts on service delivery, creating new dynamics and realities that UNRWA and its pupils have been forced to adapt to and negotiate.

The Arab-Israeli war of June 1967 is a case in point. Almost 300 UNRWA teachers were outside Gaza at the time of the war and were not permitted by the new occupying power Israel to return in time for the start of the next school year. More significantly, Israel banned the entry of most of the Egyptian textbooks used in UNRWA schools in Gaza. Israel had long been critical of these books, which in its view offered a "distorted account of the events leading up to and following the establishment of the State of Israel and tended to induce hatred of Israel in the minds of the children using them." In coordination with UNESCO, UNRWA was forced to produce its own temporary textbooks and teaching notes.

Special arrangements also had to be made to allow several thousands of students to complete secondary-school leaving examinations (*tawjihi*), a requirement for continuing education in the Arab world. Some students were permitted to travel to Jordan to complete their studies, while UNRWA and UNESCO succeeded in bringing examination papers into Gaza for the remainder. This entailed a complex logistical effort, involving a team of forty international staff, as well as hundreds of inspectors and teachers, and representatives of the ICRC and United Nations Emergency Force. These arrangements remained in place for twelve years, until the signing of a peace deal between Israel and Egypt in 1979.[31]

Two Decades of Crisis in Gaza and the West Bank

The eruption of the first Intifada in Gaza in 1988 effectively marked the start of two decades of upheaval and crisis for the education system in the occupied Palestinian territory, which continue to this day. During the first Intifada, the education system was directly targeted, with schools and students often at the centre of violent confrontations with the occupying power. In Gaza, UNRWA schools were closed on average every third day; even greater amounts of time were lost in the West Bank, where UNRWA's three training centers were also shut for more than two years from the spring of 1988.[32]

Although students and youth were less directly involved in the second Intifada, its impact on the education process has been no less devastating. Since September 2000, Israel has significantly tightened its system of restrictions on the movement of Palestinians and Palestinian goods into, out of, and within the West Bank and Gaza, with dramatic consequences for all aspects of Palestinian life.[33] The right to education for many has been systematically undermined and violated, with movement of teachers and pupils constrained by checkpoints and closure and regulated by Israeli-issued permits, which are routinely denied. Since 2004, Israel has banned Palestinian students in Gaza from studying at institutes of higher education in the West Bank and Israel. Palestinians in Gaza seeking to travel abroad to pursue disciplines not available in Gaza have also been prevented from leaving, including a number who had been awarded Fulbright scholarships to study in the United States.[34] In the West Bank, the national character of many universities is being eroded by travel and movement restrictions.

Levels of violence have spiraled, including both isolated spikes, for example, raids into refugee camps or targeted assassinations of persons wanted by Israel, and more protracted military operations such as the recent war on Gaza, Operation Defensive Shield in the West Bank in 2002, and more recent inter-Palestinian clashes in Gaza. As well as direct physical and material losses—313 children were killed in Gaza during Operation Cast Lead, according to the Palestinian Centre for Human Rights, and 181 schools partially or totally destroyed[35]—these exact high social and psychological costs for pupils, teachers and families, with deleterious immediate and longer-term consequences.

The past decade has also seen an escalation of attacks on the Palestinian national curriculum, whose introduction coincided with the start of the second Intifada. In its most legitimate form, scrutiny of the curriculum has helped to promote constructive debate on the politics of textbooks, including the appropriate framing of history for Palestinian schoolchildren and the role of education in promoting peace and shaping national identity. Unfortunately, the focus of debate has often moved beyond purely scholarly considerations, with various pressure groups framing Palestinian textbooks as a source of conflict, designed to promote violence and incite hatred of Israel. The allegations and accompanying advocacy campaigns have been used to discredit the Palestinian Authority (PA) and also formed part of an effort to undermine international support for UNRWA. This is despite the fact that independent research has concluded that allegations are based on claims that are "tendentious and highly misleading," and that, notwithstanding some elements of imbalance, the overall orientation of the Palestinian curriculum is "peaceful, despite the harsh and violent realities on the ground."[36]

In some cases, education providers have been able to negotiate some of the physical and administrative obstacles created by the second Intifada, or at least limit their effects. This includes the reassignment of teachers to schools nearer their homes, the introduction of remedial learning and recreational programmers, and the provision of free stationery and meals to poor students.[37]

Efforts to improve the quality of education have also continued. The PA has persisted with an ambitious program of reform, with the World Bank recently commending the remarkable advances made since the start of the second Intifada.[38] Despite campaigns by its detractors, independent research has also highlighted the constructive and systematic steps taken by the PA to constantly reform and improve the curriculum, including focusing on faculties of critical thinking and creative thinking and promoting concepts of human rights, democracy, and pluralism. For its part, UNRWA has introduced a human rights, conflict resolution, and tolerance curriculum in its schools, integrated into lesson plans, with children as young as five learning the principles, history, and core values of international human rights instruments.

There are also indications that Palestinian families have developed a fairly sophisticated armory of coping strategies to adapt to the new reality, reflecting a continuing, even heightened commitment to education over the past decade. Data from the Palestinian Central Bureau of Statistics show that educational attendance among both males and females has increased at every stage of the education process in Gaza and West Bank since 2000, despite the decreasing ability of parents to support their children's higher education. Research has identified an association between investment in education and the loss of unskilled wage labor opportunities in Israel due to closures.[39]

At the same time, the protracted crisis in the occupied Palestinian territory is also limiting the resources and attention that service providers can devote to education, given other competing priorities. Over the past decade, donor funding has been increasingly directed toward humanitarian relief and—in the case of the PA—the budget support that it needs to ensure its survival, at the expense of more strategic, longer-term, and productive development investment. UNRWA expenditure data in the West Bank, for example, indicates that more was spent on relief activities—including food aid, cash assistance and temporary employment programmers—than education between 2002 and 2010.

In addition, recent testing in UNRWA schools points to significant drops in educational performance. Although efforts are underway in both Gaza and West Bank to address this through remedial actions and recovery plans, the longer-term consequences of today's protracted crisis on education—those leaving UNRWA schools at the time of writing had barely begun their first grade when the Intifada erupted—will not be fully understood for several years. And while the PA and UNRWA have so far been able to successfully defend themselves against attacks on the integrity of the material used in their classrooms, these campaigns have nonetheless been extremely damaging, particularly in terms of their shaping of the negotiations agenda and diverting attention away from evidently more pressing issues.

Conclusion

The history of UNRWA's education system, and that of Palestinian education in general, is peppered with crises and emergencies that continue to the present day. The attacks on UNRWA schools in Gaza described in the opening paragraphs of this chapter echo similar destruction wrought during the 1967 war; and just as Israel banned the entry of Egyptian textbooks to Gaza in the aftermath of that war, so today it places restrictions on the passage of paper and educational materials, including those concerning UNRWA's human rights curriculum.[40] From direct obstacles such as bans on entry of supplies and enforced closure of schools to indirect hindrances created by closures and checkpoints, the education system itself has often been thrust to the very center of the conflict. This is particularly the case in the occupied Palestinian territory, where the role of education in the formation of national identity, the framing of historical narratives, and the peace process itself remains under intense scrutiny, sometimes for political ends.

Its experiences mirror those of the Palestinian population as a whole over the past sixty years, and indeed "Palestinian education" bears many of the hallmarks of dispossession and statelessness. As the relationship with both the Gulf and Israeli labor markets has shown, investment in higher education has typically been geared less toward national Palestinian economic needs than those of regional markets. The economic fruits of education have been similarly exported, leaving Palestinian families and communities exposed to exogenous and repeated shocks—most recently, the loss of access to Israeli markets and debilitating obstacles to normal economic activity has generated an employment crisis of unprecedented magnitude for Palestinians in the Gaza Strip and West Bank.

In a similar manner, the debate and very content of the Palestinian curriculum is reflective of the complexity of Palestinians' unresolved struggle for statehood and the sometimes uncomfortable relationship between on-the-ground realities and accepted principles of international law. This relationship often borders on the perverse, as shown by the notion of teaching future generations of Palestinians the value and primacy of the very rights and laws that the international community denies them on a daily basis.

When considering these constraints, challenges, and controversies, we should not allow our attention to be diverted from the transformative role played by education, and UNRWA's programs in particular, on successive generations of Palestine refugees over the past sixty years. This has ensured social, if not economic, progress that more closely resembles Western European states in the aftermath of the Second World War than that of neighboring Arab states in the immediate postcolonial period. Despite the efforts of pressure groups and detractors to shape public opinion to the contrary, education programmers have also made a significant contribution to stability and state building across the region. Ongoing national Palestinian curriculum reform efforts, as well as UNRWA's dedicated human rights and conflict resolution programs are testament to the vitality of this contribution.

These achievements should not be overlooked by those involved in the latest phase of peace-making diplomacy in the region. As the protracted socioeconomic crisis in the occupied Palestinian territory highlights, it is increasingly clear that any successful political plan must be accompanied with a development and economic plan of the vision and ambition of UNRWA's early years, founded on the successful education system that exists there. This is essential for meeting the future economic needs of Palestinians—both refugees and non-refugees—and ensuring that at times of peace as at war they are able to continue contributing to the productive development of the region.

Reflections from 2012

In recent years, education systems across the Middle East, including in the countries where UNRWA operates, have come under increasing scrutiny. Decried by policy makers, academics and economists alike as failing to equip pupils with the skills needed to compete in an increasingly global and knowledge-based economy, the poor quality of schools has been viewed as symptomatic of deeper societal and public policy failings.

International testing (Trends in International Mathematics and Science Survey—TIMSS) has given a good deal of credence to this criticism.[41] Although enrollment rates have improved dramatically in recent years, recent data suggest that the quality of schooling is often poor, with pupils in Middle Eastern countries falling behind their peers in other global regions.

Spurred on by declining quality in its own schools, in October 2011 UNRWA launched an ambitious set of reforms designed to improve the quality of its education services.[42] Their evolution coincided with a period of extraordinary transformation in the Middle East. The tumultuous events of the Arab Spring, sparked off by the self-immolation of Tunisian market vendor Mohammed Bouazizi in December 2010, have seen momentous change, in countries as far apart as Tunisia to Yemen. These upheavals have placed young people at the very heart of political and development agendas across the region.

Although Palestine refugees have not participated in the protests—directed primarily at ruling parties and state authority—we would be wise to consider their needs and aspirations through the lens of the Arab Spring. Like their peers in other Middle Eastern countries, refugee youth are often disproportionately affected by poverty, unemployment, and exclusion, socially, politically and economically disempowered.

It is therefore particularly opportune that UNRWA is seeking to reform its education programs and deepen its engagement with young refugees at this pivotal moment. In so doing, and particularly through support to refugee youth—a growing share of the Palestinian population, whose needs have sometimes been neglected in the Millennium Development Goal era—UNRWA is retreading a development path that yielded such successes during the organisation's formative years. It is vital that these reforms bear fruit.

What Can Modern Society Learn from Indigenous Resiliency?

Margareta Wahlstrom

The Global Platform on Disaster Risk Reduction in 2011 found that "a lot of knowledge about climate adaptation is not reaching those who need it the most." How much more of a challenge is it, then, to get information, good practices, and capacity-building tools into the hands of indigenous communities using non-mainstream languages, so that they can adapt what has been learned to their ways of life? This challenge is alluded to in the international blueprint for disaster risk reduction agreed and endorsed by all United Nations Member States, the Hyogo Framework for Action (HFA), which prioritizes the use of knowledge, innovation, and education to build a culture of safety and resilience at all levels. The HFA Hyogo Framework Priority No. 3 recommends "Provid[ing] easily understandable information on disaster risk and protection options, especially to citizens in high-risk areas, to encourage and enable people to take actions to reduce risk and build resilience. The information should incorporate relevant traditional and indigenous cultural heritage and be tailored to different target audiences, taking into account cultural and social factors."

It is well recognized among policymakers and academics that indigenous peoples are more vulnerable than most to the factors driving risk such as poverty, bad planning, poor governance, prejudice, environmental degradation, and forced migration to cities and towns. Indigenous people also have something to teach modern communities about resilience and practices that protect environment and the community. However, many indigenous communities, pushed to the limits of their traditional lifestyles, have changed and may also adopt harmful practices that impact negatively on ecosystems for their survival.

Another important reality check is "scaling up." In a continuous search for viable alternatives to the consumer patterns that deplete natural resources and increase vulnerability, traditional practices offer inspiration to explore methods, but on a scale that is limited in space and habitat. The challenge is to find out how and what can be scaled up to apply to today's urban communities that are different socially and economically from the indigenous communities.

Indigenous communities in many ways define resilience. How else would you describe a community that has preserved its institutions and ways of life over centuries other than as resilient? Yet, in other aspects, indigenous peoples, numbering some 370 million in ninety countries, are among the most vulnerable to natural and human-made hazards.

Some of the most disaster-prone countries in the world are also countries in which the indigenous people are a significant percentage of the overall population. The Instituto Indigenista Interamericano reckons that indigenous people constitute 66 percent of the population in Guatemala, 63 percent in Bolivia, and 40 percent in Peru and Ecuador.

The range and intensity of hazards faced by indigenous communities is increasing with climate variability and more freak and extreme weather events. The Navajo Nation, for instance, is facing one of the longest droughts in recorded history, while at the other end of the extreme, Pacific Islanders face the challenges of rising sea levels and increasingly intense typhoons.

As in all communities around the world, vulnerability to hazards among indigenous peoples is inextricably linked to socioeconomic development choices. The locations and structures that indigenous people live in may contribute to the risks. In too many indigenous communities development choices are not the community's choices. The forest fires that plague the peoples of Borneo—destroying crops and damaging health—can often be traced to large-scale land conversion. In other countries, forced relocation and dispossession has pushed people onto unfamiliar and inhospitable lands. And it is not a coincidence that indigenous lands are often selected as sites for toxic waste dumps. Socioeconomic drivers of risk such as extreme poverty, environmental degradation, and limited access to health care are pervasive in many indigenous communities.

Still it would be wrong to cast indigenous people as helpless victims because their endurance tells us that is not the case. Often theirs is the story of survival through adversity. So, how can this resilience be explained? Equipped with knowledge accumulated through generations of observation, many indigenous communities benefit from the hard-learned lessons of their ancestors. Some have resulted in resilient building designs that have withstood blowing winds and trembling earth.

The government of Bhutan, for example, has undertaken to examine their own construction practices and to learn from other cultures and share their insights internationally. In some cases, this entails blending the old with the new. In India, advice on bringing out the best of different knowledge systems and building disaster-resilient structures is available in the Guidelines for Earthquake Resistant Non-Engineered Construction report; such approaches exemplify the principal of doing more with less.[1]

In many indigenous communities, the accumulated knowledge stems from intimate observation of their environment. Native Hawaiians, for example, have long been able to identify dozens of types of winds and storms, even anticipating what we now recognize as the onset of the El Niño–Southern Oscillation. Local knowledge saved the lives of many villagers on the island of Simulue during the 2004 Indian Ocean tsunami. It is no surprise that when indigenous Dayak community leaders designed a training program for fire prevention in Borneo, they set "learning to observe local forest and temperature conditions" as the first learning objectives.

One of the distinguishing features of resilience is found in the ways that communities recover. Indigenous communities have strong adaptive capacities. Extensive and enduring social networks that bind communities provide the foundations of a social safety net. The ways that indigenous communities establish networks are translated into broader national and international settings. Grassroots and indigenous women first met in Antigua, Guatemala, for example, in 2008 and shared their experiences in making their communities less vulnerable to disasters. They drafted a document outlining their plans for increased cooperation among themselves and for greater participation in the disaster risk reduction plans of their respective governments. This is a very practical example of how indigenous knowledge can be immediately transformed into learning for the wider society.

The history of indigenous peoples includes periods of resistance and cooperation with populations that have sought to dominate them. Article 3 of the United Nations Declaration on the Rights of Indigenous Peoples states, "Indigenous peoples have the right to self-determination. By virtue of that right they freely determine their political status and freely pursue their economic, social and cultural development." Indigenous peoples have long struggled for the right to say no to shortsighted development schemes and to promote their own approaches to development. Determination of balanced approaches to growth and development is not a right held exclusively by indigenous peoples.

The cultural diversity of the world's indigenous peoples is an asset to us all in our various efforts to build resilient communities and nations. Diverse ways of life, values, and knowledge systems can reduce our collective fragility and, in fact, enrich us. It is, however, important to base this on the understanding that the right of indigenous populations to participate in the economic and social progress of countries is a fundamental one—and a necessary starting point.

PART VI

Exit Strategies

After the immediate challenges of disasters are addressed survivors need to regain a sense of security, reuniting families and rebuilding community structures. This process should begin as soon as a relief program is developed for vulnerable, displaced people, whether they are in refugee camps, forced to migrate, or, hopefully, been able to return to their own homes. It must be done with generosity of spirit and fully understanding the scars of loss. To prepare traumatized populations for the transition back to normal lives requires an enduring respect for their own customs and traditions. One must promote a sense of justice coupled, if at all possible, with forgiveness. All this is part of an exit strategy that should be part of the planning at the very start of every humanitarian assistance mission.

In this section are philosophic and practical suggestions to accomplish the goal of realizing as seamless a transition from crisis to stability.

To Bind Our Wounds

A One-Year Post-9/11 Address

Kevin M. Cahill, M.D.

Throughout the centuries, those who survive disasters have offered memorials to the dead, and they have done so with different tools and different skills: Picasso did it for the victims of Guernica with oil paints. Verdi mourned the poet/patriot Manzoni with a musical masterpiece. Graveyards and public squares are full of sculpture and architecture dedicated to those we loved and those we honor as fallen heroes. Many of us, however, still record our losses and deepest sorrows with words.

I've always been fascinated by words, by the challenge of trying to capture an essence in a well formed phrase, an image in the structure of a sentence, and then molding the flow of words so that ideas and coherent arguments emerge. There is something very satisfying—something almost inherently good—in identifying words, simple sounds with meaning, to link our most personal inner feelings with external facts and events. We create words that can withstand the pressures of reality and sustain us on our journeys of discovery into the private depths of our souls as well on our sometimes even more perilous excursions into contact with other human beings and nature itself.

I'm not sure that my memory of last September 11 and the weeks thereafter is as comprehensive as I would have liked in preparing this special memorial address. But I vividly recall the verbal reaction at the time—a moral certainty on the part of leaders summarized in words suitable for centers of religious worship, or "sound-bites" for the current church of the masses, the evening television shows. They offered a global philosophy based on words from a simpler era—a "you're either with us or against us" view of the world. But wrapping oneself in a flag, or invoking God to justify aggression and preemptive strikes, seemed to me a rhetoric disconnected from the complex world I knew, a world of diversity and rich but varying values and traditions that simply could not be forced into a single mold.

A few months ago, when I was asked to deliver this talk, I thought how apt it would be to go back 138 years and quote from the Gettysburg Address. As all of you now know, that brief, beautiful memorial is being recited today by the Governor and the President, and, it seems, by every public official of every political party in every State of the Union. So I read further in Lincoln's biography and realized that for this September 11 anniversary program at Lenox Hill Hospital, it would be far more appropriate to cite a few lines from Lincoln's Second Inaugural Address. These provide the framework for my talk.

At his Second Inaugural, as the Civil War was grinding to a bloody close, President Lincoln used the words of medicine to help prepare a battered nation for a time of healing, of reconciliation, and reconstruction. The war had been pursued with firmness, and there were many who wanted to wreak vengeance on, and demand total submission from, the vanquished. Lincoln, however, urged his audience to "bind up the nation's wounds" and "to care for him who shall have borne the battle, and for his widow and his orphans."

That is our privileged role every day in medical life—to bind wounds, to care for the afflicted. Today, it is from this solid foundation that I suggest we must develop the courage to move beyond the traditional restraints of our profession. We must share our wisdom and experience for the sake of our nation, as it once again struggles in a search for a way out of a war mentality and towards a new era of peace.

We should also learn from Lincoln that the way forward cannot be based merely on violence against violence. In fact, if our society is ever to regain security and tranquility, there is no safe way forward based on vengeance and no possible way if we fail to see—and address—the wrongs that prompted our adversaries to their actions. In that Second Inaugural Address, at the end of a bitter and long conflict, wearily but wisely, President Lincoln said that the only way forward was "with malice towards none, and with charity towards all."

For almost a century and a half after Lincoln spoke these simple, profound words, our nation was spared the physical and psychological effects of an assault on our shores. Will we listen today to the wisdom of Lincoln, to the strong, but forgiving, caring, and gentle President, or will we attempt to memorialize our dead by assuring more dead in an endless cycle of violence? Health workers are among the most respected members in our society and we have, I believe, an opportunity—as well as an obligation—to rekindle Lincoln's spirit in a scarred nation in danger of being isolated in its own pain.

In this solemn memorial, we do not gather here today only as individuals or as citizens, but as members of the Lenox Hill Hospital family, with vivid images of those tense days a year ago permanently seared in our minds. I am certain that most of you who work in this building can recall the almost surreal weeks that followed last September 11.

The streets around our hospital were filled with desperate people searching for their missing, with the walls and doors around the emergency room covered with photographs of the almost certainly dead. In the evening one could hear, as the crowds thinned, the silent cry of the anguished. And then Lenox Hill Hospital became the scene of a fatal bioterrorist assault, with pulmonary anthrax snuffing out the life of one of our own family. Most of you can also recall the lines of frightened and confused employees waiting to receive their prophylactic antibiotic supply from the Department of Health. Although the initial cutaneous anthrax cases at NBC did not require inpatient care in our hospital, many of you know that I diagnosed those first two cases and was in close contact with our medical and laboratory colleagues. Our hospital, located in the very heart of New York, cared for one sixth of the entire national number of anthrax cases.

"Ground Zero" was not merely the dramatic rubble where the World Trade Center once stood. It was a newly vulnerable city. With anthrax, we discovered how fear could paralyze a society as efficiently as missiles. Anthrax, never previously seen by most physicians, was now a topic to be taught to interns and residents. Yet, as health workers must, every day of our lives, we learned and adapted.

In fact, I believe that medicine's age old tradition to learn from failure, to constantly adapt, to modify therapies in the daily battle with disease, offers a model for a way out of our current national morass. Medicine offers a unique way of looking at problems, a way that now seems almost absent in our country's political lexicon. The discipline of medicine reflects a capacity to see and study disaster, and not to waver, but to discover new approaches—even if progress must come in the autopsy room—and to think afresh, every day, on chronic, intractable, sometimes uniformly fatal diseases.

So today, as we all remember the destruction and deaths caused by terrorists, and some sadly reflect on their own personal losses, we must also use the occasion to recommit ourselves to applying the noble heritage of medicine to the ills of society. I believe there are fundamental contributions that the medical community can offer our nation today.

Medicine and public health provide a common language, understood all over the world, and a philosophic approach that has sustained humanity's ageless search for healing without causing further damage, for respecting all wounded regardless of their affiliations or viewpoints, for creating calm and order from chaos, for promoting peace where there was war. The methodology of public health may provide a new and imaginative way to solve problems in the far less specific arenas of diplomacy and public policy. At the very least, such an approach offers a badly needed balance to the current national emphasis of trying to address our problems solely with overwhelming force. In his Nobel Prize acceptance speech, William Faulkner said the will of man is "not merely to endure but to prevail." But we need not prevail over someone else. Rather, we must learn to prevail with and through others. Only in that way will our society realize that growth and development can be achieved without destruction, and that we, in a field devoted to helping and healing, may hold the answer to a future based on mutual security and safety.

Wanton killing and brutality within supposedly sovereign borders, ethnic and religious strife, millions of starving or near starving refugees, other millions of migrants fleeing their homes out of fear for their lives or in a desperate search for a better life, human rights trampled down, appalling poverty in the shadows of extraordinary wealth, inhumanity on an incredible scale in what was supposed to be a peaceful dawn following the fall of the Berlin Wall: these are the awesome challenges that face us just as much as the hidden terrorists determined to destroy our way of life. The challenges are quite different from the nation-state rivalries and alliances that preoccupied statesmen during most of the past century. They call for earlier diagnoses and new kinds of therapy. Underlying causes have to be attacked sooner rather than later, before they become fulminating infections that rage beyond rational control or political containment.

Almost five hundred years ago, in a small book that remains a classic text, Machiavelli employed analogies with health in explaining a fundamental tenet of governance. He wrote:

> When trouble is sensed well in advance, it can easily be remedied; if you wait for it to show, any medicine will be too late because the disease will have become incurable. As the doctors say of a wasting disease, to start with it is easy to cure but difficult to diagnose; after a time, unless it has been diagnosed and treated at the outset, it becomes easy to diagnose but difficult to cure. So it is in politics.

It seems to me there are several important lessons in that quote. The shrewd and cynical Machiavelli knew that health images would help make his message clear to a skeptical public, and he wisely noted that politics is part of life. Most physicians have shied away from politics. We need not be ashamed of, and should not be hesitant to become involved in, political life. Our health profession has so much to offer that is rare in public life today. At its best, medicine, as a way of life, can provide some of those almost forgotten standards on which our fragile society must ultimately rely in its endless struggle for stability, prosperity, and peace.

Ancient principles guide the discipline of clinical medicine—qualities we take for granted such as confidentiality, discretion, honesty, integrity, respect for other's bodies and minds, whether those be beautiful or, in the eyes of the world, diseased and deformed. It is in the daily application of clinical medicine's unique mix of art and science that we win the respect and honor that is ours. And it is by using this stature and credibility that we can influence public policy above and beyond our own profession.

On this first anniversary of a terror filled day, it behooves us to remember the universality of tragedy and disaster, and also, very importantly, to recall the global outpouring of sympathy for America after September 11. That brief shared identity, a spontaneous warm international reaction, a solidarity that money couldn't buy, it seems to me, holds something precious for the future. There is nothing shameful or weak in admitting our pain. It is a reality doctors and nurses deal with every day, one that allows patient and health worker to become one in the battle against illness. So, too, can a proud nation, wounded and hurt, grow stronger and better if we recognize in tragedy the chance for new foundations. If we do not grow from our pain, all will be wasted in an arrogant selfish isolation, fueled by the evil fear of other colors and religions.

Those who suffer, and are rejected, are the predictable perpetrators of future terrorist attacks, and no amount of counterintelligence or preemptive attacks will stamp out these huge populations. If health workers have the skills to heal individuals, as well as the tools to stop epidemics and even eliminate diseases from the face of the earth, then we should not—in fact we cannot—absent ourselves from this new war on terrorism, a war with no apparent end and few definable borders. New solutions are obviously needed, and they may lie, silently and unappreciated, in the rich traditions of our profession.

Many years ago, in the midst of a raging civil war in South Sudan, I participated in humanitarian actions that opened doors to negotiated settlements. Even in the midst of armed conflict, neutral and impartial immunization efforts for children were begun. These programs created corridors of tranquility and understanding that led to de facto cease-fire periods and, eventually, became permanent bridges to peace.

Since that time I have worked with humanitarian and diplomatic leaders around the world, and today there is a growing consensus that the failed approaches of the past will inevitably fail again. Power politics and military actions may provide transient solutions; but, to be lasting, these efforts must be coordinated with health and human rights and educational improvements. Health workers are, therefore, major partners if peace is to be realized, and we must assume new responsibilities in a world where another failure may prove to be the final act of civilization. In my book *Preventive Diplomacy*, the somewhat immodest subtitle is *Stopping Wars Before They Start*. But, for everyone's sake, that is what we must try.

In a small examining room in my medical office there is a painting of an American flag done by an Irish artist. Many years ago, the artist, sitting on the porch of our home and looking at our national flag, suddenly said "do you not see the heart in the stars?" I share this image because it captures so much of what I feel today.

America demonstrated its heart in remarkable ways in the period after the September 11 attacks. We all know the stories of those who rescued the disabled and then went back into the burning World Trade Center buildings to save their fellow workers. We know of the heroic work of police and firefighters, and one had only to see, as I did, the people in the command center and down at the Ground Zero site to know that America has a very big heart indeed. We saw this spirit at Lenox Hill Hospital after the anthrax attacks.

America demonstrated a heart that we may have always known was there but, as is our fashion, was too rarely exposed. It is critically important today that the world understand that America is a nation of caring and compassion. If we are perceived as only a military power that will seek only vengeance, then violence and retribution will inevitably continue. For many years, I have been, as my wife sometimes suggests, obsessed with the idea that health and humanitarian affairs ought to be central in our foreign policy, not peripheral afterthoughts. We have failed, as a great nation, to let the outside world understand the goodness of our people, to be as proud of America's "heart in the stars" as we are of our undoubted strength.

Persisting in our current national responses to the attacks of last September 11, responses that are predictable, and even understandable, but tragically limited, will assure a perpetuation of threats and violence against Americans everywhere. Is it not obvious that we must expand our options, create bold new initiatives that address all aspects of a complex crisis that is now endangering America's heart and soul as well as its physical body?

We can, as Lyndon Johnson once said, walk and chew gum at the same time. An earlier President, Harry Truman, noted that he was good at making decisions when there were no alternatives. Choosing to continue reacting with only military might, abandoning the very foundations on which this great nation was built, indulging in gross violations of human rights and dignity for the illusion of safety is not—and should not—be an alternative. We have lived through an incredible year, one that has bound us together as never before. It is important that we go forth in confidence, and in love, using the power of the mind and the heart, and the mores of medicine, to secure a more united and safe America and a better world.

I have been honored by your invitation to speak at this memorial ceremony among my colleagues and friends. May God bless all of you, especially this hospital family, and may God bless America.

—Lenox Hill Hospital, New York, 9/11/2002

The Transition from Conflict to Peace

Richard Ryscavage, S.J.

Humanitarian assistance workers may find themselves hopelessly confused by the range of problems facing a society struggling to move from war to peace. These problems can be approached from many directions: the shift from emergency relief into longer-range development assistance; the religious, cultural, and psychosocial models for dealing with trauma, recovery, and reconciliation; conflict management and conflict resolution methods; the place of civil society organizations; the challenges of refugee repatriation and internally displaced people; the role of international peacekeepers and outside military forces; the connection between peace, democracy, and development.

This chapter will survey the various approaches and try to organize them into levels and "lenses" that, depending on where the humanitarian actor is in the process, he or she may find a helpful starting point for analysis and action.

Conflict to Peace: Some Basic Questions

Most humanitarian actors make the basic assumption that peace is good and war is bad. By all means, at certain levels a peaceful world seems preferable to a planet torn by violence. Yet too much emphasis on peace for its own sake can block the paths to peace. Many people, not just rich people, profit immensely from war. Economics on a wartime footing can be much more productive than peacetime economies. So simply from the socioeconomic perspective, a quick transition from war to peace may not be in the best interests of a society. It is always useful to stand back from a violent conflict and do a cost-benefit analysis. Who benefits from this war? Who bears the most costs?[1]

More importantly, the process of moving from war to peace is almost never a straight line. The process has a more cyclical nature characterized by one step forward and two steps back. Large-scale violent conflict might end, but smaller sporadic outbursts of violence can continue for many years. A fragile peace agreement can quickly break down, and an even more violent stage of conflict erupts. So in general it is not very useful to view the transition from war to peace as a continuum. In some senses peace begins to emerge in the midst of violence, and violence can emerge even when peace seems rather secure. This is the reason Johan Galtung and other peace theorists have argued for years that peace-building must begin before the conflict ends.[2]

How one builds peace in the midst of violence can be addressed only by looking at the various actors or potential actors: military, guerillas, governments, UN, local nongovernmental organizations, international nongovernmental organizations. Peace-building actions must be tailored to the nature of the specific actor. For example, the military is not trained for nation building and strengthening democracy. Similarly, a humanitarian NGO should not be expected to provide security or disarm warring parties.

From the perspective of most UN Member States and most nongovernmental humanitarian actors, the transition from violent conflict to social peace requires international assistance designed to strengthen local socioeconomic and cultural development. It does this by helping societies recover from war and limiting future violence.

This mission seems more straightforward than it actually is. The approach rests on the assumption that socioeconomic and cultural development is good. Many ecologists would challenge that assumption. "Sustainable development" can damage the local small market economy and make people more, not less, vulnerable.[3] The policy also presumes some rather long-term commitments and relationships with the international community.

Most international politicians and military people are hesitant to lock themselves into a long-range development for peace strategy. Overall, though, the current consensus seems to be that the transition from violent conflict to peace must be addressed through a development perspective.

Relief to Development Model

In the classic vocabulary of humanitarian assistance there are three phases: relief, rehabilitation, and development. These three phases often involve different goals, skills, agendas, and ways of operating. Yet there is much controversy over the actual boundaries between the three phases. Conflict resolution, education and peace strengthening can be aspects of all phases, but the limits of each phase must be respected if the peace activity is to have any chance of success.

Relief

Relief usually means the earliest operations phase of assistance. Sometimes the term is qualified by saying "emergency relief." Although the development phase might be characterized by considerable governmental controls and the involvement of multilateral organizations, the relief phase is dominated by private international and local voluntary organizations. A high-profile crisis can generate millions of dollars in government and private donations for immediate relief. Hundreds—even thousands—of NGOs will try to jockey for a piece of the relief money.[4] This relief aid may not often fit well with the longer-range development needs of a country.

Beginning in the early 1990s governments and private donors began shifting most of their humanitarian assistance away from development into relief aid.[5] Not only were the emergency needs in places like Rwanda and the Balkans enormous, but also they were well publicized. So large amounts of private short-term donations reduced the perceived need for long-term budgetary commitments.

It was in the context of post-genocide Rwanda and the war in the Balkans that the term "complex emergency" arose. It is a useful term because it highlights the fact that certain humanitarian disasters are multidimensional. In essence it refers to civil war, manmade disasters, political chaos, and power struggles that accompany and cause a humanitarian crisis. Because the need for emergency food or water exists in the middle of violent conflict and complicated political and military maneuvering, the road out of that emergency stage will be equally complex.[6]

Rehabilitation

Rehabilitation is a kind of midway stage between relief and development activities. It has a very important role to play in peace-building. Rehabilitation usually means activities that restore basic services (water, electricity, schools, and health clinics), rebuilding houses and roads, and restoring some agricultural production and normal economic life.[7]

In many situations the most important rehabilitation activity will be the process of demilitarization, including de-mining. To strengthen a budding peace process and to proceed with social and economic reconstruction, it is essential to neutralize weapons stocks, disarm the irregular forces, and find jobs for the demobilized army youth. For medical, agricultural, and social reasons, de-mining becomes an urgent need. It has been shown that mine clearance is an activity that tends to foster national reconciliation by involving formerly hostile parties in the mutually beneficial task of identifying and clearing mines. De-mining is an example of how building peace can be integrated into social reconstruction during the period of rehabilitation.[8]

It is within the rehabilitation phase that human rights and legal issues of land ownership and justice can also begin to be addressed more systematically. This is particularly important where there is a problem of large-scale refugee repatriation or a situation where citizens have been displaced by war and now want to go home. If the "right of return" is not faced squarely, the fragile structures of peace will be threatened.

Sometimes coming home means rebuilding houses; more often it involves complicated legal, ethnic, and political issues, especially if people have been gone for a long period. One point is very clear: a refugee camp, by its nature, is not a place for social reconstruction and development. Refugee camps are set up for the convenience of governments, UN agencies and humanitarian workers. Camps are never in the long-term interest of the refugees themselves. One way or another, refugees and displaced people need to settle permanently somewhere before lasting peace can be established.

Development

In recent decades, thanks to globalization and with little thanks to traditional foreign aid, global poverty has been falling quite rapidly in many parts of the world. Globalization is primarily an economic process supported by new technology that allows a country or a region to participate in a global capital market. Despite its clear success in raising billions of people out of poverty, globalization faces some of the same challenges as the older approaches to development.

Full-blown development stage has traditionally involved multilateral institutions such as the World Bank, International Monetary Fund, and the United Nations Development Program, which emphasize material assistance, building infrastructures, and sustaining bureaucracies. This approach tends to reinforce and strengthen the role of the state as the chief agent for development. But if the state is corrupt and poorly managed, development can be turned to the political and personal advantage of the leadership.

Certain forms of development that stress money, infrastructure, and state regulation may not contribute at all to the reconciliation of groups previously at war. On the other hand, turning over development responsibilities to the international nongovernmental organizations may result in greater accountability and transparency. But by circumventing the country government's ministries of education, health and state development external development aid will only weaken the state's long-term ability to provide essential national services.

Traditionally most economists have defined development as showing sustained economic growth over a period of time, which includes consistent improvement in living standards for the whole society. More recently, a broader concept of development has emerged that captures a multidimensional, more sophisticated understanding of development. Economic development is still a key factor but political, cultural, and spiritual development also become essential for full integral human development.[9] Through the wider lens, development would include promotion of democracy, human rights, protection of the environment, and social justice.[10]

Within the development stage, more direct attention is needed on psychological, cultural, and religious determinants of violence. Attention to behavior that disrupts peace and the continual reinforcement of confidence and trust building measures will be equally important. Even years after a war has ended, if peacebuilding does not continue, a new social cycle of violence can form, undermining everything that has been achieved.

The relief-rehabilitation-development continuum is a way of organizing our thinking about social problems. In reality the pure continuum does not exist.[11] In some cases these "phases" can be taking place at the same time in the same country. One section of the country—less touched by war—might be ready for some prime large-scale development programs while another section is still without clean water or enough food. Within the rehabilitation phase are activities that might be considered both relief and development.

The most important point for a humanitarian actor to consider is that the introduction of humanitarian assistance, no matter what phase, can have a direct long-term impact on the achievement of peace. Humanitarian assistance is never neutral. It always has political, social, economic, and cultural consequences. Peace-strengthening approaches can be consciously built into any humanitarian assistance action—even at the very earliest emergency phase. But peace-building measures must never be introduced uncritically.

Approaches to Peace

Over the past thirty years, the academic fields of peace research and conflict resolution studies have grown enormously. Diplomats, politicians, and humanitarian actors have been using methods derived from this research to facilitate the transition from violent conflict to peace.[12]

One can roughly divide the research into two approaches. One approach concentrates on the social psychological aspects of overcoming conflict. Emphasis is placed on the attitudes and perceptions of the parties to the conflict. Changing perceptions—usually though small group work—characterizes the methodology. Theoretically the participants then feed the changed perceptions back into the political and decision-making process. The other approach tends to concentrate on the operational environment. Changing structures can change behavior. By shifting the way we give assistance, peace can be strengthened.[13]

If evaluated carefully, both approaches can suggest ways of building peace during a period of transition. Churches, for example, have been active in convening small groups of people from opposing sides in order to foster reconciliation and reduce misperceptions. Sometimes referred to as "Track II" diplomacy, nongovernmental organizations have become involved in creating problem-solving "workshops" that bring together community leaders from various parties to a conflict. The long-term benefits and cultural relevance of these "workshops" are not yet clear. In the wrong hands they can also be heavily manipulative.[14]

Using a more structural approach, some humanitarian relief workers have been able to change the food distribution system in such a way that the more marginalized and least powerful members of a community are helped. The assumption often is that by "empowering" certain people, a more just social order can be promoted and, therefore, a stronger base on which to build peace. But there is also the inherent danger of "social engineering" by outsiders who do not understand the culture and who can inadvertently create tensions and promote violence.

The Role of Civil Society and the Military

"Civil society" is a term rarely used before 1990. But with the collapse of communism, the weakening of state governments, and the phenomenal growth of nonstate actors and nongovernmental organizations, the term has taken on a new salience in the field of social and political development, including peace-building. Most simply, civil society refers to the social "space" that lies between relationships derived from family obligations and relationships derived from obligations to the state. Civil society is the mediating structures between the family and the state. Like the term "nongovernmental organization," civil society is so broad a concept that it can mean anything from organized crime groups and labor unions to church congregations and women's social clubs. Everything that is not family and not state can fit into the category of civil society.[15]

Many observers believe that the hopes for peace in a society or region rest less with governments and more with members of civil society. The approaches to conflict resolution described in the following section are all based on the importance of activating civil society in the search for peace.[16]

The military has become an increasingly important actor in large complex humanitarian emergencies. Typically the political-diplomatic actors concentrate on prevention and peace settlements; the NGOs and the UN humanitarian agencies focus on delivering humanitarian assistance; and the military are charged with providing security and logistical support. Such a neat division of labor has often been more muddled.

The nature of modern warfare has changed. The classic wars were between sovereign states. More common today are so called "asymmetrical wars," where nation-state military forces are fighting nonstate actors such as Al Qaeda. Consequently applying the traditional international laws of war that were endorsed by sovereign states in order to protect civilians and to provide access to prisoners of war have become much more difficult.

Military presence and mandates can radically differ from place to place. The classic UN peacekeepers—as they still exist in places like Cyprus today—are there to separate the conflicting parties, at the request of the parties. But even as early as 1960 in the Congo, the UN peacekeepers took up a more aggressive role in deterring the secession of Katanga. The peacekeepers became peacemakers. But in the humiliations suffered by the UN peacekeeping force in Bosnia in the 1990s, where eventually NATO military had to step in, showed the confusion that exists around the use of UN military troops for purposes of peace. Sexual abuse and other scandals have clouded the reputation of UN peacekeeping forces. Yet it is hard to see how the use of some kind of military force can be avoided in complex violent situations. Even in the transition from war to peace, some form of military presence is often essential for maintaining security, monitoring cease-fires, clearing mines, and reopening bridges, roads, and airports.

For the humanitarian worker there is a continual problem of how to relate to the military in such a transitional situation. Humanitarian agencies have a very different organizational culture from the military. The potential for bad communications between them is high. There is a long and distinguished history of military involvement in humanitarian issues. Coordination is perhaps the most challenging aspect of the relationship between the military and humanitarian work. The military are used to a highly disciplined centralized operation; the NGOs often cannot speak with one voice or require a participatory decision-making process that is cumbersome. Efforts at peace-building can be stymied by this asymmetry unless conscious steps are taken to bridge the divide.[17] Regular communication and information sharing are critical.[18]

Although the military cannot be expected to take on major "nation-building" tasks, it can provide some important peace supports. Ideally, transnational rehabilitation activities should be planned with the military and within a long-term development context that includes strengthening local civil society groups that can contribute most to the peace. [19]

Spiritual Transformations and Reconciliation

Any serious social transition from war to peace must involve psychological, cultural, and spiritual transformation. In the secular realm of social psychology there is considerable literature in the West on recovery from social trauma.[20] Much less attention has been paid to the religious, cultural, and spiritual dimensions of the transition from war to peace. How, for example, does a deep-seated "culture of violence" become a "civilization of love"? Is such a transformation ever possible?[21] Cultures do change. Indeed, some would say that they are in the constant process of change. But to what extent should the promotion of cultural change be integrated into the plans and programs for transitional peace-building?

International humanitarian workers might feel uncomfortable even discussing these questions because someone outside the specific culture can never answer the questions. Yet sometimes it takes an outsider who has some "emotional distance" from the conflicts who can initiate a dialogue on reconciliation and forgiveness. Unfortunately most international humanitarian actors, even if they work for a faith-based organization, are rarely prepared to enter into this arena of peace-building.

Reconciliation is a profound multidimensional process that does not lend itself to easy analysis because often it involves very personal transformations. Sometimes in a postconflict situation the move toward reconciliation seems much too rushed and premature. Reconciliation does not replace the need for justice. Earlier I mentioned the workshops sponsored by churches that try to move a community toward the goal of reconciliation. But there is a need for more evaluative research on how successful these attempts have been.

Peace-Building Through Democracy

The thesis that democracies do not wage war against other democracies has received increased academic attention. It is sometimes referred to as the "democratic peace proposition." The causal link between democracy and peace may not be direct, but if the proposition is basically valid, then it would follow that the promotion of democracy should be a constitutive element of peace-building in a transitional society. What this practically would mean is the promotion of participatory institutions and processes both within the state governmental structure as well as in civil society.

External intervention, however, rarely succeeds in establishing a democratic culture. The impetus and the work must come from the society itself. Building the institutional structures for democracy may take decades. It is not something that can be imposed.[22] But humanitarian assistance in the transitional stage can in small incremental ways try to introduce some participatory decision making at the local level. International NGOs, for example, by establishing full-fledged partnerships with indigenous local NGOs can begin to support and spread participative institutions in a society.[23]

Conclusion

There is an endless supply of specific proposals for how best to anchor peace in a postwar society. Many projects, from "self-esteem" classes in Bosnia to "computer connectivity" sessions for children, have been suggested or tried. Sometimes, however, the success of a specific project or approach diverts us from the fact that most large-scale efforts at international peace-building over the past forty years have been miserable failures. The United States has spent trillions of dollars trying to establish secure environments and peaceful transitions to democracy in such places as prewar Vietnam, Somalia, Haiti, Iraq, and Afghanistan.[24] The government acted in partnership with hundreds of NGOs working on specific aspects of the transition. Although certain efforts may have contributed on a micro-level to peace-building, the overall effort did not fully succeed in any of these countries. What conclusion must we draw from these experiences?

Some major research argues that the transition to peace and the democratization of a country is almost entirely the product of domestic internal factors. Other analysts suggest that proactive forms of humanitarian and military intervention do not in any way prevent the recurrence of conflict in a postwar society.[25]

It would appear that externally engineered, even highly vigorous, peace-building programs are not enough to transform a country into a peaceful democratic, economically healthy society. Other conditions must be present. The people must truly want such social change and the culture must be ripe to receive it. As we witnessed in the "Arab Spring" uprisings in the Middle East, the people themselves must become the primary engine for change. As Harrington and Huntington put it in their book *Culture Matters*, "The core values of a society are what finally shape human progress. Those values can change and be changed, but that type of change comes slowly, and, though heavily influenced by international developments, the change must finally come from within the culture itself."[26]

We must face the challenges of humanitarian assistance in the transition from war to peace with a stronger sense of realism and a bigger dose of cultural humility.

Humanitarianism's Age of Reason

Ghassan Salamé

In postconflict situations, the first challenge is to identify the sequence of events preceding conflict resolution, and how one classifies what has apparently ended is of utmost importance. Was it really a conflict? Then, what kind of conflict was it? An international police operation, a foreign aggression, a regional war, a civil war, a state collapse, all of the above, none of the above? Depending on the answers to these questions, humanitarian conditions, popular perceptions, and the kind of postconflict settlement one should work to devise and implement are substantially different in each case.

The Germans at the end of World War II were in a completely different mindset from, say, the Somalis after the collapse of President Siad Barre's regime in 1991. Both cases could equally qualify as postconflict situations; actual needs and perceptions were, however, extremely different in an industrialized country, the epicenter of a world war, from what they were in a marginal underdeveloped one, torn apart by small armed gangs.

One of the most common misunderstandings that confound postconflict resolution is perspective: How do humanitarian agencies assess postconflict situations versus how do the nationals describe what they have been going through? We think our interlocutors are coming out of a civil war while they view themselves as victims of a foreign aggression; or we think they are happy because a dictatorship has fallen while they complain about the collapse of a reassuring order. We are compassionate with their past sufferings, but they seem happy to have won their battle against some enemy group. We are motivated by the immediate past, but they have a better, deeper, somehow obsessive, grasp of history. And, looking for immediate remedies to pressing problems, we easily become fed up with history, while our interlocutors seem to have made of it their single, possessive, teacher!

Hence one of the most immediate and unnerving challenges one faces, paradoxically, deals more with the past than with the future: How far in history must we walk back and which lessons should we draw, and for what use, today and tomorrow? The easiest answer I hear is, "let bygones be bygones, we are here to help you build another, brighter, future." Although such a stand is politically correct and definitely pragmatic, individuals and groups may think humanitarian workers despise their past, because they do not want to take it into consideration. Especially following civil wars, where to start in one's narrative is crucial because at some point one group was dominating the other, before having the latter take revenge. Once, in 1975, while visiting a small Christian village in a mainly Druze area in Mount Lebanon where the people were being asked to avoid buying arms and to eschew any kind of military confrontation with their (more numerous and better equipped) neighbors, I was told, "Last time we did not arm ourselves and we lost seventeen victims." "When was that?" I asked. A chorus of village dwellers replied, "In 1860!"

Given this information, three attitudes are thus possible for humanitarian agencies to assume. One can consciously or unconsciously listen too much to one party and end up adopting its narrative. In fact, I have encountered dozens of peacekeepers and humanitarian activists who are sometimes consciously, and at other times unconsciously, pure partisans of one party, repeating its narrative without restraint. This is a recipe for disaster that strips us of our credibility and makes us a party to the conflict. The second, opposite, attitude is to ignore the past, and concentrate on the future by basically telling your interlocutors, "Your past is your property, you deal with it as you wish, we are here to help you build your future." This is certainly a more prudent stand, but somehow naïve (in view of the groups' attachment to and pride in their own past) and somehow patronizing ("We are modern and you indulge in archaism"). The third and best attitude, in my view, though the most difficult as well, is to be as knowledgeable as possible about the past.

Making the effort to comprehend the history of the conflict sends a clear message that we really care about them, that we are able not only to listen, but able to develop solutions to partisan narratives of the past, that we know enough of what happened before we arrived to prevent a repetition of past tragedies. Such a perspective gives us a much better standing with the various parties. Being respectful and wise enough to study their history lends to a determination to help them build a new history, not because one is ignorant of key events but precisely because one knows them too well.

This has been confirmed by many studies on postconflict situations. A knowledge of history will help identify local actors, beyond the present, troubled circumstances, and improve our understanding of their reactions to our proposals, as well as improve our facilitation efforts. How many times have we been faced with local leaders shouting at us, "But here it is different!" Too much reliance on past experiences in conflict resolution can become an impediment in dialogue with

357

local actors. They may be ready to acknowledge that we have accumulated experience from other conflictual situations, but we also have to modestly acknowledge that no postconflict situations are really similar, that local conditions are crucial, and that our experience drawn from past involvements all over the world is only of relative value. Packages built on our past experiences are to be tested against the peculiarities of the local conditions and possibly forgotten when faced with a new challenge.

Our characterization of the latest conflict to date is therefore crucial. Those who went to Afghanistan in 1988 and described the situation there as mainly a post-foreign-occupation situation missed the complexities of the Afghan domestic tensions and rivalries underlying the occupation/liberation paradigm. Those who went to Iraq and missed the complex history of that country and their even more complex fabric of society remained prisoners of the dictatorship/democracy paradigm. This is important to realize, but is certainly not the exclusive or even the most important paradigm needed to build a better future for Iraq. The durability of the settlement will depend on a number of variables drawn from each country's history. Has there been a tradition of authoritarian rule or, on the contrary, a competition between an authoritarian rule and a parallel tradition of mutual accommodation among the warring groups? Were alignments dominated by ideological factors (as in the Greek or Spanish civil wars), by social and economic interests (as in many African civil wars), by identity issues (often the case in the civil wars in the Balkans and the Caucasus) or, more generally, by a sui generis combination of all these ingredients?

Politically, in Iraq, a postconflict situation was officially declared the day a statue of the past president fell down in one Baghdad square. But it soon appeared that, from a military point of view, Iraq was entering into a state of (geographically concentrated but nationally disrupting) insurgency that was to take the lives of many more Iraqis and foreign troops than the war itself. From a humanitarian point of view, Iraq was neither in a new conflict nor in a postconflict situation. Rather the conflict was in a stage of post-sanctions. One's view depends, of course, on perspective. I believe that politically, sanctions have been much more harmful to daily life than the successive wars that have hit the country or dictatorship itself.

Iraqis have known the taste of wars, harsh repression, and authoritarian nepotism long before Saddam, although he had practically three decades to excel in each of these fields, especially in his last decade in power. Still, the long years of UN-imposed sanctions appear to have been the most destabilizing factor in the Iraqis' daily life, public values, professional activity, and view of the world. Sanctions deconstructed a rather thriving economy and, more importantly, a lively, talented, upward-moving society. Sanctions produced a new, flawed, almost cynical and substantially arbitrary relationship between state and society.

Ask Iraqis when their country's infrastructure began to collapse. Ask them when their salaries lost 90 percent of their value. Ask them when lawlessness became rampant, when tribalism began to surge. Ask them when civil administration became widely inefficient and corrupt. Ask them when social ills such as prostitution, disinterest in education, and lack of solidarity among family members became evident. In all cases, they would answer almost invariably, "When the sanctions were imposed on our country." I dare to add that, twenty years from now, collective Iraqi memory will probably keep sanctions as the worst source of modern misery and sadness. They may differ on the identity of who to blame for that sudden misery: the fallen regimes, world powers, and even the UN. Iraqis still have yet to see how external, government and nongovernmental actors are integrating this factor in their approach to present-day Iraq.

Again, any generalization would be dangerous. Elsewhere sanctions might have been more useful in bringing about positive change without having the same devastating effects on the society (South Africa, for example). Mentioning sanctions leads to a wider issue—the proper characterization of the fallen regime. When leaders have been around for ten, twenty, or thirty years, they tend to operate within developed successive forms of rule and control. How many times were we told that the post-Kuwait, post-sanctions Saddam Hussein was radically different from the pre-1990 Saddam?

One has to develop a clear idea of the evolution of the fallen regime. In Iraq, Ba'athists would be the first to recognize that the regime that fell on April 9, 2003, was very different from the one their party had built in 1978 and even farther from the one they thought they would be building. The regime's last decade in power was indeed marked by a rapid, deep, disturbing deterioration of the state/society contract. The regular army had been sidelined and the regime was relying instead on a number of competing praetorian guards to protect itself. The party was weakened by tribal and semi-religious forms of mobilization that utterly contradicted the principles upon which the Ba'ath party had been established. Saddam's sons, too young to play a role before 1990, became the pillars of the latest configuration of power. Sectarianism, muted for a long time in view of the regime's secular orientation, became devastating after the savage quelling of the 1991 Shi'a intifada. Kurdish nationalism, for which Hussein himself was willing to give substantial concessions in the 1970 Status (something for which he had been criticized by many in the Ba'aths' own ranks), became radically different after the attack on Halabdja and the 1991 campaign of repression.

By ignoring the crucial fact that the regime that fell in 2003 was radically different from the one prewar American and British propaganda portrayed, as well as from what the regime had been at its inception, very serious major mistakes have been committed by the Coalition in the postwar era. These include a reckless disbandment of the army at a time when it could have been used in imposing law and order; a sweeping, indiscriminate, revengeful de-Ba'athification that fed the insurgency with new recruits and aggravated sectarian feelings; and a poorly inspired *tabula rasa* policy in public administration that disrupted the daily life of a weakened population.

Then comes a second, no less crucial question: When does a conflict *really* end and when does a postconflict situation *effectively* start? Of course, the line is blurred and there very rarely is a conflict that suddenly stops at a single point of time to be followed by peace. Uncertainty about the mere beginning of a postconflict situation is an organic ingredient of such a situation, and that is why we are generally unable to name it and content ourselves by saying, "This is the period that comes after a conflict is apparently over." Still, the question begs to be asked in Congo as well as in Sierra Leone, in Burundi as well as in Iraq. Is what we call postconflict a mere lull in the fighting? Is it only the passage from one sequence to the next in a chain of wars? Is an ongoing insurgency a mere sequel of the past or the first steps in a future wide-scale rebellion?

I witnessed a fifteen-year conflict in my home country of Lebanon. It was the case over and over that we would falsely think that we had reached a postconflict situation when militias were, in fact, preparing themselves for the next phase in their fighting, when foreign powers were preparing themselves for a new kind of interference, when arms dealers were secretly making new juicy contracts. I tend to believe that being truly in a postconflict situation should remain an open-ended question and not a foregone conclusion. More often than not, a postconflict situation is viewed by local actors as one in which winning parties try to consolidate their grip on power and resources and defeated groups prepare themselves for a new round of conflict, while neighboring countries reassess the situation. And, if any of the actors think that the new status quo is detrimental to their interests, they try to favor acts of destabilization directly or through proxies, which is why a postconflict situation for some may be seen as a preconflict one, as well.

Such a contrast in perceptions, of course, affects our willingness to invest in infrastructure rehabilitation, the selection of local interlocutors, and the timeframe of our mission, not to mention the very essence of that mission. Are we doing what can be done before the country enters a new phase of a protracted conflict or are we, on the contrary, starting to rebuild the country because fighting is over? Our analysis will have crucial personnel, financial, and programmatic effects.

But our analysis should always take into consideration the way nationals view their situation. Having ignored that in the past, a number of humanitarian missions have ended up indirectly, though substantially, helping armed groups prepare themselves for the next battle. This has especially been the case in Africa. For having mistaken a truce for a postconflict situation, a lot of people looked naïve to the local population and/or wasted precious resources on already doomed projects. Any humanitarian mission, in such uncertain times, needs to prepare for the worst while trying to persuade the communities that conflict, like all human endeavors, is not a fatality. Working with local communities, especially when people think that foreigners are better informed, means telling them the truth while encouraging them to seek and long for more peaceful times.

One should, however, never underestimate the fact that while reconstruction is important in and for itself, it is also a message of confidence in the future of peace. Postponing reconstruction does not only mean a delay in the rehabilitation of equipment or in restoring basic public services and utilities, it also implicitly means that foreigners (governments, international organizations, NGOs) are too skeptical concerning the country's immediate future or the chances for peace to invest energy and resources.

If only to avoid giving the locals such an impression, taking an uncertain bet on the future of peace is never too expensive: even in doubt about Israeli intentions, rebuild Gaza airport; even in fear of new fighting, build roads to connect cities in Congo; even when Taliban are active again, build the Kabul-Kandahar highway. A balance is, of course, to be found between available resources and the need to reassure locals of confidence in their immediate future. A haste to do things may squander one's funds, but too much reluctance will certainly fuel more pessimism and despair.

What is the situation in Iraq? Yes, it is a postconflict situation, which means that an invasion took place and that a regime change has been imposed. There are, however, reasons to believe that resisting the invasion was merely postponed by the fallen regime until the occupation was completed, because it knew it did have the means to oppose the progress of the US troops. Its leaders chose instead to make the invader's stay extremely costly, waiting to absorb the initial shock before launching counterattacks. The Coalition war on Iraq was not a conflict but a regime change by force. The regime collapsed and the Coalition tried to impose a post-Saddam order. In the process they unleashed new forms of insurgency against the new order, incited new forms of external interference by state and nonstate actors, and possibly opened the door to new forms of domestic instability. To be in a postconflict situation is an assumption, a bet on the Coalition's capabilities of imposing a post-Saddam order as well as a regime change that will benefit the Iraqis and produce a stable, prosperous new Iraq.

Hence a nagging issue: Should we in the UN help in imposing that order at the risk of antagonizing those who oppose foreign occupation? How do we label those who challenge the new order: resistors; insurgents; armed groups; terrorists? The same pointed question has been asked in post–Idi Amin Uganda, post-Taliban Afghanistan, and not to mention post-Saddam Iraq. Here again some conciliation between one's beliefs and the population's feelings is always necessary. One does not want to adopt their vocabulary but one can also not hurt them. I understand that humanitarian action seeks to avoid such issues as much as possible, but one has to understand that local communities can be highly interested in national politics and that this is, after all, a basic right of theirs.

They may think nationally, but one needs to work locally and expect some tension between the two outlooks, especially when rejection of a fallen regime does not automatically translate into an acceptance of foreign occupation, as is largely the case in Iraq. Those who thought that these two concepts were synonymous are still paying for their mistake. Anyone given the responsibility of managing a postwar situation should ask every morning, "Am I doing the right thing so that one conflict is not replaced by another? Am I stabilizing the country or helping fuel another war?" Poor postconflict management in Colombia (1957) led to a new civil war a few years later. Poor management of unity in Yemen between 1990 and 1994 led to a bloody North–South military confrontation. The conclusion of the Taïf Agreement in Lebanon induced an intra-Christian civil war in its wake. Poor management in Iraq led to fueling the insurgency ad infinitum. Most important is to remind oneself that past exclusion prone, predatory elites can sometimes be replaced by equally exclusion prone, predatory groups. Mobilization clichés against a rogue regime are of no use in dealing rationally with postconflict situations.

Reconciling differences of perspective between the victors of the conflict and the people who live in the supposed postconflict situation leads naturally to another concept. I have strong reservations on "creating leadership and governance." A more modest, and certainly more efficient, way of approaching local communities is first and foremost to identify forms of leadership that are already there. One may not be aware of existing leaders, may not like them, or may not share their views, but they are always there and often where unexpected: heads of tribes, clerics, recycled warlords, traditional urban notables. What does one do with them? Recognize them although one hates their politics? Challenge them by supporting contenders closer to one's heart? Try to weaken their impact among those one is helping?

A conceptual issue is central in this respect: Civil society is never exactly the one you think of. There has been a wide, and very debatable, infatuation with the concept that strengthening civil society institutions is, for many, the remedy to all ills. But is this really the case? In situations of state collapse (and many states are more or less in this situation), the most urgent task, precisely in order to protect the society, is to rebuild a state apparatus or at least to maintain the existing one and gradually, patiently, reform it.

No peaceful society can survive without a minimum of state institutions and politically recognized legitimate order. Many societies, torn apart by years of civil war, long principally for the restoration of legitimate authority as a prerequisite for the restoration of civil peace. What happened in Central and Eastern Europe cannot be transplanted everywhere. Where the state apparatus has been strong, well entrenched and totalitarian in nature, building up civil society organizations in postconflict eras is the primary task.

Elsewhere, indeed in most conflictual cases in Asia and Africa, the State's weakness is much more of a problem than an asset. Reinforcing the State becomes a popular demand and an objectively urgent task, as well. There is a thirst for a regularly operational, efficient, clean state that is somehow omnipresent in postconflict situations in the developing world. External helpers, too much obsessed with civil society, often tend to ignore this. "Bring the State back in," is a rallying cry some are still not ready to hear. It is time they do.

The most crucial challenge is to distinguish between the State apparatus and the political regime, avoiding an all too common temptation to identify one with the other in a *tabula rasa* approach. Conflating the two would paradoxically vindicate the fallen regime, which often tries to legitimize itself by identifying its rule with the proper, neutral, nonpolitical functioning of a public administration. A more exhausting, time-consuming, but certainly better approach is to impose a clear difference between party and government, regular army and intelligence agencies, national police and praetorian guard, etc. Postconflict emerging elites may not help in this endeavor, because like their nemesis, they have learned to mistake a political regime for a legitimate State. Hence the looting of public offices once a regime falls, from Mogadishu to Monrovia, and from Kinshasa to Baghdad.

A third party should distance itself from these easy, dangerous associations. An effort to gradually patch up elements of the defeated elites with elements of the emerging ones should then begin, as a first step toward national reconciliation. Government agencies, by allowing bureaucrats, experts, and civil servants to somehow merge in order to produce a new order that is based on some continuity of the state apparatus and on the introduction of new blood, should be a pioneering example for the society to start thinking about peaceful coexistence of various groups in a stabilized country. One common error is to mistake the management of postconflict situations for an all-encompassing revolution. No one has a mandate to help run Iraq the way Republicans ran France in 1789, or Maoists ran China in 1949, or Khomeinists ran Iran in 1979!

Next comes the issue of determining the first thing one should think of doing in matters of governance. Holding elections is the answer most often heard. But this is not (more precisely, not in most cases) my view. First, because people usually do not call for elections as an urgent task to perform and, second, because elections are often very hard to organize in a proper way during the initial phases of a postconflict situation. Poorly timed, improperly prepared, or insufficiently credible elections are the source of tensions and new forms of exclusion. Elections may mean a proper way of leadership selection to some, while others may consider them as a way of pursuing the conflict by other means. In cases such as Iraq, elections are primarily perceived as a way of transforming a sociological majority into a political one. That is fine with any democrat, but often it is hard to convince other groups that elections are not primarily a way to consolidate and aggravate their exclusion.

It is crucial that a number of measures be taken to instill a democratic definition of the election process and to introduce safeguards that prevent elections from becoming synonymous with a rampant coup d'état (e.g., Algeria, 1991, where the army reacted by brutally stopping the process) or with a collective punishment of a previously dominant group. As Arend Lijphart, Theodor Hanf, and many others have convincingly written, multiconfessional, multiethnic, multilinguistic societies cannot be ruled through elections by a mere application of the one-man, one-vote principle.[1] Westminster is great where it is; it is not necessarily a successful ready-made product.

To elaborate, ethnocentrism can be fatal. In societies where individualism has been the dominant political and social value for centuries, the Western type of democracy easily fits. In other societies, where recently emerging individualism is still in competition with well-entrenched forms of family, tribal, or other bonds of collective solidarity and mutual help, one has to balance individual human (and voting) rights with the group's fear of losing their political standing, or even their mere existence. To organize electoral systems that prevent an automatic, brutal transformation of an ethnic majority into a legally dominant hegemonic group through the electoral process, one needs time, subtle yet often complex legal techniques, and visionary, cooperative local leaders. These essentials are not necessarily available the very first day, or year, the guns fall silent. Elections can be facilitated quickly, but only if they are part of the solution and not part of the old problem or the source of a new one.

Governance often means the drafting of a new constitution. Constitutions and other basic laws can be written in a few hours, as we are often told by "experts," but here the process is almost as important as the product. That is why it is crucial to help create the proper conditions for a truly national, transparent process by which a consensus can emerge gradually so that the drafting process of a constitution acts as a unifying, rather than divisive, process. A truly legitimate process cannot be rushed.

Various political and/or ethnic factions, leading and recognized legal experts, secular and religious leaders, and the population at large should be given a real chance to appropriate the process. Haste to impose drafts by winning groups, exclusion of large sectors of the society, drafting in closed rooms by unknown local and foreign experts, and brutal transposition of models adopted elsewhere often mar a constitutional process, affect its durability, and can incite new forms of armed rebellion.

One important factor is to be humble enough to let nationals devise their own political future. Do not underestimate the quality of professional expertise in legal and other matters one finds in most war-torn countries. We should not rush to propose our own expertise in constitution drafting, or in other topics, in countries with an educated elite, and politicized population. They need us to amplify their influence on events, but they know the country's needs much better than we do.

We can offer expertise if requested, play the neutral facilitator, and/or help devise a proper drafting process if locals feel they have reached an impasse. Those who invaded Iraq with an already written constitution in their pocket while entering Baghdad were adding insult to injury in the home country of many notable jurists, some of whom had been helping build legal regimes in neighboring countries. I fully understand that the days of absolute sovereignty are behind us and I applaud the most recent evolution in our interpretation of the concept. Still, this evolution should never reach the point where the sovereign right of a people to choose a political regime of their liking is denied, a position even less acceptable than the absolute exercise of sovereignty by authoritarian leaders.

The fine line between "old" regime change and "new" regime imposition by force was not really crossed in Afghanistan. It probably was in Iraq. While regime change as a superpower's policy is highly debatable, the imposition of a new political regime, constitutional arrangements included, is a clear violation of a people's right to self-determination. Persuasion, facilitation, and mediation by foreign actors are acceptable in constitution drafting. Beyond that, a foreign actor is merely imposing a foreign will.

In many postconflict situations, of much more immediate relevance than the organization of elections or the drafting of a new constitution, are three tasks, equally essential for civil peace. The *first* is to ensure the establishment or the reform of national police. In order to push for an early, peaceful start of the reconstruction effort, security of the civilian population is of the essence in the immediate postconflict period. What about existing national police? What about the role given to the military in domestic security? What role should occupying and/or peacekeeping forces play in ensuring urban security? What about dealing with spontaneous ad hoc organizations practicing a police role on the local level? It is dangerous to employ a one-size-fits-all formula in view of the substantial differences one finds from one country to the next. Sometimes there is no such a thing as a national police. In other cases, the police have been so tainted with past illegal practices and/or human rights violations that there is no other solution than to disband them. In some cases, police can be salvaged with other leadership and, more importantly, another code of conduct.

If there is one single rule in this respect, it would be to take the civilian population's fear of aggression, looting, theft of property, kidnapping, seriously. It is not enough to put the blame on the past regime, competing militias, or even the supposedly "natural right" of some to express their newly acquired freedom by attacking their neighbors. Of course, politically motivated saboteurs may have a free run; professional criminals and recently liberated prisoners can wreak havoc in uncertain times. Still, human nature being what it is, normal people, with no crime antecedents, can and do behave inappropriately in transitional times.

In Iraq, "transitional" has a name: Farhoud, a time when anyone may do anything. Postconflict transitions have a history and, fearful of these special days, Islamic legal experts of the past have come to the conclusion that "a hundred years of arbitrary rule are better than one single night without a ruler." Poorly inspired attacks on government buildings have to do with a deeply flawed confusion of a fallen regime with public-sector property. By taking revenge on the state, people ignore the fact that they are hurting their future more than punishing their fallen rulers. Attacks on private property are even less excusable. Hence the importance of rapid police redeployment, a task that must be tackled empirically depending on the case, but one that should always be given the highest priority.

A *second* immediate task is justice—that is, regular, ordinary tribunals. Civil peace often depends on the rapid reactivation of the judicial system in order to settle civil disputes on property: disappearances of heads of families, inheritances, pensions, labor conflicts. Clear examples showing that tribunals are operational, that justice is no longer constrained by vested interests, or political pressure, are important early on in the process. This rebuilds confidence in the state and does not rely upon private justice or illegal (re)appropriation of property. This challenging task may be much less spectacular than the prosecution of war criminals, but it is much more vital in the rapid rewriting of a new social contract between state and society.

Grandiloquent speeches on rule of law remain useless if the population does not develop a rapid, sincere, confidence in its country's judicial system. Although repression and authoritarianism are the curses of many a country in the developing world, the failure to provide proper civil judicial courts is much more common, even in relatively peaceful and/or democratizing countries. And while the quality of the political regime is of the highest concern to those who are politically motivated, the quality of the judicial system is of utmost importance for every single citizen. It is particularly sensitive in matters of real estate ownership.

In so many conflicts, personal property issues are intertwined with political/ethnic considerations. Sometimes personal lust has prevailed, and with others, it is collective punishment against a group. These are issues for which people are ready to die, or kill. A very prudent approach should be followed (although I am not sure all international organizations were very prudent in Iraq). Real estate is not going to disappear, so a gradual, slow, approach is important, with a growing involvement of the national reconstituted judiciary in settling individual cases and, later, collective cases.

Transitional justice is equally important, even on the local level. Postconflict situations are full of acts of revenge. The reality is one cannot entirely prevent people from taking revenge on those who harmed them, but one needs, on the other hand, to develop a spirit of reconciliation. Things are much easier when national institutions are still operational and can take care of these issues. But if this is not the case, acts of revenge can incite the frightening climate of collective indiscriminate punishment, or create new ethnic tensions.

Skepticism envelops transitional justice in most postconflict situations. In most cases, it is viewed as the victor's justice. Hence the crucial importance of international norms, so crime is not followed by revenge and the doors to reconciliation are left open. In general, international tribunals are hotly debated, and it is not my purpose to engage those debates here. One thing, though, is certain. These issues are much less important for most people than the settlement of judicial civilian cases that are much more vital to them. A reconstituted independent civilian judiciary, a less spectacular endeavor indeed, is a much more urgent task.

A *third* immediate task is the preservation of civil society's acquired rights. While one crucial challenge in Afghanistan has been to reintroduce women's rights, suppressed under the Taliban, the main challenge in today's Iraq is to preserve the substantial progress in women's rights acquired in the past five or six decades, now challenged by some opposition forces. Civil society is not necessarily made up of liberated women, or modernistic, multilingual intellectuals. Civil society leadership is mainly made up of people who have influence unrelated to their position in the power structure. One has to be sure that a civic culture is not thrown away with a fallen regime.

Many regimes have had the ambition to modernize their societies while imposing their own authoritarian rule—two mutually supportive tasks. Authoritarianism was used to destroy, or at least weaken, traditional loci of influence or power, which had the perverse effect of strengthening dictatorial rule while opening venues for nontraditional forms of group solidarity. Infatuated with their "creative chaos approach," postmodernists tend to reject both modernity and authoritarianism. The gender issue points to a wider problem. The real challenge is to maintain and reinforce the modern sectors of the society—even if they were introduced by authoritarian leaders—while also introducing democratic reforms to the political domain.

While no two cases are absolutely similar, it is natural and useful to learn from past experiences. But, then, which past experiences should we learn from, as often the references are so distant that we add to the problems rather than settling them. The obsession with 1945 Germany in understanding present-day Iraq is one case among many. Mistaking Baghdad for Berlin is one of the most important US blunders in Iraq. This simplistic approach has led to a number of unfortunate decisions such as the indiscriminate de-Ba'athification that weakened the state apparatus and disrupted public services, and the disbanding of the army, which increased the ranks of the insurgency with disgruntled officers.

I do not think that civilizations really exist as political actors, that cultural identities remain static, or that cultural, linguistic, or religious borders are able to prevent the dissemination of human ideas, values, or institutions. Cultural borders are real, but they keep moving. They are always relative and have a strong tendency to collapse before new ideas. Cultural identities are real but they are never reduced to one religious, professional, or cultural ingredient. They are a combination of all these. Identities are also in a permanent flux of deconstruction and reconstruction and they tend to admit, in such a process, foreign as much as domestic inputs. Cultural boundaries are thus flexible, always reshapable and easy to cross. To present anybody as Shi'a or Tutsi or Berber as a self-explanatory qualification is, in my view, utterly stupid. As a corollary, to entirely ignore the fact that one is Shi'a or Tutsi or Berber is utterly naïve.

Humanitarian action cannot rely on instant anthropologists, the way Iraq has produced instant Iraqologists and the war in Afghanistan, instant Islamologists. It is not because something is daily repeated in the media that it is true. Iraq is not made up of Sunnis, Shi'a, and Kurds—people who have reduced the secular fabric to only one of these categories. Iraq is made up of Iraqis. The identity of each of them is extremely complex and, more disturbingly, flexible. It is deconstructed and reconstructed daily, taking into consideration factors such as their many-generations socialization as national Iraqis, their professional occupation, the urban/rural cleavage, their tribal affiliations, ethnic-linguistic divide, and sectarian denomination.

That is what makes their society rich and fascinating—that tribes are often divided along sectarian lines, that sects are divided along ethnic or tribal lines, that many families have shifted their tribal or sectarian or geographic allegiances more than once in the past two centuries, yet many have learned to forget all this and define themselves as Iraqis.

I never knew the sect of my driver in Iraq. I never asked, and he never told me. Most importantly, from listening to him, I clearly understood that his sect ties were irrelevant to him, as it is irrelevant to many Iraqis I have met. The shift, in many Western opinion-makers' minds, from where traditional loyalties are utterly ignored in the name of nation building to a position where modernization (and its effects) is utterly ignored to the benefit of some postmodernistic infatuation with ethnicity is really disturbing. Does the author of *The Clash of Civilizations* (Huntington, 1994) still remember the fine political scientist who wrote *The Soldier and the State* (Huntington, 1957), the eloquent proponent of (even authoritarian) modernization? Should fashion and/or political agendas prevent us from simultaneously taking the two issues in consideration?

One should never become an accomplice in the ongoing process of overestimating the attachment of people to their religion or the strength of their sectarian, tribal, and other traditional affiliations. I am indeed struck by the easiness with which so many Westerners tend to underestimate the strength of modern, Western-inspired nationalism in Third World societies. A form of amateurish orientalism, or rather anthropologism, dominates the field, and so many people think they have found an answer to their questions by the mere mention of some traditional piece of identity they guess in their interlocutor. What you think, or what you say, is now less relevant than what I think you are because I guessed you are Tamil, Sikh, Sunni, or God knows what. Peacemakers would be well advised not to blindly follow these intellectual fashions. We live in a world where modernity is often deeply intertwined with resilient tradition; to ignore either one of these two is to make peace even less likely.

Humanitarianism has hopefully reached its age of reason. It started as a noble sentiment, entered the body of international law a century ago, exploded during the past century's decades into a widely shared ideal, drifted into a full-fledged universalistic ideology. And now it is back to what could be a long-term status, not a substitute to politics, nor an appendix of it, but a useful, indeed indispensable, complement to economic rationality and political activity. Humanitarianism is now a mature self-confident human activity, operating in what still is basically a world of States, now slightly nuanced by limited areas of accepted world governance and of transnational norms.

Healing with a Single History

Richard J. Goldstone

There is no democracy in which justice and the rule of law are not axiomatically assumed to be foundational principles. In 1895, Professor A. V. Dicey, the great English legal philosopher, defined the principles of the Rule of Law. One of them, he declared, was that "no man is punishable or can be made to suffer in body or goods except for a distinct breach of law."[1] Almost a century later, Professor Archibald Cox expressed the opinion that it is "the genius of American constitutionalism which supports the Rule of Law."[2]

The South African Constitution of 1996 was the product of the experience of other democratic constitutional states and South Africa's own painful history of oppression and discrimination. In the Preamble, it is stated that:

> We the people of South Africa, Recognize the injustices of our past;
> Honour those who suffered for justice and freedom in our land;
> Respect those who have worked to build and develop our country;
> and Believe that South Africa belongs to all who live in it, united in our diversity.
> We therefore, through our freely elected representatives, adopt this Constitution as the supreme law of the Republic so as to—
> Heal the divisions of the past and establish a society based on democratic values, social justice and fundamental human rights
> Lay the foundations for a democratic and open society in which government is based on the will of the people and every citizen is equally protected by law . . .

The Constitution goes on to make respect for human dignity, justice, and the rule of law central principles. In one of the oldest as well as in one of the most recent democratic constitutions, there is the recognition of the fundamental nature of justice and the rule of law.

During South Africa's transition, there was much debate as to the appropriate manner in dealing with the sordid past of racial oppression. Nelson Mandela and the African National Congress would have wished for Nuremberg-style prosecutions for the political and security force leaders. If then President F. W. de Klerk had his way, there would have been blanket amnesties for the apartheid leaders. The compromise, and it was a political compromise, was a form of truth commission.

Soon after South Africa elected its first democratic legislature, it decided to establish the Truth and Reconciliation Commission (TRC). The experience of other truth commissions played an important role in that endeavor, especially that of Chile. However, unlike its Chilean counterpart, the South African model provided for public hearings and the "naming of names." There was also no restriction on the kind of serious human rights violations that were investigated.

More than 20,000 victims gave their testimony to the TRC, and so, too, did some 7000 perpetrators. Amnesty, both criminal and civil, was granted only to those perpetrators who made full confessions of the crimes in respect of which they sought the amnesty. The result was an outpouring of evidence of the heinous human rights violations that were perpetrated in the execution of the apartheid policy.

There has been much debate, both in South Africa and in the global community, about the successes and failures of the TRC. The extent to which individual perpetrators benefited is a complex subject about which there are many contradictory views. It is clear that some victims left the TRC angry and frustrated, while others were able, through their testimony, to begin a healing process.

Whatever the effect of the TRC on individual victims, in my opinion, there can be no doubt that the general South African society has been a beneficiary of the TRC process. During the apartheid era, the majority of white South Africans believed the denials of human rights violations that were put out by the government's security forces. It was more comfortable for those denials to be accepted by the people who felt they were benefiting from them. But for the work of the TRC, that acceptance of the truth of those denials would have continued into the post-apartheid era. The mass of evidence made public by the TRC has given South Africa a single history of the apartheid era—and the denials have disappeared. My grandchildren and their black friends are being taught the same history of apartheid, and so too will their children.

Much of the violence in our contemporary world is the result of the partial history that groups believe. That is certainly the position in the Balkans, where too many Serbs, Croats, and Bosniacs believe that they are the victims and the others are the perpetrators. It is those false denials that provide the toxic fuel that enable evil leaders of the ilk of Slobodan Milosevic to appeal to the nationalism of extreme groups and embark on programs that result in ethnic cleansing.

The cancer of such false denials has been removed in South Africa by the TRC. Not only does this militate against future racism in our country, but it also facilitates the acceptance by the white minority of government programs designed to benefit the majority of our people who were so grievously disadvantaged by hundreds of years of racist oppression. The fairness and morality that require such programs has become manifest. While not suggesting that there is no opposition to such programs, they attract substantially less criticism than would have been the case without the work of the TRC.

If we are ever to live in peace and harmony and prevent the cycles of bloody wars that dominated the twentieth century, the global community will also have to accept that justice and the rule of law are the values that should govern the relationship between sovereign states.

I propose, in this chapter, to undertake an overview of human rights today, examining the attitude of the United States to international law, its behavior and that of some other countries since September 11, 2001, and the relationship between peace and justice. The last mentioned topic illustrates compromises between conflicting objectives—essentially the kind of compromise that needs to be undertaken in respect of national security and human rights.

The Development of Human Rights

Between the end of World War II and September 11, 2001, there was an impressive and even awesome development of the rule of law within nations and, in some areas, in the governance of the global community. In the domestic arena, that development has been evident in the flowering of democratic forms of government in a number of regions of the world. It is foundational to the structure of the European Union (EU) and has been an explicit goal of the Organization of American States (OAU), the African Union (AU), and the Commonwealth of Nations.

Over the first half century of the life of the United Nations, a fundamental contradiction has emerged with regard to the protection of fundamental human rights. Article 2(4) of the UN Charter obliges all Members to refrain from using force against the territorial integrity or political independence of any State. Article 2(7) prohibits the UN from intervening in matters that are essentially within the domestic jurisdiction of any State. It was the latter provision that enabled South Africa to object to attacks by Member States on the evil system of apartheid. Despite that objection, in 1946 India requested the General Assembly to investigate the treatment of Indian nationals in South Africa. The resolution passed but with the opposition of the United States and the United Kingdom (UK).

As colonialism came to an end and it became less acceptable for democratic states to discriminate against their citizens on grounds of race or sex, so it became more acceptable for governments and international organizations to concern themselves with serious violations of human rights wherever they might occur. The provisions of Article 2(7) of the Charter were no longer recognized as a protection even when the UN or its Members took punitive steps in an attempt to end such violations.

The recognition of universal jurisdiction for the most heinous international crimes further eroded the strict application of sovereignty.[3] Citizens of any country could be placed on trial before the courts of any other country for such international crimes even in the absence of a connection between the crime and such nation.

These developments reached their zenith when, in 1993, the Security Council established the International Criminal Tribunal for the former Yugoslavia and, in the following year, the International Criminal Tribunal for Rwanda. Then there was the 1999 bombing of Serbia by the members of NATO in order to protect the Kosovar Albanians from ethnic cleansing. Even though Security Council authority was absent, and the intervention thus illegal, there was no condemnation of the action. Russia attempted to have the Council condemn the intervention but failed miserably. Instead, a UN administration was set up to govern that province of Serbia.

The contradiction in the UN system between respecting state sovereignty and protecting human rights is also illustrated in Security Council Resolution 1244 of June 10, 1999, which established the terms of the UN administration in Kosovo. It reaffirmed "the commitment of all Member States to the sovereignty and territorial integrity of the Federal Republic of Yugoslavia." It also reaffirmed the call in previous resolutions for "substantial autonomy and meaningful self-administration for Kosovo." It went on to decide on the deployment, under UN auspices, of an international civil presence and authorized Member States to establish an international security presence in Kosovo.

This formula was bound to lead to contradictory policies. When members of the Independent International Commission on Kosovo met with the Foreign Affairs Committee of the Russian Duma, we were handed a long list of complaints against the UN administration in Kosovo. For example, there was a strong feeling that the UN replacing Yugoslavian currency with the German mark as the currency of Kosovo was inconsistent with the recognition of the sovereignty of the Federal

Republic of Yugoslavia. So, too, Russia objected to the issuing by the UN of visas to persons visiting Kosovo. When Russians visit Kosovo, they make a point of traveling there from Belgrade with appropriate travel documents issued by the Yugoslav government.

The developments to which I have referred were unthinkable a little more than a decade ago. It was the widely accepted view that an international criminal court could only be treaty based. And humanitarian intervention was a theory thought unlikely to be implemented in practice.

The consequences of these developments, whether within nations or in the global community, have been significant. Democratic ideals have spread around the world, and especially to states of the former Soviet Union, many of which are ever more enthusiastic to be accepted as members of the European Union.

Even less anticipated was that an International Criminal Court would be established early in the new millennium, that by the end of 2003 some ninety-three nations would have ratified its founding treaty, that eighteen judges would have been elected, and that that Court's Prosecutor would be preparing to launch his first investigation into serious war crimes allegedly committed in the Democratic Republic of the Congo.

Who would have thought a little more than a decade ago that the work of international criminal courts would have a profound effect on humanitarian law—that the somewhat irrational distinction with regard to the protection of innocent civilians caught up in international and non-international armed conflict would be reduced almost to the point of extinction? Who would have thought that an international criminal court would hold that systematic mass rape could be held to constitute genocide? And who would have anticipated that in wars fought by democracies, their military leaders would take the requirements of humanitarian law seriously?

Insufficient attention has been given to this last mentioned development. In World War II, civilians became the target of warfare. Cities on both sides were firebombed, and the atomic bomb was dropped with the intention of devastating whole cities in Japan. In the wars in Korea and Vietnam, deaths of civilians outnumbered those of troops by about 90 percent. It was only in the post-international criminal tribunal world that the military leaders of Western nations became committed to attacking only military targets and taking all reasonable steps to protect nonbelligerents. The consequence in the war over Kosovo was a relatively low number of civilian deaths—fewer than 2,000 after 78 days of massive bombing.

Before the establishment of the war crimes tribunals, humanitarian law was a subject taught at some army colleges. Since 1993, when the Yugoslavia Tribunal was established, humanitarian law has become a subject of daily discussion in the media and is taught in thousands of law schools around the world.

I wish that the story ended on this high note. It does not. At the levels of both domestic law and international law, justice and the rule of law have been dealt grievous blows. How much permanent damage has been done, only time will tell. The tragedy is compounded by the fact that these blows have been dealt by the democratic nations of the world, and none more so than by the United States.

The United States and International Law

The United States has been regarded and has regarded itself as the leader of the democratic world. It earned that reputation because of its concern for the human rights of all people. The annual State Department report on human rights discussed the manner in which human rights were respected or violated in just about every country of the world. The US played the leading role in the establishment of the UN war crimes tribunals and in calling the diplomatic conference that led to the treaty under which the International Criminal Court was established.

I know from my own experience that without the political and financial power of the United States neither the Yugoslav nor the Rwandan tribunals would have become viable institutions. In their early years, the US government bent the UN's financial rules in order to ensure that appropriate experts and resources reached The Hague, Kigali, and Arusha. When governments such as Croatia's were tardy in cooperating with the Yugoslav Tribunal, it was US financial pressure that virtually compelled the surrender of indicted war criminals. It was the US ambassador to Cameroon who assisted me in making the crucial official contacts that, in turn, led to the surrender of leaders indicted for the 1994 genocide to the Rwandan Tribunal.

All this was to change. In recent years, the attitude of the United States to the United Nations has been problematic. It has been tardy in paying its dues to the world body. In the 1990s this almost brought the UN to the point of insolvency. In relation to the war against Iraq, it decided to act outside its Charter obligations. When it later welcomed an international effort to bring democracy to Iraq, the nations that opposed the war were none too keen to have their nationals become involved in the ongoing conflict.

The US government's approach to ratifying international treaties has been patchy at best. It took forty years to ratify the Genocide Convention and is the only nation failing to ratify the Convention on the Rights of the Child. More recently, it refused to ratify a protocol to the Torture Convention, which would allow inspections of the prisons of nations suspected of violating the provisions of that Convention.

US ambivalence to international law and international organizations became ever more exceptional. It refused to accept that any of its nationals should ever be brought before an international court, out of fear that such moves might be politically motivated and biased against the United States. It demanded that the jurisdiction of the International Criminal Court should be subject to the approval of the Security Council and thus enable it, and the other four permanent members, to control where the Court could operate. When the overwhelming majority of nations assembled in Rome rejected that approach, the US government demanded that jurisdiction be restricted to nationals of nations that ratified the Rome statute. That too was rejected, and the United States joined only six other countries that voted against the adoption of the Rome Treaty while 120 nations voted in favor of it.

The US approach to the International Criminal Court has become even more hostile under the second Bush administration. While former President Bill Clinton signed the Rome Treaty, President George W. Bush "withdrew" that signature and has actively campaigned against the institution. The United States has threatened or cajoled a number of nations to enter into bilateral agreements undertaking not to hand its citizens to the international court. It has withdrawn military cooperation from some nations that have refused to enter into such agreements.

This recalcitrant attitude of the US government has seriously retarded the building of international justice and the rule of law. If the most powerful nation in the world does not regard itself bound by those laws it *has* ratified, on what basis can it be expected that less powerful nations will remain law-abiding?

The Effect of September 11

I turn to consider the effect of the events of September 11, 2001, on domestic justice and the rule of law. Again, the United States is unfortunately the democracy so visibly denying civil liberties of persons under its control, whether they are citizens or noncitizens. I refer to the resort by the US government to secret deportation hearings; the detention of citizens and noncitizens without trial and without access to a lawyer or to any court; the prospect of trials on capital crimes by military commissions from which there is no appeal to any civilian court; the indefinite detention of persons presumed by the Third Geneva Convention to be prisoners of war, without the benefits of those Conventions and again without access to lawyers or courts. A flicker of hope has been kindled by the US Supreme Court's agreeing to hear an appeal from some of those detained in Guantanamo Bay who question the lawfulness of that detention.

Other democracies have also not fared too well. Prior to September 11, the UK enacted wide-ranging measures to counter terrorism. It did so predominantly in the face of IRA terrorist activities. After September 11, a new antiterrorism statute was enacted. Its most controversial provision is that providing for the internment, without trial, of a "suspected international terrorist" if the Home Secretary reasonably believes that such person's presence in the UK is a risk to national security and suspects that such person is a terrorist. If the person is not a UK citizen, he or she can be detained for an unspecified period without charge or trial. There is no appeal to the ordinary courts but only to a government-appointed commission. It was this provision that led the UK government to derogate from the human rights provisions of the European Convention on Human Rights.

These denials of justice and acts inconsistent with the rule of law are having serious consequences in other countries. If powerful nations can act in such a way, what stops weaker nations from acting in a similar fashion in their regions of the world? Of course, there is a knock-on effect.

Recent Indian legislation invades the privacy of persons in material respects and allows detention of terrorist suspects without trial for periods of up to ninety days. Pending South African legislation also provided for detention without trial. The cruelty and abuses that accompanied detention without trial during the apartheid era led to protests and these contentious provisions have now been removed.

In a recent report by the Lawyers Committee for Human Rights,[4] one reads that Egypt has passed even more draconian laws allegedly to fight terrorism. Egypt's President Mubarak declared that the new US policies "proved that we were right from the beginning in using all means, including military tribunals, to combat terrorism.The United Nations Security Council itself was tardy in making an effort to ensure that civil liberties were respected in legislation that Member States were peremptorily required, by Resolution 1373, to enact. The attitude, as conveyed to me by the first chairman of the Counter-Terrorism Committee, Sir Jeremy Greenstock, was that human rights are not the concern of the Security Council.

In the same Human Rights Watch report, there is reference to an instruction given to US ambassadors. They were to report human rights violations to the State Department in preparation for the 2002 report (issued in March 2003). According to the instruction, "Actions by governments taken at the request of the United

States or with the expressed support of the United States should not be included in the report."

There is no doubt that the events of September 11 created a new concept of democracy that differs from the one that Western states defended before those events took place, and especially so with respect to the freedom of the individual. There is no better illustration than the Bush administration's attempting to justify the indefinite detention of citizens and noncitizens without any court intervention. This is based primarily on the President's declaration that such persons are "unlawful combatants."

The oppressive former dictator of Liberia, Charles Taylor, before he ignominiously left his country and accepted asylum in Nigeria, used the American "unlawful combatant" formula to justify the arrest and torture of innocent journalists. In November 2001, President Robert Mugabe of Zimbabwe claimed that foreign correspondents, including American correspondents, were terrorist sympathizers for reporting on political attacks against white Zimbabweans. His spokesman insisted that it was an open secret that such correspondents were assisting terrorists and distorting the facts. He then said: "As for correspondents, we would like them to know that we agree with the United States President Bush that anyone who in any way finances, harbors, or defends terrorists is himself a terrorist. We too will not make any difference between terrorists and their friends and supporters. This kind of media terrorism will not be tolerated."[5]

A third illustration from the Human Rights Watch report relates to Indonesia. The government of that nation announced in May that it was intending to build a Guantanamo Bay–like island detention camp to house prisoners in its long-standing struggle against armed separatists in northern Sumatra.

I am not suggesting that these evil leaders are doing what the US government is doing. What I am saying is that when the most powerful nation in the world fails to respect its own great values, other nations will become less restrained in the manner in which they treat their own people.

During 2002, I co-chaired a Task Force established by the International Bar Association to report on international terrorism and the role of lawyers in helping combat it.[6] The Task Force included members from Africa, Asia, Europe and the Americas. In our unanimous report we recognized the right, and indeed the duty, of all governments to protect their citizens. Obviously that is one of the most important obligations of government. The challenge that international terrorism presents to justice and the rule of law is to balance the means taken to combat it and the invasion of the civil liberties of citizens. There can be no warrant for the wholesale casting aside of the freedoms for which leading democracies have fought so hard and for so long.

Peace and Justice

Soon after he assumed office as the UN High Commissioner for Human Rights, Sergio Vieira de Mello remarked:

> [M]easures must be taken in transparency, they must be of short duration, and must respect the fundamental non-derogable rights embodied in our human rights norms. They must take place within the framework of the law. Without that, the terrorists will ultimately win and we will ultimately lose—as we would have allowed them to destroy the very foundation of our modern human civilization. I am convinced that it is possible to fight this menace at no cost to our human rights. Protecting our citizens and upholding rights are not incompatible: on the contrary, they must go firmly together lest we lose our bearing.

We are involved in a clash of values and rights that contradict one another. In order to combat international crime, policing authorities in democracies require additional, nontraditional powers. They need to be equipped to foil the plans of sophisticated criminals who do not hesitate to use modern technology and who might have access now or in the near future to weapons of mass destruction. The right balance between national security and the protection of human rights is an excruciatingly difficult one to find, but nonetheless one that can be found.

The Way Forward

These problems illustrate that leaders should recognize clashes of values and make every effort to find a balanced solution in the policies that are adopted. What concerns me is that in the aftermath of September 11, politicians in too many countries feel that they have to be seen to be taking steps to combat terrorism regardless of the efficacy of those measures and regardless of the invasion of fundamental rights that they might cause. A fearful electorate becomes an acquiescent electorate.

I would suggest that governments in democratic nations should be encouraged to set up their own civil liberties monitoring departments. In other words, governments should have senior officials responsible for monitoring and reporting on violations by their own legislatures and executives of fundamental human rights. This is especially appropriate where those rights are protected by their own constitutions or by international conventions to which they are bound. This kind of public oversight would unquestionably act as an effective brake on excessive and unjustified encroachments of human rights.

If democracies lose respect for justice and the rule of law, it will bode ill for the future of the human race. Not only are oppressive dictators relying on the US concept of "unlawful combatants," but it has even become acceptable in some democracies to speak publicly of killing unpopular leaders of other nations or groups.

The powerful nations of our world have a responsibility to set an example for others to follow. That is the obligation that comes with leadership.

Afterword

This chapter was written toward the end of 2003. It is remarkable how international criminal justice has advanced and matured since then. The 93 States that had then ratified the Rome Statute on the International Criminal Court are now risen to 121. All of the persons indicted by the International Criminal Tribunal for the former Yugoslavia have been apprehended and sent for trial to The Hague. This includes Karadzic, Mladic, and Gotovina. A popular uprising in Egypt toppled Mubarak and Charles Taylor, the former President of Liberia, has been found guilty of serious war crimes by the Special Court for Sierra Leone. There are now seven situations before the ICC, three of them referred by governments and two by the Security Council. The US government's policy with regard to the ICC has changed from outright hostility to friendly cooperation. While the road ahead is not an easy one, happily the prophets of doom regarding the future of international justice have been proven wrong.

PART VII

Epilogue

This *Reader* concludes, as the International Humanitarian Affairs Book Series began, with a short essay combining dreams, hopes, and reality, and then with a poem. This chapter offers some philosophic reflections drawn from personal experiences in a career that has linked my own profession in clinical tropical medicine with periods of intensive scientific field research; public health appointments; international humanitarian assistance, especially in complex emergencies; government and United Nations service; and academic responsibilities in both medical schools and the university. It is hoped that this final section will allow the reader to share the many joys and inordinate satisfactions that sustain those who deal with the great problems posed by international humanitarian crises.

The sixteenth-century poem/prayer by Sir Francis Drake captures, I believe, in four short stanzas, major themes of this *Reader*. All the contributors took risks in their professional careers to help define an emerging profession, one that aims at translating times and places of tragedy and chaos into peaceful and stable communities. And they have done their work with, as the poet notes, "courage, hope and love."

The Evolution of a Tropicalist

Kevin M. Cahill, M.D.

The eighth Jubilee Edition of *Tropical Medicine: A Clinical Text* concludes with some personal reflections on my own professional journey. When the initial chapters of my first book were serialized in the *New York State Journal of Medicine* in 1961, I was a young physician who had been introduced to tropical infections on a fellowship in Calcutta, India. I was fascinated by the history of epidemic diseases, by the dramatic clinical presentations, and by the diagnostic and therapeutic challenges they pose.

In Calcutta, I fell in love with a way of life, seeming to find romance in settings that others might—quite legitimately—see only as dirty, broken-down wastelands. Surely those negatives existed in Calcutta. But amidst the fetid stenches of Indian urban decay, I mainly recall the strong aroma of exotic spices. I close my eyes and see saffron robes rather than soiled rags. I hear music in the cacophonous sounds of the slums and in the long silence of a city drenched in the humid heat that comes with the monsoon rains.

Over the next four months I attended, every morning, clinical rounds at the All India Institute of Tropical Medicine. But being young and indefatigable, I also spent every afternoon helping to tend the dying in a gutter with a then-unknown Albanian nun whom the world now remembers as Mother Teresa. I was immersed in a wonder-filled, strange culture, and I faced utterly new challenges and, just as important, new opportunities.

One of the most important lessons of India that has remained with me for life and helped determine what I have tried to do, and how, was the realization that one must stay calm and focused in the midst of chaos if one wanted to help others. There was no time for self indulgent, personal concerns. The petty needs that so often dominate our lives distract us from getting critical tasks accomplished. One quickly learned that our own individual cares simply did not matter much in the face of what others were suffering every day, all day, in the disaster that life offered them.

Fortune continued to bless my nascent career in tropical medicine. At the beginning of the 1960s, due to the ever-expanding war in Vietnam, doctors in the United States were drafted into military service. I was assigned to the US Navy Medical Corps and, blessedly, was first allowed to complete a degree at the London School of Hygiene and Tropical Medicine before being sent to Naval Medical Research Unit 3 in Cairo, Egypt. As the Unit's Head of Epidemiology and Director of Clinical Tropical Medicine, I undertook, over the next few years, field investigations in Sudan, Somalia, Ethiopia, Egypt, Turkey, and across the Middle East. Once again, I discovered beauty in areas that are most often described as desolate. The arid deserts and harsh bush of Somalia and the even more difficult, sodden, mosquito-laden swamps of South Sudan became my favored places for epidemiologic exploration. These journeys gave direction to my own medical and academic career as a tropicalist.

During this period, I became increasingly aware of the extramedical, complex demands one faced in dealing with the trauma of natural and man-made disasters in areas where there were few resources. These developing, often newly independent nations could barely cope in relatively stable times. In the face of famine, drought, floods and civil wars, these societies—and their very basic health services—quickly collapsed.

On my discharge from the Navy in the mid-1960s, I established a career pattern that included daily clinical work, teaching, and continued field research. Since then, I have been Director of the Tropical Disease Center at Lenox Hill Hospital in New York City and Clinical Professor of Tropical Medicine and Molecular Parasitology at the NYU Medical School. For thirty-six years (1969–2006), I was also the Chairman of the Department of International Health and Tropical Medicine at The Royal College of Surgeons in Ireland, and have served as the Consultant in Tropical Medicine for the United Nations Health Service and for numerous international corporations and nongovernmental organizations (NGOs).

I was able to maintain close contact with the realities of life in the tropics through semiannual research trips to Somalia, the Sudan, and Nicaragua, and by responding to complex humanitarian crises, particularly in conflict zones, or after devastating national disasters such as earthquakes. This latter work slowly became my primary interest. I gradually changed my focus from individual diagnosis and therapy to the far broader challenges of providing emergency care to refugees and internally displaced persons.

It is at times of great calamity and suffering—in humanitarian crises—where the developed and developing worlds most intimately interact. These occasions, if mismanaged, cause further divisions in an ever more polarized world between the "haves" and the "have-nots." But, if managed correctly, with forethought and planning, with sensitivity and clinical efficiency, then something profoundly good may emerge. There may be no more important arena in which academic standards need to be urgently applied than in the repetitive humanitarian crises that shame our so-called civilization.

There are obvious, cruel realities in humanitarian fieldwork, and no amount of diplomatic sophistry can dehumanize the horrors of conflict and the waste of innocent lives. These are human beings, not dull statistics, who suffer and die in such situations. In the sad settings of refugee camps where I have worked, mothers and children are the disposable refuse of global insecurity; becoming a child soldier or a sex slave are terribly realistic options for innocent youngsters.

In humanitarian crises, one also struggles with the dark and tangled roots of hatred and the incipient revenge that blossoms in such unrelenting misery. One quickly becomes aware that there are no simple answers in such situations. Solutions, when they can be constructed, draw on many, many disciplines. It is essential to extend the professional standards that prevail in tropical medicine to the less-disciplined field of humanitarian affairs. Disaster management is an evolving science, embracing every stage: from prevention and preparedness, through rapid assessment and cluster assignments, to the final phases of reconstruction and development.

When I was young, and very innocent, I thought I was inordinately important as a medical doctor in a refugee camp. But it did not take long to look around and realize, with growing humility, that those in charge of water or food or shelter or security or sanitation or education were essential partners. It did not take long to realize that no one could accomplish very much working alone. I came to understand that if there were to be any progress in restoring a semblance of stability for those who had lost almost everything, we had to overcome our own restrictive professional barriers.

One had to develop a radically different perspective regarding those treasured academic distinctions we had been taught were so important during medical training. One also had to learn not to be afraid to venture afield as circumstances demanded. Diplomas and degrees can easily become artificial boxes that prevent flexibility. In providing humanitarian assistance, flexibility is an indispensable and absolute necessity.

Rigid definitions of duty cripple programs in the field. There is that inevitable time when, at least in my experience, one must move beyond the traditional confines of any discipline. There had been no courses—except possibly in philosophy, anthropology, or comparative literature—that prepared me for the almost bizarre demands one faces in attempting to establish and manage camps for tens, and sometimes hundreds, of thousands of frightened, ill and endangered people, the vast majority being extremely vulnerable women and children. Three examples demonstrate different challenges that expanded my traditional role as a physician:

> Early in my career, I found myself in Southern Sudan, responsible not only for health concerns, but also for providing other basic human services, including security. It certainly was of little help to a young girl to tell her that her malaria was cured if she was raped every time she went foraging for firewood.

> In 1972, an earthquake destroyed Managua, Nicaragua. I served as Chief Medical Adviser, sharing a tent with the then-President. There, I learned how politics and corruption can pollute so-called relief missions. A significant percentage of the international aid was openly looted by the President's cronies, and donors did not even complain for "diplomatic" reasons. One sadly realized the limitations of altruism in the face of evil.

> Retraining and resettling large numbers of refugees was essential in Somalia after the Sahel drought caused a mass migration across Africa. I was directing camps with almost 1 million refugees, and the only outlet was the Indian Ocean. Trying to teach nomads to abandon an age-old dependency on camels and cattle to seek survival as fishermen was an interesting exercise for an evolving tropicalist. The experiment worked, at least for a while.

There were also obvious diplomatic possibilities in our tropical public health work, and these could—and needed to be—exploited. Medicine offered an almost ideal platform for preventive diplomacy. Almost fifty years ago, in the midst of a raging civil war in Southern Sudan, "corridors of tranquility"—so-called immunization breaks—were established. These were de facto ceasefire zones, and they eventually became temporary bridges to understanding and peace. That peace didn't last, but the effectiveness of those "corridors" is still recalled today by those who struggle to find the elusive common ground in the blood-soaked sands of Sudan.

My responsibilities in this field inevitably grew, particularly in the chaotic reality that is far too often, the norm around the globe, especially in conflict prone zones where poverty and aggression prevail. One had to devise new, imaginative, and innovative paths forward. Managing complex humanitarian emergencies, particularly in the midst of conflicts and disasters, is not a field for amateurs. Good intentions are a common, but tragically inadequate, substitute for well-planned, efficiently coordinated, and carefully implemented operations that must have a beginning, a middle, and an end. Compassion and charity are only elements in humanitarian assistance programs; alone, they are self-indulgent emotions that for a short time may satisfy the donor, but will always fail to help victims in dire straits.

When I first began working in complex humanitarian crises, there were almost no standards of training. In fact, there was not even a common vocabulary. What was desperately needed was the creation of a new profession, one that could embrace the many areas of expertise required to provide an overall response. This is where academia had to enter the picture. More than twenty years ago, new, practical, university-level programs geared to the unique needs of international aid workers were developed. At Fordham University in New York, we now have more than 2,000 graduates from 133 nations, and one can earn a postgraduate master's degree or pursue an undergraduate minor in the field.

It is primarily in the university where knowledge is analyzed and defined, where good—and bad—practices are studied, where the lessons of the past are distilled in a continuing search for wisdom and understanding. Humanitarian assistance is an ideal area for academic interest. It presents a multidisciplinary challenge, drawing on, among others, the fields of public health and medicine, law and politics, logistics and security, technology and anthropology; indeed, all the social, physical, moral, economic, and philosophic arts and sciences.

In trying to establish the broadest possible base for programs in humanitarian assistance, much depends on how one approaches problems, and troubled areas. The multiple causes of and difficult solutions to humanitarian crises require an arena for the free, unfettered exchange of ideas where the development of new initiatives to overcome the failed status quo is encouraged. That is the essential environment of a good university. The university should be—and usually is—the last bastion where open discussions, and respect for differing ideas, prevail. It is society's ultimate refuge from bias and prejudice, and these are among the most significant causative factors in humanitarian crises. The search for answers cannot be limited to the medical school, or the law school, or any other specialized school. It involves all the many, linking disciplines that are the foundation of a true university.

During a very full, joyous career—if that is an appropriate description for a journey where there were few guideposts along the way—I have worked in sixty-five countries, mostly in refugee camps and war zones. I have seen plenty of tragedy during those travels. Many scenes are still seared into my soul: the appalling waste of life and human dignity; pain that I was often unable to relieve; the stares of starving children, and the dying gasps of too many mothers after childbirth. Yet I have always realized how privileged I have been to serve, to share, and even begin to identify with those caught in the crossfire of conflicts not of their making. A spiritual solidarity develops in just being with them. They are my brothers and sisters.

But that realization was obviously not enough. I had to construct solutions to problems that, at least for me, were without precedent. I soon came to understand that tradition and culture were as essential as aspirin or bandages in running a basic medical program. One quickly realized that prejudice and economic exploitation, pride and politics, racism and religion, weather and witchcraft, corruption and incompetence, were all integral parts of the problems one had to address. It is necessary to appreciate the cry of the oppressed, and the burden of ignorance, fear and poverty, if one is to practice medicine in a developing land, especially during—and after—periods of disaster.

In the most sordid situations, I have always felt inordinately humbled to see, often with amazement, always with admiration, the courage and resiliency of the downtrodden, those who seem to have been totally overwhelmed, but then, like the Phoenix, rise again from the ashes. I have always returned—although part of me never returned—from refugee camps grateful to be allowed to participate in their valiant efforts.

I have helped, even healed, many desperate victims in humanitarian crises, but they in turn, helped, healed, instructed, and changed me. I have been the recipient of their kindness: They who had so little gave their meager supplies to me, and, on more than one occasion, offered to protect me with their lives. I learned much about the values of clan loyalty and family love around campfires in the deserts of Somalia and Sudan, with elders who were guided by values as noble as my Judeo-Christian traditions.

I have been caught behind the lines in armed conflicts, and seen senseless slaughter from Beirut to Managua, and all across the scarred landscape of modern Africa. Somehow in the twisted wreckage of war, and in the squalor of refugee camps, the incredible beauty of humanity prevailed for me, as it does for most of those privileged to work in humanitarian assistance. It is that perspective that sustains us on what otherwise may seem like a journey through hell on earth. It takes time to refocus the romance of youth into reflective, lasting programs in humanitarian crises, to change the passion of love into healing projects. One learned from errors and failures, and then struggled ahead, with more hard work. As Samuel Beckett once wrote, we must "Try again. Fail again. Fail better."

It would certainly have been easier—and safer—to reap the rewards assured by a predictable medical practice at home. However, that was not what fate offered. My wife and I discovered a new world—and ourselves—in politically volatile areas where change and revolution were in the air, and on the streets. Some were planned in our living room. Medicine allowed unusual access, even for a Western stranger, in closed, often hostile, societies. We were able to share in the dreams and aspirations of men and women in the developing world who were fighting for freedom, equality, basic human rights, and often their very survival.

In such situations, silence and isolation are simply not viable options. In this era of instant communications, basic moral values make it impossible for any of us to hide from massive sufferings. And mere compassion is an utterly inadequate response. We simply are not free to stay in some blissful state of denial, or to think that expressions of concern, or endless discussions, will suffice.

The discipline of tropical medicine has taken me in uncharted directions with multiple crisscrossing yet mutually supportive paths: from the isolation of a research laboratory through the examining room and the lecture hall, to epidemiologic field work in remote areas, and to the rough and tumble of refugee camps.

There is no substitute in a medical career for the legitimacy and credibility earned in the daily care of individual patients. One must provide the technical basis for that critical continuity of clinical service. But revisions and additions in successive editions of this textbook clearly reflect a personal commitment to developing a new, and fully recognized, profession of international humanitarian assistance.

My concluding hope is that this effort may also offer a foundation for those who dare to broaden the horizons of a discipline and strive in new—yet unknown—ways to help the poor and oppressed masses in the tropics realize a safer, more just and healthy world.

Disturb Us, O Lord

Sir Francis Drake

As with previous books, we end this volume with a poem. This one, from 1577, seems appropriate, citing both challenge and hope.

> Disturb us, Lord, when
> We are too well pleased with ourselves,
> When our dreams have come true
> Because we have dreamed too little,
> When we arrived safely
> Because we sailed too close to the shore.
>
> Disturb us, Lord, when
> With the abundance of things we possess
> We have lost our thirst
> For the waters of life;
> Having fallen in love with life,
> We have ceased to dream of eternity
> And in our efforts to build a new earth,
> We have allowed our vision
> Of the new Heaven to dim.
>
> Disturb us, Lord, to dare more boldly,
> To venture on wider seas
> Where storms will show your mastery;
> Where losing sight of land,
> We shall find the stars.
>
> We ask You to push back
> The horizons of our hopes;
> And to push into the future
> In strength, courage, hope, and love.

Appendix: The IIHA Resource Library

Humanitarian action requires a diverse set of skills and knowledge. Resources do not sit in any one body of literature, but across a multitude of disciplines and languages. More suited toward the modern student, the IIHA has developed a comprehensive resource library that has its foundations in electronic links. These links allow access to the fundamental principles, standards, Conventions, Treaties, Charters, guidelines and basic reference handbooks that a humanitarian student might require for background information. The IIHA Resource Library also contains all of the books sourced in this *Reader*.

Visit the IIHA Resource Library at www.fordham.edu/iiha.

Notes

Paul Grossreider, Humanitarian Action in the Twenty-First Century: The Danger of a Setback

Originally published in Kevin M. Cahill, M.D., ed., *Basics of International Humanitarian Missions* (New York: Fordham University Press, 2003), 3–17.

1. Christianity is understood here to refer to the religion and the sociological reality, and not to the Christian faith as the transcending religion.

2. As François Bugnion wrote in a 1991 ICRC memo: "The Cold War therefore weighed heavily on relation between the ICRC and the USSR, on the ICRC's possibility to act in the conflicts stemming from rivalry between the two blocs, in particular in Korea, Indochina, and Afghanistan. . . . It was not until January 1992, after the break-up of the USSR, that the ICRC was authorized to contact the newly independent governments and offer them its services" (original in French).

3. Frantz Fanon, *Les damnés de la terre* (Paris, 1961); Samir Amin, *Le développement inégal* (Paris, 1973).

4. J.C. Rufin, *Mondes rebelles* (Paris: Michalon, 1996), p. xiii.

Michel Veuthey, Humanitarian Ethical and Legal Standards

Originally published in Kevin M. Cahill, M.D., ed., *Basics of International Humanitarian Missions* (New York: Fordham University Press, 2003), 113–141.

1. Yersu Kim, "Global Problems and Universal Values," available at http://www.unesco.org/opi2/philosophyandethics/pronpro.htm. "The last decade of our century is witness to a rising demand for a universal ethics. Against the backdrop of the positivistic abstinence on questions of value and of the relativism of values of the preceding decades, there is an increasing search for universal values and principles that could serve as the basis for collective efforts toward peace and development, as well as for peaceful and productive interaction among nations and societies. . . . In 1993, representatives of more than 120 religions of the world, meeting for the first time in one hundred years in the Parliament of the World's Religions in Chicago, adopted a Declaration toward Global Ethics. . . . In 1996, some thirty former heads of state and government who constitute the InterAction Council made an appeal for a set of 'Global Ethical Standards' needed to deal with the global problems facing humanity in the twenty-first century." Yersu Kim, Director, Division of Philosophy and Ethics, UNESCO.

2. Michael Renner, "Breaking the Link Between Resources And Repression," chap. 7 in *World Watch Institute State of the World* 2002: *Special World Summit Edition* (New York: Norton, 2002).

3. *Ethics & International Affairs*, vol. 13 (New York: Carnegie Council on Ethics and International Affairs, 1999), contributions from Thomas G. Weiss, Cornelio Sommaruga, Joelle Tanguy, Fiona Terry, David Rieff, and others; http://www.cceia.org/lib_volume13.html.

4. See H. E. J. Cowdrey, "The Peace and the Truce of God in the Eleventh Century," *Past and Present* (1970): 42–67; Georges Duby, "The Laity and the Peace of God," *The Age of Chivalry*, trans. Cynthia Postan (London: Edward Arnold, 1977); *The Peace of God: Social Violence and Religious Response in France Around* 1000 *A. D.*, ed. Thomas Head and Richard Landes (Ithaca, N.Y.: Cornell University Press, 1995). See also http://www.mille.org/people/rlpages/paxdei.html.

5. See Semichon, *La paix et la treve de Dieu* (Paris, 1869); Huberti, *Gottes und Landfrieden* (Ansbach, 1892), The Catholic Encyclopedia, vol. 10. http://www.newadvent.org/cathen; see also http://www.hillsdale.edu/dept/History/Documents/War/Med/1063-peace.htm and http://www.bartleby.com/65/tr/truceGod.html.

6. New Testament Matt. 7:7–12; but also Muhammad 13ᵉ Hadiths de Nawawi; Mahavira: Yogashastra 2, 20; Bouddha Sutta Pitaka, Udanagavva 5, 18; Confucius; Analecta 15, 23; Mahabaharata 5: 15, 17; Talmud bab, Shabbat 31a; Baha'u'llah: Kitab-i-aqdas 148; Isocrate: Nicocles 61. *Calendrier inter religieux* 2001–2002 (Geneva: Enbiro Lausanne & Plate-Forme inter religieuse, 2000).

7. Platon, *La Republique*, trans. R. Baccon (Paris, 1966), pp. 224–227. See also Andre Bernand, *Guerre et violence dans la Grece antique* (Paris: Hachette, 1999); Pierre Ducrey, *Le traitement des prisonniers de guerre dans la Grece antique* (Paris, 1978); and Jacqueline de Romilly, *La Grece antique contre la violence* (Paris: Ed. De Fallois, 2000).

8. Frank Keitsch, *Formen der Kriegfuhrung in Melanesien* (Bamberg, 1967), p. 380.

9. Maurice R. Davie, *La guerre dans les societies primitives. Son role et son evolution. Traduit de l'anglais par M. Guerin* (Paris: Payot, 1931) (*The Evolution of War: A Study of Its Role in Early Societies* [New Haven: Yale University Press, 1929]).

10. E. E. Evans-Pritchard. *The Nuer: A Description of the Modes of Livelihood and Political Institutions of a Nilotic People* (Oxford: Oxford University Press, 1940).

11. Buddhism contains two fundamental principles, maître (friendliness, benevolence) and karuna (mercy, compassion), closely related to the principle of humanity.

12. For Hinduism, numerous rules on the kind treatment to be granted to the vanquished are found in the *Mahabharata* (XII, 3487, 3488, 3489, 3782, 8235), which also prescribes loyalty in combat (XII, 3541, 3542, 3544–51, 57-60, 64, 3580, 3659, 3675, 3677). See also the famous Laws of Manu, VII: 90–93 (*The Laws of Manu* [Oxford, 1886]).

13. On Taoism, see Gia-Fu Cheng, and Jane English, trans., *Lao Tse: Tao Te Ching* (New York: Vintage, 1972), in particular no. 68 ("a good winner is not vengeful") and no. 38.

14. See Barbara Aria and Russell Eng Gon, *The Spirit of the Chinese Character* (San Francisco: Chronicle Books, 1992), p. 47.

15. On Bushido, see Sumio Adachi, "Traditional Asian Approaches: A Japanese View," *Australian Yearbook of International Law* 9 (1985): pp. 158–167; and, by the same author, "The Asian Concept," *International Dimensions of Humanitarian Law* (Paris: UNESCO, 1986): pp. 13–19, which also considers Buddhism.

16. On Judaism, see Erich Fromm, *You Shall Be As Gods* (New York: Holt, Rinehart and Winston, 1966).

17. On Christianity, Max Huber, *The Good Samaritan: Reflections on the Gospel and Work of the Red Cross* (London: Gollancz, 1945). See also Joseph Joblin, *'L'église et la guerre. Conscience, violence pouvoir* (Paris, 1988) and in particular, for *jus in bello,* page 193 and onward; Alfred Vanderpool, *La doctrine scolastique du droit de la guerre* (Paris, 1919).

18. On Islam, see, among others, Hamed Sultan, "The Islamic Concept," *International Dimensions of Humanitarian Law* (Geneva/Paris: UNESCO/Nijhoff, 1988): 29–39; Marcel Boisard, *'L'humanisme de l'Islam* (Paris, 1979); Jean-Paul Charney, *L'Islam et la guerre. De la guerre juste a la revolution sainte* (Paris, 1986). See also M. K. Ereksoussi, "The Koran and the Humanitarian Conventions," *International Review of the Red Cross* (May 1962); Ameur Zemmali, *Combattants et prisonniers de guerre en droit islamique et en droit international humanitaire* (Paris: Pedone, 1997).

19. See Geoffrey Best, *Humanity in Warfare, The Modern History of International Law of Armed Conflicts* (London: Weidenfeld and Nicolson, 1980).

20. See Eric Fromm, *The Anatomy of Human Destructiveness* (New York: Holt, Rinehart and Winston, 1973), p. 168.

21. The full text, available at http://www.mtholyoke.edu/acad/intrel/kant/kant1.htm, is: "No State shall, during War, permit such Acts of Hostility which would make mutual Confidence in the subsequent Peace impossible: such are the employment of assassins ("percussores"), poisoners ("venefici"), breach of Capitulation, and Incitement to Treason ("perduellio") in the opposing State."

22. http://35.1911encyclopedia.org/L/LA/LAS_CASAS_BARTOLOME_DE.htm.

23. See Giulio Basetti Sani, *L'Islam et St Francois d'Assise. La mission prophetique par le dialogue* (Paris: Publisud, 1987).

24. World Conference on Religion and Peace. Mission Statement available at http://www.wcrp .org/RforP/MISSION_MAIN.html.

25. Protocol for the Prohibition of the Use of Asphyxiating, Poisonous or Other Gases, and of Bacteriological Methods of Warfare, Geneva, June 17, 1925.

26. Declaration Renouncing the Use, in Time of War, of Certain Projectiles, Saint Petersburg, November 29/December 11, 1868.

27. The Fourth Convention respecting the Laws and Customs of War on Land and Its Annex: Regulations Concerning the Laws and Customs of War on Land, The Hague, October 18, 1907.

28. See Jean Pictet, *Humanitarian Law and the Protection of War Victims* (Leiden, 1975).

29. This was the term used by the Diplomatic Conference on the Reaffirmation and Development of International Humanitarian Law applicable in Armed Conflicts (CDDH), which met at Geneva from 1974 to 1977 to adopt the two Additional Protocols to the Conventions of 1949.

30. "Laws of war" is the expression still most widely used today in military circles. Cf Frederic de Mulinen, *Handbook on the Law of War for Armed Forces* (Geneva: ICRC, 1987); or Thomas B. Baines, "The Laws of War and the Rules of Peacekeeping," presented to the Joint Services Conference on Professional Ethics, January 30-31, 1997, at the National Defense University, Washington, D.C. Available at http://www.usafa.af.mil/jscope/JSCOPE97/Baines97.htm.

31. "Law of Geneva" is sometimes used with the intention of stressing aspects relating to the protection of victims of war, as opposed to the regulation of conduct as regards methods and means of destruction between combatants, designated by the expression "Law of The Hague."

32. The Protocols of 1977 have to some extent merged the Law of Geneva and the Law of The Hague; this was merely the culmination of a trend that began when the rules of The Hague relating to the treatment of prisoners of war were incorporated and expanded upon in the Second Geneva

Convention of 1929, and later the Third Convention of 1949; similarly, the Fourth Convention of 1949 incorporated most of The Hague Regulations of 1907 on military occupation. All this is of considerable significance: apart from the historical memory, it is the customary nature of the rules of The Hague (and hence of the provisions incorporated in 1949 and 1977) that should be emphasized.

33. This was the term used by the United Nations for almost ten years after the International Conference on Human Rights held in Teheran (April 22–May 13, 1968). Numerous resolutions of the United Nations General Assembly, advocating further codification and describing how this was to be done, were adopted under the heading of "Respect for Human Rights in Armed Conflicts," as well as reports by the Secretary-General of the United Nations (A/7720 in 1969, A/8052 in 1970, A/8370 in 1971, A/8781 in 1972, A/9123 in 1973, A/9669 in 1974, A/10195 in 1975).

34. See Georges Abi-Saab, "The Specificities of Humanitarian Law," in *Studies and Essays on International Humanitarian Law and Red Cross Principles in Honour of Jean Pictet*, ed. Christophe Swinarski (Geneva: ICRC, 1984), pp. 265–280.

35. See Henry Dunant, *A Memory of Solferino* (Geneva: ICRC, 1939).

36. Geneva Convention for the Amelioration of the Condition of the Wounded and Sick in Armed Forces in the Field, August 12, 1949; Geneva Convention for the Amelioration of the Condition of the Wounded, Sick, and Shipwrecked Members of the Armed Forces at Sea, August 12, 1949; Geneva Convention Relative to the Treatment of Prisoners of War, August 12, 1949; Geneva Convention Relative to the Protection of Civilian Persons in Time of War, August 12, 1949.

37. Protocol Additional to the Geneva Conventions of August 12, 1949, and relating to the Protection of Victims of International Armed Conflicts (Protocol 1); Protocol Additional to the Geneva Conventions of August 12, 1949, and relating to the Protection of Victims of Non-International Armed Conflicts (Protocol 2).

38. See *Commentary on the Additional Protocols of June 8, 1977, to the Geneva Conventions of August 12, 1949* (Geneva: ICRC, 1987), p. 381, ¶ 1364.

39. The International Tribunal for the Prosecution of Persons Responsible for Serious Violations of International Humanitarian Law Committed in the Territory of the Former Yugoslavia since 1991 was established by the Security Council on May 25, 1993.

40. The International Criminal Tribunal for the Prosecution of Persons Responsible for Genocide and Other Serious Violations of International Humanitarian Law Committed in the Territory of Rwanda and Rwandan Citizens Responsible for Genocide and Other Such Violations Committed in the Territory of Neighboring States between January 1 and December 31, 1994, was established by the Security Council on November 8, 1994.

41. See the Tadic Case: International Criminal Tribunal for the Former Yugoslavia, *Prosecutor v. Dusko Tadic a/k/a "Dule"*: Decision on the defence motion for interlocutory appeal on jurisdiction. Decision of October 2, 1995, case no. IT-94-1-AR72. Two articles written on this case: John Dugard, "Bridging the Gap Between Human Rights and Humanitarian Law: The Punishment of Offenders," *International Review of the Red Cross* 324 (September 1998): 445–453; and Thomas Graditzky, "International Criminal Responsibility for Violations of International Humanitarian Law Committed in Non-international Armed Conflicts," *International Review of the Red Cross*, no 322 (March 1998): 29–56.

42. See I. William Zartman, ed., *Collapsed States: The Disintegration and Restoration of Legitimate Authority* (Boulder: Lynne Rienner, 1995), p. 301; and the Preparatory Document Drafted by the ICRC for the First Periodical Meeting on International Humanitarian Law, "Armed Conflicts Linked to the

Disintegration of States Structures," mentioning Resolution 814, ¶ 13 (Somalia), Res. 788, ¶ 5 (Liberia), Geneva, January 19-23, 1998.

43. See Robert Fox, "On the Age of Postmodern War. Beyond Clausewitz: the Long and Ragged Conflicts of the Coming Millennium," *The Times Literary Supplement*, 15 May 1998.

44. As Martin Van Crefeld puts it in *The Transformation of War* (New York: Free Press, 1991), "Once the legal monopoly of armed force, long claimed by the State, is wrestled out of its hands, existing distinctions between war and crime will break down."

45. ICRC Commentary III, Article 1. Available online at http://www.icrc.org/ihl.nsf/b466ed681d dfcfd241256739003e6368/49cfe5505d5912d1c12563cd00424cdd?OpenDocument.

46. International Court of Justice, Case Concerning the Military and Paramilitary Activities in and Against Nicaragua (*Nicaragua v. United States of America*), Judgement of June 27, 1986 (Merits), vo. 114, ¶ 218. On this case, see Rosemary Abi-Saab, "The 'General Principles' of Humanitarian Law According to the International Court of Justice," *International Review of the Red Cross* (July–August 1987): 367–375.

47. The United Nations Convention on the Prohibition of Military or Any Other Hostile Use of Environmental Modification Techniques (ENMOD), adopted on December 10, 1976.

48. Convention on the Rights of the Child, adopted by Resolution 44/25 of the United Nations General Assembly on November 20, 1989.

49. See Michael Ignatieff, "The Attack on Human Rights," *Foreign Affairs* (November–December 2001).

50. See the interesting article by Chih-yu Shih, "Opening the Dichotomy of Universalism and Relativism," *Human Rights and Human Welfare. International Review of Books and Other Publications* 2, no. 1 (January 2002), reviewing Linda S. Bell, Andrew J. Nathan, and Ilan Peleg, eds., *Negotiating Culture and Human Rights* (New York: Columbia University Press, 2001); and Daniel A. Bell, *East Meets West: Human Rights and Democracy in East Asia* (Princeton: Princeton University Press, 2000).

51. See Amartya Sen, *Development as Freedom* (New York: Random House, 2000).

52. Paragraph 2 of the Proclamation of 1968 Tehran reads as follows: "The Universal Declaration of Human Rights states a common understanding of the peoples of the world concerning the inalienable and inviolable rights of all members of the human family and constitutes an obligation for the members of the international community."

53. Paragraph 1of the 1993 Vienna Declaration states that: "The World Conference on Human Rights reaffirms the solemn commitment of all States to fulfill their obligations to promote universal respect for, and observance and protection of, all human rights and fundamental freedoms for all in accordance with the Charter, other instruments relating to human rights, and international law. The universal nature of these rights and freedoms is beyond doubt . . .

All human rights are universal, indivisible, and interdependent and interrelated. The international community must treat human rights globally in a fair and equal manner, on the same footing and with the same emphasis. While the significance of national and regional particularities and various historical, cultural, and religious backgrounds must be borne in mind, it is the duty of States, regardless of their political, economic, and cultural systems, to promote and protect all human rights and fundamental freedoms."

54. I. C. J. Reports (1951), p. 12. See Christa Rottensteiner, "The Denial of Humanitarian Assistance as a Crime Under International Law," *International Review of the Red Cross* 835 (1999): 555–582.

55. See the Web site dedicated to the Charter: http://www.europarl.euint/charter/default_en.htm. The text was published in the Official Journal of the European Communities, C 364/1 (2000).

56. For this "third generation of human rights," see Karel Vasak, "Pour une troisieme generation des droits de l'homme," in *Studies and Essays on International Humanitarian Law and Red Cross Principles*, ed. Christophe Swinarski (Geneva: ICRC, 1984), pp. 837–845; Karel Crawford and Hans Kruuk, *The Rights of Peoples* (Oxford: Oxford University Press, 1992).

57. See: Edith Brown Weiss, ed., *Environmental Change and International Law: New Challenges and Dimensions* (Tokyo: The United Nations University, 1992); http://www.unu.edu/unupress/unupbooks/uu25ee/uu25ee0k.htm; and especially Alexandre Kiss, "An Introductory Note on a Human Right to Environment," http://www.unu.edu/unupress/unupbooks/uu25ee/uu25ee0k.htm; "The Fundamental Right to Life at the Basis of the Ratio Legis of International Human Rights Law and Environmental Law," http://www.unu.edu/unupress/unupbooks/uu25ee/uu25eeop.htm. See also "Report of the Joint OHCHR-UNEP Seminar on Human Rights and the Environment," January 16, 2002, E/CN.4/2002/WP. 7 (March 22, 2002), submitted to the Fifty-eighth Session of the Commission on Human Rights; http://www.unhchr.ch/huridocda/huridoca.nsf/Documents?OpenFrameset.

58. Declaration on the Right to Development, G.A. res. 41/128, annex, 41 UN GAOR Supp. (no.53) at 186, UN Doc. A/41/53 (1986). Available at the University of Minnesota Human Rights Library Web site: http://www1.umn.edu/humanrts/instree/s3drd.htm; and on the UN Web site: http://www.un.org/documents/ga/res/41/a41r128.htm. See also Arjun Sengupta "The Right to Development as a Human Right," on the Francois-Xavier Bagnoud Center for Health and Human Rights, Harvard University, Web site: http://www.hsph.harvard.edu/fxbcenter/FXBC_WP7-Sengupta.pdf.

59. See the Web site of the Office of the High Commissioner for Human Rights: http://www.unhchr.ch/html/menu2/10/e/rtd_main.htm; and the Report of the High Commissioner for Human Rights, submitted in accordance with Commission on Human Rights resolution 1998/72. E/CN.4/2002/27 (November 27, 2001) available at http://www.unhchr.ch/huridocda/huridoca.nsf/Documents?OpenFrameset.

60. Statement in January 1997. http://www.unesco.org/general/eng/whatsnew/decl.eng.html.

61. See the WHO Web site "Health as a Human Right," http://www.who.int.archives/who50/en/human.htm; and the interdisciplinary discussion held at Harvard Law School in September 1993, http://www.law.harvard.edu/programs/HRP/Publications/economic1.html; and Henrik Karl Nielsen, *The World Health Organisation—Implementing the Right to Health*, as well as "Health and Human Rights. An International Journal" published by the Francois-Xavier Bagnoud Center for Health and Human Rights, Harvard University, since 1994; http://www.hsph.harvard.edu/fxbcenter/journal.htm.

62. See the FAO Website: http://www.fao.org/Legal/rtf/rtfood-e.htm.

63. See *The Fundamental Principles of the Red Cross and Red Crescent Movement*, 2nd ed. (Geneva: ICRC, 1996).

64. See Jean Pictet, *The Fundamental Principles of the Red Cross: Commentary* (Geneva, 1979).

65. Text available at http://www.doctorswithoutborders.org/about/charter.shtml.

66. See the following Websites: http://www.tandf.co.uk/journals/tfs/15027570.html (*Journal of Military Ethics*); http://dir.yahoo.com/Government/Military/Ethics, http://www.usna.edu/Ethics (Center for the Study of Professional Military Ethics); http://plato.stanford.edu/entries/war (Stanford Encyclopedia of Philosophy); http://www.iihl.org (International Institute of Humanitarian Law).

67. See Cees de Rover, "Police and Security Forces. A New Interest for Human Rights and Humanitarian Law," *International Review of the Red Cross* 835 (September 1999): 637–647; and C. de

Rover, *To Serve and to Protect Human Rights and Humanitarian Law for Police and Security Forces* (Geneva: ICRC, 1998).

68. The Hippocratic Oath (available at http://classics.mit.edu/Hippocrates/hippooath.html) and the following document of the World Medical Association: "World Medical Association Resolution on Human Rights" (adopted by the Forty-second World Medical Assembly, Rancho Mirage, California, U.S.A., October 1990, and amended by the Forty-fifth World Medical Assembly, Budapest, Hungary, October 1993, the Forty-sixth General Assembly, Stockholm, Sweden, September 1994, the Forty-seventh General Assembly, Bali, Indonesia, September 1995).

"Having regard to the fact that:

1. The World Medical Association and its member associations have always sought to advance the cause of human rights for all people, and have frequently taken actions endeavoring to alleviate violations of human rights;

2. Members of the medical profession are often among the first to become aware of violations of human rights;

3. Medical Associations have an essential role to play in calling attention to such violations in their countries.

The World Medical Association again calls upon its member associations:

1. To review the situation in their own countries so as to ensure that violations are not concealed as a result of fear of reprisals from the responsible authorities, and to request strict observance of civil and human rights when violations are discovered;

2. To provide clear, ethical advice to doctors working in the prison system;

3. To provide effective machinery for investigating unethical practices to physicians in the field of human rights;

4. To use their best endeavors to ensure that adequate healthcare is available to all human beings without distinction;

5. To protest alleged human rights violations through communications that urge the humane treatment of prisoners, and that seek the immediate release of those who are imprisoned without just cause; and

6. To support individual physicians who call attention to human rights violations in their own countries." http://www.wma.net/e/policy/20-2-90_e.html.

69. See the Code accepted in 1954 by the World Congress of the International Federation of Journalists (IFJ), and amended in 1986: http://www.ifj.org/ifj/codee.html; and the Databank for European Codes of Journalism Ethics: http://www.uta.fi/ethicnet.

70. See http://www.unglobalcompact.org/un/gc/unweb.nsf/content/thenine.htm.

71. Common Article 1 to the 1949 Geneva Conventions.

72. ICRC, *ICRC Commentary on the Additional Protocols* (Geneva: ICRC, 1987), p. 35, ¶ 39.

73. ICRC Commentary 3, p. 18 (Article 1). See Luigi Condorelli and Laurence Boisson de Chazournes, "Quelques remarques a propos de l'obligation des Etats de 'respecter et faire respecter' le droit international humanitaire 'en toutes circonstances,'" in *Studies and Essays on International Humanitarian Law and Red Cross Principles*, ed. Christophe Swinarski (Geneva: ICRC, 1984), pp. 17–35; and Umesh Palwankar, "Measures Available to States for Fulfilling Their Obligaiton to Ensure Respect for International Humanitarian Law," *IRRC* 298 (1994): 9–25.

74. The 1949 Geneva Conventions as well as Additional Protocol 1, for the States Party to this Protocol. See the ICRC *Commentary on the Protocols*, ad Article 1 of Protocol 1, pp. 35–38.

75. Article 7 ("Meetings"): "The depositary of this Protocol [Switzerland] shall convene a meeting of the High Contracting Parties, at the request of one or more of the said Parties and upon the approval of the majority of the said Parties, to consider general problems concerning the application of the Conventions and of the Protocol." Such a meeting was convened by Switzerland on December 5, 2001 in Geneva ("Conference of the High Contracting Parties to the Fourth Geneva Convention").

76. *ICRC Commentary on the Additional Protocols*, p. 36, ¶ 43. See also Michel Veuthey, "Pour une politique humanitaire," in Swinarski, *Studies and Essays on International Humanitarian Law and Red Cross Principles*, pp. 989–1009.

77. Training is an obligation according to the Four 1949 Geneva Conventions. Article 47 of the First Convention states the following: "The High Contracting Parties undertake, in time of peace as in time of war, to disseminate the text of the present Convention as widely as possible in their respective countries, and, in particular, to include the study thereof in their programs of military and, if possible, civil instruction, so that the principles thereof become known to the entire population, in particular to the armed fighting forces, the medical personnel and the chaplains." The Second Convention contains a similar provision (Article 48). Article 127 of the Third Convention ads the following paragraph: "Any military or other authorities, who in time of war assume responsibilities in respect of prisoners of war, must possess the text of the Convention and be specially instructed as to its provisions." Article 144 ¶ 2 of the Fourth Convention reads as follows: "Any civilian, military, police or other authorities, who in time of war assume responsibilities in respect of protected persons, must possess the text of the Convention and be specially instructed as to its provisions." Additional Protocol 1: (a) Reaffirms the duty to disseminate (Article 83—Dissemination); and (b) Adds the obligation to ensure that legal advisers are available (Article 82—Legal Advisers in armed forces). Additional Protocol 2, applicable in non-international armed conflicts, simply states that "This Protocol shall be disseminated as widely as possible" (Article 19—Dissemination).

78. Article 36 ("New Weapons") of Protocol 1 reads as follows: "In the study, development, acquisition, or adoption of a new weapon, means, or method of warfare, a High Contracting Party is under an obligation to determine whether its employment would, in some or all circumstances, be prohibited by this Protocol or by any other rule of international law applicable to the High Contracting Party."

79. The Four 1949 Conventions contain common provisions on the "Repression of Abuses and Infractions:"

> First Convention: Article 49–51
>
> Second Convention: Article 50–52
>
> Third Convention: Article 129–131
>
> Fourth Convention: Article 146–148
>
> Article 85 of Additional Protocol 1 reaffirms those provisions, adds a few acts to be considered as grave breaches (especially attacks against civilians and civilian objects), and classifies grave breaches of the 1949 Conventions and Protocol 1 as war crimes.

See also Maria Teresa Dutli and Cristina Pellandini, "The International Committee of the Red Cross and the Implementation of a System to Repress Breaches of International Humanitarian Law," *IRRC* 300 (May 1994): pp. 240-254.

80. See George A. B. Peirce, "Humanitarian Protection for the Victims of War: The System of Protecting Powers and the Role of the ICRC," *Military Law Review* 90 (1989): 89–162; and D. P.

Forsythe, "Who Guards the Guardians? Third Parties and the Law of Armed Conflict," *American Journal of International Law* 70 (1976): 41–61.

81. H. Coulibaly, "Le role des puissances protectrices au regard du droit diplomatique, du droit de Geneve et du droit de La Haye," in *Implementation of International Humanitarian Law*, F. Kalshoven and Y. Sandoz, eds. (Dordrecht: Martinus Nijhoff, 1989), pp. 69078. C. Dominice and J. Patrnogic, "Les protocoles additionnelles aux Conventions de Geneve et le systeme des puissances protectrices," *Annales de Droit International Medical* 28 (1979): 24–50. J.-P. Knellwolf, "Die Schutzmacht im Volkerrecht unter besonderer Brucksichtigung der schweizerischen Verhaltnisse" (Dissertation Bern, Bern: Ackermanndruck, 1985). B. Laitenberger, "Die Schutzmacht," *German Yearbook of International Law* 21 (1978): 180–206.

82. It was used in Suez in 1956, in Goa in 1961, and between India and Pakistan in 1971. For a more recent example, see the State Department Press Briefing, Thursday, April 1, 1998: "The United States Government is contacting authorities in Belgrade through our Protecting Power, Sweden, in regard to the illegal abduction of three American servicemen who were serving in non-combatant status in Macedonia. There is no basis for their continued detention by the Belgrade authorities. We insist that they be provided any necessary medical assistance and treated humanely and in accordance with all prevailing international agreements and standards. We will hold Belgrade authorities responsible for their safety and treatment." http://www.aiipowmia.com/inter/in040299e.html.

83. Protocol 1, Article 2, Letter C.

84. Third Geneva Convention, Article 126.

85. Fourth Geneva Convention, Article 143.

86. Fourth Geneva Convention, Articles 59 and 61.

87. Third Geneva Convention, Article 123.

88. Fourth Geneva Convention, Article 140.

89. First Geneva Convention, Article 23.

90. Fourth Geneva Convention, Article 14.

91. Fourth Geneva Convention, Article 30.

92. Article 9 of Conventions 1, 2, and 3; Article 10 of the Fourth Convention.

93. Common Article 3 to the 1949 Conventions.

94. The Web site of the Commission: http://www.ihffc.org.

95. See Patrick Healy and Kimberly Prost, "International Criminal Law" McGill University Faculty of Law: http://www.law.mcgill.ca/academics/coursenotes/healy/intcrimlaw, and the following links mentioned there: Nuremberg Trials, London, Agreement of August 8, 1945 (http://www.yale.edu/lawweb/avalon/imt/imt.htm); Charter of the International Military Tribunal (http://www.yale.edu/lawweb/avalon/imt/imt.htm); Judgment of the IMT for the Trial of German Major War Criminals (http://www.yale.edu/lawweb/avalon/imt/imt.htm).

96. See the following links, quoted by Patrick Healy and Kimberly Prost, *Jurisdiction of the Yugoslavian and Rwandan Ad Hoc Tribunals,* Security Council Resolution 827 (1993), May 25, 1993 (http://www.un.org/Docs/sc.htm); Security Council Resolution 955 (1994), November 8, 1994 (http://www.un.org/Docs/sc.htm); Statute of the International Criminal Tribunal for the Former Yugoslavia ("ICTY"), Articles 6, 8, 9 (http://www.un.org/icty/basic.htm); Statue of the International Criminal Tribunal for Rwanda ("ICTR"), Articles 5, 7, 8 (http://www.ictr.org); ICTY, Rules of Procedure and Evidence, Rules 7–13 (http://www.un.org/icty/basic.htm); ICTY, *Prosecutor v. Dusko Tadic a/k/a "Dule,"* Appeals Chamber Decision on the Jurisdictional Motion, October 2, 1995, ss. 9–48, 9–64

(http://www.un.org/icty/cases-ae2.htm); *Substantive Law and the* Ad Hoc *Tribunals,* Statute of the ICTY, Articles 2–5, 21 (http://www.un.org/icty/basic.htm); Statute of the ICTR, Articles 2–4, 20 (http://www.ictr.org) ; ICTY, *Prosecutor v. Drazen Erdemovic,* Appeals Chamber, Joint separate opinion of Judge McDonald and Judge Vohrah, ss. 32058, 66, 73–91; Separate and dissenting opinion of Judge Cassese, ss. 11–12, 40–51 (http://www.un.org/icty/cases-ae2.htm); ICTR, *Prosecutor v. Jean-Paul Akayesu,* Trial Chamber, Judgment, ss. 5.5 and 7 (http://www.ictr.org); *Evidence, Procedure, and the* Ad Hoc *Tribunals,* ICTY, Rules of Procedure and Evidence, Rules 39–43, 54–61, 89–98 (http://www.un.org/icty/basic.htm); ICTY, *Prosecutor v. Dusko Tadic a/k/a/ "Dule,"* Judgment on evidentiary matters (http://www.un.org/icty/cases-te.htm); Judgment on Corroboration in section V(c), Judgment on Hearsay in section Voh), ICTY, *Prosecutor v. Blaskic,* Judgment on the request of The Republic of Croatia for review of the decision of Trial Chamber 2 of July 18, 1997, ss. 25–60 (http://www.un.org/icty/blaskic/ace14.htm).

97. See *Jurisdiction of the ICC: Trigger Mechanisms and the Exercise of the Court's Jurisdiction* (http://www.un.org/ic/backinfo.htm); Rome Statute of the International Criminal Court, Articles 11–15, 17–18 (http://www.un.org/icc); *Substantive Law and the ICC: Crimes within the Court's Jurisdiction* (http://www.un.org/icc/backinfo.htm); Rome Statute of the International Criminal Court, Articles 5–9, 21, 22-23, 55, 67, 69 (http://www.un.org/icc); Preparatory Commission for the International Criminal Court; Results of Working Groups on the ICC Rules of Procedure and Evidence; Most recent laws (http://www.un.org/law/icc/prepcomm/docs.htm).

98. ICRC, *International Criminal Court: A Reality at Last* (Geneva: ICRC, April 11, 2002).

99. See the Website of the CPT: http://www.cpt.coe.fr.

100. Elisabeth Kardos-Kaponyi, "The Charter of Fundamental Human Rights in the European Union," p. 139, mentions the Office for Democratic Institutions and Human Rights (ODHIR), the High Commissioner of National Minorities and the Representative on Freedom of the Media, Document available online: http://www.lib.bke.hu/gt/2001-1-2/kardos-kaponyi.pdf.

101. Ibid., pp. 140–170.

102. The ICRC can offer its good offices to facilitate the establishment of hospital zones (according to Article 23 of the First 1949 Convention) and safety zones (Article 14, First Convention). Other institutions or persons could offer their good offices. See B. G. Ramcharan, *Humanitarian Good Offices in International Law: The Good Offices of the United Natiosn Secretary-General in the Field of Human Rights* (The Hague: Martinus Nijhoff, 1983).

103. See Roy W. Gutman, "Spotlight on Violations of International Humanitarian Law. The Role of the Media," *IRRC* 325 (December 1998): 619–625; Urs Boegli, "A Few Thoughts on the Relationships Between Humanitarian Agencies and the Media," *IRRC* 325 (December 1998): 627–631, and, more generally, Yael Danieli, ed., *Sharing the Front Line and the Back Hills: International Protectors and Providers—Peacekeepers, Humanitarian Aid Workers and the Media in the Midst of Crisis* (Amityville, N.Y.: Baywood, 2002).

104. See the open letters sent to public officials in Washington, D. C., and in Europe after September 11, 2001, in order to promote the application of international humanitarian law and fundamental human rights guarantees. See also the open letter sent to the Revolutionary Armed Forces of Colombia-People's Army (FARC-EP) on May 8, 2002, denouncing the use of indiscriminate weapons (gas cylinder bombs) as contrary to international humanitarian law. A copy of the letter sent to Commander Marulanda can be found at http://www.hrw.org/press/2002/05/colombia0508.pdf.

105. See Rainer Hofmann and Nils Geissler, eds., "Non-State Actors as New Subjects of International Law—From the Traditional State Order Toward the Law of the Global Community,"

Proceedings of an International Symposium of the Kiel Walther-Schucking Institute of International Law, March 25 to 28, 1998 (Berlin: Duncker & Humblot, 1999); Daniel Byman, Peter Chalk, Bruce Hoffman, William Rosenau, and David Brannan, *Trends in Outside Support for Insurgent Movements* (Washington, D.C.: Rand, 2001).

106. See the "Guidelines for Engaging Non-State Actors in a Landmine-Ban," at http://www .icbl.org/wg/nsa/library/draft%20guidelines.html; Claude Bruderlein, "The Role of Non-State Actors in Building Human Security: The Case of Armed Groups in Intra-State Wars," Policy Paper for the Centre for Humanitarian Dialogue, Geneva, Switzerland (prepared for the Ministerial Meeting of the Human Security Network in Lucerne), May 2000; http://www.hdcentre.org/NewsEvents/1999/ Policy%20paper.doc.

107. Safeguarding human rights is not only the concern of governments and international organizations. Representatives of other international and local players, like human rights defenders, drawn from civil society, have also felt committed to this issue for a long time. See "The 'Human Security Network' Commitments," at the Second Ministerial Meeting in Lucerne, Switzerland, May 11-12, 2000. http://www.humansecuritynetwork.org/commit-e.asp.

108. See the following Human Rights Watch appeals: "Israel/Palestinian Authority: Protect Civilians, Allow Independent Reporting," HRW Press Release, April 3, 2002, at http://hrw.org/ press/2002/04/isr-pa040302.htm; "Jenin: War Crimes Investigation Needed: HRW Press Release, May 3, 2002, at http://hrw.org/press/2002/05/jenin0503.htm.

109. See Daniel L. Smith-Christopher, ed., *Subverting Hatred: The Challenge of Nonviolence in Religious Traditions* (New York: Orbis Books, 1998).

110. See http://www.santegidio.org/ and Andrea Riccardi, *Sant'Egidio, Rome et le monde,* Beauchesne editeur (Paris, 1996); and Philippe Leymarie, "Les batisseurs de paix de Sant'Egidio," *Le Monde Diplomatique* (September 2000): 16–17.

111. See the Executive Summary of the Global Report at http://www.icrc.org/icrceng.nsf/5cacfdf 48ca698b641256242003b3295/be5298c00339e340c1256af4004efaf3?OpenDocument.

112. "Human rights is a complex idea with differing emphases even as between various Western societies. Only with appropriate humility and self-doubt can true dialogue be encouraged." Stephen J. Toope, "Cultural Diversity and Human Rights" (F. R. Scott Lecture). http://collections.ic.gc.ca/ tags/cultural.html.

113. Paul Grossrieder, "Humanitarian Standards and Cultural Differences," in ICRC, *Seminar for Nongovernmental Organizations on Humanitarian Standards and Cultural Differences.* Summary Report, ICRC & The Geneva Foundation to Protect Health in War, Geneva, December 14, 1998.

114. See Umesh Palwankar, "Measures Available to States for Fulfilling Their Obligation to Ensure Respect for International Humanitarian Law," *IRRC* 298 (1994): 9–25. http://www.icrc.org/ Web/Eng/siteeng0.nsf/iwpList113/35289C31F0187A41C1256B6600591427.

115. Such as the U.S. Foreign Assistance Act, which forbids security assistance to any government that "engages in a consistent pattern of gross violations of internationally recognized human rights" [22U.S.C. Secs 2034, 2151n].

116. Mary Griffin, "Ending the Impunity of Human Rights Atrocities: A Major Challenge for International Law in the Twenty-first Century," *IRRC* 838 (2000): 369–389.

117. Resolution 827.

118. Article 2 of the Statute.

119. Article 3.

120. Article 4.

121. Article 5.

122. See Iain Guest (Overseas Development Council) on National Public Radio ("All Things Considered"), Friday April 16, 1999. "The Hague Tribunal was established by the UN Security Council in May 1993, ostensibly to deter war crimes, but the [Security] Council squabbled over funding and even delayed appointing a prosecutor for a year" (on July 8, 1994, Resolution 936, appointing Richard J. Goldstone).

123. See Patricia Grossman, "Bring Warlords to Justice," *International Herald Tribune,* March 9–10, 2002, p. 10.

124. See the following recommendations by Amnesty International:

   1. Ratify the Rome Statute of the International Criminal Court and enact effective implementing legislation to cooperate fully with the Court.

   2. Enact and use universal jurisdiction legislation for the crimes of genocide, crimes against humanity, war crimes, torture, extrajudicial executions and "disappearance," in order that their national courts can investigate and, if there is sufficient admissible evidence, prosecute anyone who enters its territory suspected of these crimes, regardless of where the crime was committed or the nationality of the accused or the victim.

   3. Enact legislation to ensure effective cooperation with the International Criminal Tribunals for the Former Yugoslavia and for Rwanda and any other international criminal court created in the future.

125. International humanitarian law is one of the many legal, political, ethical instruments, in today's global disorder, to deal with our "genocidal mentality" and to "become healers, not killers, of our species." Robert Jay Lifton and Eric Markusen, *The Genocidal Mentality: Nazi Holocaust and Nuclear Threat* (New York: Basic Books, 1990), p. 279.

126. See http://www.guardian.co.uk/waronterror/story/0,1361,583028,00.html; Dr. Scilla Elworthy, "Conflict Resolution in the Twenty-first Century," Tuesday, October 30, 2001; and Michel Veuthey, "Remedies to Promote the Respect of Fundamental Human Values in Non-International Armed Conflicts," *The Israeli Yearbook on Human Rights* 30 (2001): 37–77.

127. The March 2002 issue of Democracy Issues, an electronic journal published by the United States Department of State, is dedicated to human rights education. It includes some interesting contributions, including articles by Felisa Tibbitts ("Emerging Models for Human Rights Education") and Nancy Flowers ("Human Rights Education in U.S. Schools"); an interview with human rights educators from South Africa ("Human Rights Education in Divers, Developing Nations: A Case in Point—South Africa"); and an article on training for judges, prosecutors, attorneys, and the police ("International Human Rights Training" by Michael Hartmann). The journal also features a short bibliography and related Websites. The full text of the journal can be found at http://usinfo.state.gov/journalsitdhr/0302/ijde/ijde0302.htm.

128. Including by campaigns for a universal ratification of human rights and international humanitarian law treaties. See Hans-Peter Gasser, "Steps Taken to Encourage States to Accept the 1977 Protocols," *IRRC* 258 (May 1987). Another example is the campaign conducted in February 2002 to recommend to the U.S. Senate that it ratify the Optional Protocol to the Convention on the Rights of the Child on the Involvement of Children in Armed Conflict; http://world.pylduck.com/02/0212.html

129. See the ICRC's "Woza Africa! Music Goes to War." This was the slogan adopted by six popular African musicians who, responding to the ICRC's call, led a campaign in 1997 to help curb the

indiscriminate violence that has long plagued their continent. The musicians strove to reach people's hearts and minds through a series of original songs, which they performed live and recorded.

130. See "commitment to Global Peace," The Millennium World Peace Summit of Religious and Spiritual Leaders, New York, August 2000; http://global-forum.org/research/globalpeace.html.

131. See the educational programs of the International Committee of the Red Cross (ICRC) (http://www.icrc.org), Red Cross and Red Crescent National Societies, as well as by UNESCO (http://www.unesco.org) and human rights NGOs such as Human Rights Watch, Human Rights Internet, and academic institutions such as the International Institute of Humanitarian Law in San Remo (Italy) with courses on laws of war for military personnel, on refugee law, and on international humanitarian law (http://www.iihl.org).

132. It is not only needed to stop the use of child soldiers (http://www.hrw.org/campaigns/crp/index.htm), but also to reintegrate them into society. See Mike Wessels, "Child Soldiers," *Bulletin of Atomic Scientists* (November–December 1997) (http://pangaea.org/street_children/africa/armies .htm); and the Website of the Office of the SRSG for Children and Armed Conflict (http://www.undp .org/erd/recovery/ddr/organizations/osrg.htm); and UNICEF, "Children at Both Ends of the Gun," http://www.unicef.org/graca/kidsoldi.htm.

133. See *Amnesty International Handbook*, 7th ed., available online, at http://www.amnesty-volunteer.org/aihandbook, especially chap. 4 ("Campaigning") and chap. 5 ("AI Action—Advice and Guidelines"); as well as the excellent *Human Rights Education Handbook* (University of Minnesota Human Rights Resource Center, 2000), available online at http://www.hrusa.org/hrmaterials/hreduseries/hrhandbook1/toc.html.

134. See Morton Winston, "NGO Strategies for Promoting Corporate Social Responsibility," *Ethics & International Affairs* 16, no. 1 (spring 2002). According to Morton Winston, there is a basic divide between NGOs:

    a. Engagers try to draw corporations into dialogue in order to persuade them by means of ethical and prudential arguments to adopt voluntary codes of conduct, while confronters believe that corporations will act only when their financial interests are threatened, and therefore take a more adversarial stance toward them.

    b. Confrontational NGOs tend to employ moral stigmatization, or "naming and shaming," as their primary tactic, while NGOs that favor engagement offer dialogue and limited forms of cooperation with willing MNCs.

135. See William Hartung, "The New Business of War: Small Arms and the Business of Conflict," *Ethics & International Affairs Annual Journal of the Carnegie Council on Ethics and International Affairs* 15, no.1 (2001). The author's argument is the following: The proliferation of internal conflicts fueled by small arms poses a grave threat to peace, democracy, and the rule of law. The weapons of choice in today's conflicts are not big-ticket items like long-range missiles, tanks, and fighter planes, but small and frighteningly accessible weapons ranging from handguns, carbines, and assault rifles on up to machine guns, rocket-propelled grenades, and shoulder-fired missiles. In conflict zones from Colombia to the Democratic Republic of the Congo, picking up a gun has become the preferred route for generating income, obtaining political power, and generating "employment" for young people, many no more than children, who have little prospect of securing a decent education or a steady job. Ending the cycle of violence fueled by small arms must become a top priority for the international community. No single treaty or set of actions, however, will "solve" the problem of light weapons proliferation. What is needed is a series of overlapping measures involving stricter laws and regulations, greater transparency, and innovative diplomatic and economic initiatives.

136. See Anna Segall, "Economic Sanctions: Legal and Policy Constraints," *IRRC* 81, no. 836 (December 1999): pp. 763-784; and Claude Bruderlein, "UN Sanctions Can Be More Humane and Better Targeted," *Public Affairs Report* (University of California, Berkeley) 41, no. 1 (January 2000) http://www.igs.berkeley.edu/publications/par/Jan2000/Bruderlein.html; Arthur C. Helton and Robert P. DeVecchi, "Human Rights, Humanitarian Intervention and Sanctions," http://www .foreignpolicy2000.org/library/issuebriefs/IBHumanRights.html; and H. C. Graf Sponeck, "Sanctions and Humanitarian Exemptions: A Practitioner's Commentary," *European Journal of International Law* 13, no. 1 (2002): 81–87. Full text available at http://www3.oup.co.uk/ejilaw/current/130081.sgm .abs.html.

137. See Michel Veuthey, "The Contribution of the 1949 Geneva Conventions to International Security," *Refugee Survey Quarterly* 18, no. 3 (1999): 22–26.

138. See Antonia Cassese, "The Martens Clause: Half a Loaf or Simply Pie in the Sky?" *EJIL* 11, no. 1 (2000): 187–216; Theodor Meron, "The Martens Clause, Principles of Humanity, and Dictates of Public Conscience," *AJIL* 94, no. 2 (2000): 78–89; Shigeki Miyazaki, "The Martens Clause and International Humanitarian Law," in *Etudes et essais sur le droit international humanitaire et sur les principes de la Croix-Rouge en l'honneur de Jean Pictet*, ed. C. Swinarski (Geneva: ICRC, 1984), pp. 433–444.

Nicola Smith and Larry Hollingworth, Humanitarian Vignettes

Originally published in Kevin M. Cahill, ed., *Technology for Humanitarian Action* (New York: Fordham University Press, 2005), 40 and 138.

Valerie Amos, Humanitarian Response in the Era of Global Mobile Information Technology

Originally published in Kevin M. Cahill, M.D., ed., *More with Less: Disasters in an Era of Diminishing Resources* (New York: Fordham University Press, 2012), 110–122.

1. A video of the creation of this volunteer map is viewable at http://vimeo.com/9182869.

2. See (SBTF team member) Patrick Meier, "The [unexpected] Impact of the Libya Crisis Map and the Standby Volunteer Task Force." Available at http://blog.standbytaskforce.com/sbtf-libya-impact.

3. One of several accounts of the intervention can be found on the SBTF website: http://blog .standbytaskforce.com/unhcr-somalia-latest-results.

4. Internews, *Dadaab, Kenya: Humanitarian Communications and Information Needs Assessment among Refugees in the Camps* (Washington, D.C.: Internews, 2011). Available at http://www.internews .org/sites/default/files/resources/Dadaab2011-09-14.pdf.

5. Statement by WFP.

6. Linus Bengtsson, Xin Lu, Richard Garfield, Anna Thorson, and Johan von Schreeb, *Internal Population Displacement in Haiti: Preliminary Analyses of Movement Patterns of Digicel Mobile Phones: 1 January to 11 March 2010* (Karolinska Institute and Columbia University). Available at http://haiti .humanitarianresponse.info/LinkClick.aspx?fileticket=ZPH8pFFkMnU%3D&tabid=149&mid=1045.

7. See, for example, Concern Worldwide, Oxford Policy Management, and the Partnership for Research in International Affairs and Development, *New Technologies in Cash Transfer Programming and Humanitarian Assistance* (Oxford: Cash Learning Partnership, 2011), 57.

Alain Destexhe, M.D., Neutrality or Impartiality

Originally published in Kevin M. Cahill, M.D., ed., *Preventative Diplomacy: Stopping Wars Before They Start* (New York: Routledge, 2000), 101–117.

1. H. Dunant, *Un souvenir de Solferino* (Geneva, 1862).

2. A. Destexhe, *L'humanitaire impossible ou deux siècles d'ambiguité* (Paris: Armand Colin, 1993).

3. J. C. Favez, *Une mission impossible? Le CICR, les deportations et les camps de concentration Nazis* (Lausanne: Editions Payot, 1988).

4. J. de Saint Jorre, *The Nigerian Civil War* (London: Hodder & Stoughton, 1972).

5. A. Destexhe, "Why Famine?" in *Populations in Danger*, ed. F. Jean and A. M. Huby (London: John Libbey/Médecins Sans Frontières, 1992).

6. R. Lemkin, *Axis Rule in Occupied Europe* (Washington, D.C.: Carnegie Endowment for International Peace, 1994).

7. United Nations Convention on the Prevention and Punishment of the Crime of Genocide, approved December 9, 1948, in effect since January 12, 1951.

8. A. Destexhe, "The Third Genocide," *Foreign Policy* 97 (Winter 1994–95); A. Destexhe, *Rwanda and Genocide in the Twentieth Century* (New York: New York University Press, 1995).

9. *The Shorter Oxford English Dictionary* (Oxford: Oxford University Press, 1992).

10. William Shawcross, *The Quality of Mercy: Cambodia, Holocaust and Modern Conscience* (New York: Simon & Schuster, 1984).

11. On several occasions, Bosnia's leaders made it known that if they were given the choice between humanitarian aid and arms (or the lifting of the arms embargo), they would prefer the latter option.

Timothy W. Harding, M.D., Torture

Originally published in Kevin M. Cahill, M.D., ed., *Traditions, Values, and Humanitarian Action* (New York: Fordham University Press, 2003), 191–211.

1. J. Swain, *A History of Torture* (London: Tandem Books, 1986).

2. E. Peters, *Torture* (Oxford: Blackwell, 1985).

3. D. Forrest. ed., *A Glimpse of Hell* (London: Amnesty International/Cassel, 1996).

4. S. Milgram, "Behavioural Study of Obedience," *Journal of Abnormal Social Psychology* 67 (1963): 277–285.

5. Y. Tanaka, *Hidden Horrors: Japanese War Crimes in World War II* (Boulder, Colo.: Westview, 1996).

6. K. Farrington, *History of Punishment and Torture* (London: Hamlyn, 2000). See also M. Kerrigan, *The Instruments of Torture* (Guilford, Conn.: Lyons Press, 2001).

7. For the relationship between the terms "torture" and "cruel, inhuman, or degrading treatment," see chapter 3 of N. Rodley, *The Treatment of Prisoners Under International Law* (Oxford: Oxford University Press, 1987).

8. P. Tavernier, "Article 15" in L-E. Petititi, E. Decaux, and P-H. Imbert, *La Convention européenne des droits de l'homme: Commentaire article par article* (Paris: Economica, 1995).

9. Human Rights Watch, *Torture Archipelago: Arbitrary Arrests, Torture and Enforced Disappearances in Syria's Underground Prisons since March 2011* (New York: Human Rights Watch, 2012).

10. Rita Maran, *Torture: The Role of Ideology in the French-Algerian War* (New York: Praeger, 1989).

11. International Committee of the Red Cross, *Report on the Treatment by Coalition Forces of Prisoners of War and Other Protected Persons by the Geneva Conventions in Iraq during Arrest, Internment and Interrogation* (Geneva: ICRC, 2004).

12. Neil A. Lewis, "Red Cross Finds Detainee Abuse in Guantanamo," *New York Times*, November 30, 2004.

13. The full judgment can be found at http://www.hudoc.echr.coe.int.

14. Editorial, "Doctors and Torture," *British Medical Journal* 319 (1999): 397–398.

15. British Medical Association, *Torture Report* (London: Tavistock, 1986).

16. British Medical Association, *Medicine Betrayed: The Participation of Doctors in Human Rights Abuses* (London: Zed Books, 1992).

17. R. J. Lifton, *The Nazi Doctors: The Psychology of Medical Killing* (London: Papermac, 1986; new edition available from Basic Books with the modified title *The Nazi Doctors: Medical Killing and the Psychology of Genocide*, 2000).

18. E. Staub, "The Psychology and Culture of Torture and Torturers," in *Psychology and Torture*, ed. P. Suedfeld (New York: Hemisphere, 1990).

Judy A. Benjamin, Issues of Power and Gender in Complex Emergencies

Originally published in Kevin M. Cahill, M.D., ed., *Emergency Relief Operations* (New York: Fordham University Press, 2003), 153–179.

1. UNHCR report, *On Sexual Violence and Exploitation in West Africa*, Note for Implementing and Operational Partners by UNHCR and Save the Children U.K., April 26, 2002.

2. Caroline Moser, *Gender Planning and Development: Theory, Practice and Training* (New York: Routledge, 1993).

3. In this chapter the terms "refugee women" and "displaced women" are for the most part interchangeable.

4. Universal Declaration of Human Rights (UDHR), General Assembly, A/RES/17 A (III), December 10, 1948.

5. The Convention on the Elimination of All Forms of Discrimination against Women (CEDAW), A/RES/34/180, December 18, 1979.

6. The Convention against Torture and Other Cruel, Inhuman or Degrading Treatment or Punishment (Torture Convention), General Assembly, A/RES/39/46, December 10, 1984.

Larry Hollingworth, Terrorism: Theory and Reality

Originally published in Kevin M. Cahill, M.D., ed., *Traditions, Values, and Humanitarian Action* (New York: Fordham University Press, 2003), 226–241.

1. Alex P. Schmid and Albert J. Longman, et al., *Political Terrorism: A New Guide to Actors, Authors, Concepts, Data Bases, Theories and Literature* (Amsterdam: North Holland, 1988).

2. Noam Chomsky, "International Terrorism: Image and Reality," in *Western State Terrorism*, ed. Alexander George (New York: Routledge, 1991).

3. U.S. State Department, Annual Review of Global Terrorism 2002.

4. Igor Primoratz, "State Terrorism and Counterterrorism," Center for Applied Philosophy and Public Ethics, University of Melbourne.

5. Rakesh Gupta, "Changing Conceptions of Terrorism," JNU: http://www.idsa-India.org.

6. Primoratz, "State Terrorism and Counterterrorism."

7. Jacques Ellul, *Violence* (London: Mowbrays, 1978).

8. Ibid., 56.

9. Chomsky, "International Terrorism."

10. Extracts from Rudolph Peters, *Jihad* (Lanham, Md.: Marcus Weiner, 2005).

11. Edward S. Herman and David Peterson, "The Threat of Global State Terrorism: Retail versus Wholesale Terror," *Z Magazine* (January 2002).

12. William Blum, *Killing Hope* (Monroe, Maine: Common Courage Press, 1999).

13. William Blum, *Rogue State* (Monroe, Maine: Common Courage Press, 2000).

14. "Lethal Hypocrisy—John Pilger on State Terrorism," John Pilger Pacific Media Watch, 2002.

15. Primoratz, "State Terrorism and Counterterrorism."

16. Irving Kristol, "Where Have All the Gunboats Gone?" *Wall Street Journal*, December 13, 1973.

17. Lev Grinberg, "State Terrorism in Israel?" *Tikkun* (May–June 2002).

18. Chomsky, "International Terrorism."

19. "Israel, the Occupied West Bank and Gaza Strip, and the Palestinian Authority Territories. Jenin: IDF Military Operations," *Human Rights Watch* 20, no. 10 (May 2002): 10.

20. Grinberg, "State Terrorism in Israel?"

21. "Israel and the Occupied Territories," *Amnesty International* (November 2002).

Irene Khan, A Human Rights Agenda for Global Security

Originally published in Kevin M. Cahill, M.D., ed., *Human Security for All* (New York: Fordham University Press, 2004), 15–27.

Francis Deng, The Limits of Sovereignty

Originally published in Kevin M. Cahill, M.D., ed., *Preventative Diplomacy: Stopping Wars Before They Start* (New York: Routledge, 2000), 119–142.

1. The working definition of the internally displaced used by the 1992 analytical report of the UN Secretary-General considers them "persons who have been forced to flee their homes suddenly or unexpectedly in large numbers, as a result of armed conflict, internal strife, systematic violations of human rights or natural or man-made disasters; and who are within the territory of their own country" (*Analytical Report of the Secretary-General on Internally Displaced Persons*, E/CN.4/1992/23(1992), pp. 4–5). IDP figure cited in 1999 GA report at par. 1. Refugee figure (actual figure is 11, 491, 710) cited in UNHCR's *Refugees and Others of Concern to UNHCR-Statistical Overview* (Table 1.4, "Indicative number of Refugees, 1989–1998").

2. Statement by Mrs. Sadako Ogata to the World Conference on Human Rights (Vienna, June 15, 1993), 3.

3. UNHCR, *The State of the Word's Refugees: In Search of Solutions* (London: Oxford University Press, 1995), 8–10.

4. Ogata, Statement to the World Conference on Human Rights, 3.

5. M. Toole, Centers for Disease Control, Department of Health and Human Services, testimony before the U.S. Senate, April 3, 1990, as quoted in Refugee Policy Group, "Internally Displaced Women and Children in Africa" (1992).

6. Boutros Boutros-Ghali, Report of the Secretary-General on the Work of the Organization, A/50/60; S/1995/1, 3.

7. Ibid., 5. Evidently, because there are no reliable statistics, estimates for both refugees and internally displaced vary considerably.

8. L. Minear and T. Weiss, *Humanitarian Politics* (Washington D.C.: Foreign Policy Association, 1994).

9. Statement by Mrs. Sadako Ogata on the occasion of accepting the Human Rights Award from the international Human Rights Law Group, Washington, D.C., June 8, 1994.

10. Ibid.

11. Ibid.

12. B. Boutros-Ghali, Report of the Secretary-General, par. 27, pp. 7–8.

13. H. Hannum, *Autonomy, Sovereignty, and Self-Determination: The Accommodation of Conflicting Rights* (Philadelphia: University of Pennsylvania Press, 1990); G. M. Lyons and M. Matastanduno, *Beyond Westphalia?* (Philadelphia: University of Pennsylvania Press, 1995), 6; and T. G. Weiss and J. Chopra, "Sovereignty Is No Longer Sacrosanct: Codifying Humanitarian Intervention," *Ethics and International Affairs* 6 (1992): 95.

14. J. Austin, *Lectures on Jurisprudence*, ed. Robert Campbell, 1885, 225–226. Extracts reproduced in D. Lloyd, *Introduction to Jurisprudence* (London: Stevens and Sons, 1959), 134–37; and W. M. Reisman and A. M. Schreiber, *Jurisprudence: Understanding and Shaping Law* (New Haven, Conn.: Yale University Press, 1987), 270–280. See also W. Friedmann, *Legal Theory*, 4th ed. (London: Stevens and Sons, 1960), 211–13.

15. Friedmann, *Legal Theory*, 211.

16. L. L. Fuller, "Positivism and Fidelity to Law: A Reply to Professor Hart," *Harvard Law Review* 71 (1958): 634; see also H. L. A. Hart, "Positivism and the Separation of Law and Morals," *Harvard Law Review* 72 (1958): 593–629.

17. Weiss and Chopra, "Sovereignty," 103. See also F. H. Hinley, *Sovereignty*, 2d ed. (Cambridge: Cambridge University Press, 1986).

18. W. M. Reisman, "Through or Despite Governments: Differentiated Responsibilities of Human Rights Programs," *Iowa Law Review* 72, no. 2 (January 1987): 391–399.

19. Richard B. Lillich, "Sovereignty and Humanity: Can They Converge?" in *The Spirit of Uppsala* 406–407, ed. A. Grahl-Madsen and J. Toman (Hawthorne, N.Y.: De Gruyter, 1984). Quoted in Lewis Henkin et al., *International Law: Cases and Materials,* 3rd ed. (St. Paul, Minn.: West, 1993), 19.

20. Lyons and Mastanduno, *Beyond Westphalia,* 6.

21. W. M. Reisman, "Humanitarian Intervention and Fledgling Democracies," *Fordham International Law Journal* 18, no. 3 (1988): 794–805, 795. See also W. M. Reisman, "Coercion and Self-Determination: Construing Charter Article 2(4)," *American Journal of International Law* 624 (1984): 78; and "Sovereignty and Human Rights in Contemporary International Law," *American Journal of International Law* 866 (1990): 84.

22. W. M. Reisman, "Haiti and the Validity of International Action," *American Society of International Law* 899, no.1 (January 1995): 82–84, 83.

23. UN press release SG/SM/4560, April 24, 1991. Cited in Lyons and Mastanduno, *Beyond Westphalia,* 2. Portions of the statement also cited in David J. Scheffer, "Toward a Modern Doctrine of Humanitarian Intervention," 23 *University of Toledo Law Review* 253 (1992): 262.

24. J. Perez de Cuellar, *Report of the Secretary-General on the Work of the Organization* (1991), 12, 13.

25. Ibid.

26. B. Boutros-Ghali, *An Agenda for Peace,* June 17, 1992, UN Document A/47277-S/2411, p.5.

27. B. Boutros-Ghali, "Empowering the United Nations," *Foreign Affairs* (Winter 1992/93): 91–101, 99.

28. Scheffer, "Toward a Modern Doctrine of Humanitarian Intervention," 262–263.

29. Council of Ministers, *Report of the Secretary-General on Conflicts in Africa: Proposals for an OAU Mechanism for Conflict Prevention and Resolution,* CM/1710 (L. VI) Addis Ababa: Organization of African Unity, 1992).

30. Ibid.

31. United Nations, Note by the President of the Security Council, S/25344 (February 26, 1993).

32. United Nations, *Analytical Report of the Secretary-General on Internally Displaced Persons,* E/CN.4.1992/23.

33. See R. Cohen and J. Cuenod, "Improving Institutional Arrangements for the Internally Displaced," Brookings Institution/ Refugee Policy Group Project on Internal Displacement, October 1995.

34. Statement by Mrs. Sadako Ogata, United Nations High Commissioner for Refugees, to the 52nd Session of the United Nations Commission on Human Rights, Geneva, March 20, 1996, p.5.

See Economic and Social Council, Commission on Human Rights, *Internally Displaced Persons: Report of the Representative of the Secretary-General,* Mr. Francis M. Deng, E/CN.4/1995/50 (New York: United Nations, 1995); and Chris J. Bakwesegha, "The Role of Organization of African Unity in Conflict Prevention, Management and Resolution," paper prepared for the Organization of African Unity/United Nation High Displacement in Africa, Addis Ababa, September 1994.

Statement by Mrs. Sadako Ogata, United Nations High Commissioner for Refugees, to the 52nd Session of the United Nations Commission on Human Rights, Geneva, March 20, 1996, p. 5.

Alec Wargo, The Child Protection Viewpoint

Originally published in Kevin M. Cahill, ed., *Even in Chaos: Education in Times of Emergency* (New York: Fordham University Press, 2010), 26–43.

1. For the purposes of this chapter, "education" is defined as the individual persons that make up an education system who can feasibly be engaged in protection activities, including but not limited to administrators, teachers, parent-teacher associations, and, with safeguards, children themselves.

2. Under Security Council Resolutions 1612 (2005) and 1882 (2009), grave rights violations during armed conflict include recruitment or use of children by armed forces or groups, killing and maiming of children, sexual violence perpetrated against children, attacks on schools and hospitals, abduction of children and denial of humanitarian access for children. Of course, these are not exhaustive, but they are often indicative of a wider range of abuse suffered by children during wartime.

3. The UN-accepted definition of a child soldier is any child, girl or boy, recruited or used by an armed force or group in any capacity including, but not limited to, combatants, sexual slaves, porters, cooks, spies, and the like.

4. It is the viewpoint of the United Nations that children under legal age of recruitment are, by their very minority, unable to make a mature choice on what harm may befall them if they are recruited and used in armed conflict.

Peter Hansen, Preserving Humanitarian Space in Long-Term Conflict

Originally published in Kevin M. Cahill, M.D., *Human Security for All* (New York: Fordham University Press, 2004), 147–164.

1. D. Warner, "The Politics of the Political/Humanitarian Divide," *International Review of the Red Cross* 833 (March 31, 1999): 109–118.

2. A. Donini, "The Future of Humanitarian Action: Implications of Iraq and Other Recent Crises—Issues Note (workshop organized by the Feinstein International Famine Center and the Friedman School of Nutrition Science and Policy, Tufts University, Boston, October 9, 2003), 3.

3. Warner, "Politics of the Political/Humanitarian Divide."

4. "Annual Report of the Secretary-General on the work of the Organization" (annual report, United Nations, New York City, 1995), http://www.un.org/docs/sg/sg-rpt.

5. B. Megevand Roggo, "After the Kosovo Conflict, a Genuine Humanitarian Space: A Utopian Concept or an Essential Requirement?" *International Review of the Red Cross* 837 (March 31, 2000): 31–47.

6. Warner, "Politics of the Political/Humanitarian Divide."

7. C. Eguizabal et al., "Humanitarian Challenges in Central America: Learning the Lessons of Recent Armed Conflicts" (Occasional Paper, no. 14, Thomas J. Watson Jr. Institute for International Studies, Brown University, 1993), 17.

8. Australian Council for Overseas Aid, "Guiding Principles for Civil Military Action," http://www.acfoa.asn.au/emergencies/cimic_interaction.htm.

9. International humanitarian law regulates the conduct of armed conflict between states and nonstate actors. Many of its principles exist in customary international law. In conventional form, this

body of law is best exemplified by the Geneva Conventions of 1949, the fourth of which concerns the protection of civilian persons in time of war. Examples of how the concept of humanitarian space is incorporated into the Fourth Geneva Convention abound, and include, *inter alia*, the designation of civilians as "protected persons" (Article 4); the establishment of "hospital and safety zones" (Article 14) as well as "neutral zones" (Article 15); the protection of the "wounded and sick, as well as the infirm, and expectant mothers" (Article 15); the protection of "hospital staff" (Article 20); protection of medical convoys (Articles 21–22) and free passage of "medical supplies, food and clothing" (Articles 23 and 55); protection of children (Articles 24 and 50); protection against "collective penalties" (Article 33); protection of real and personal property (Article 53); and protection against "willful killing," "torture or inhumane treatment," "unlawful deportation or transfer," "unfair trials," "taking of hostages," and "extensive destruction and appropriation of property" (Article 147).

See United Nations, Geneva Convention for the Amelioration of the Condition of the Wounded and Sick in Armed Forces in the Field, August 12, 1949, 6 U.S.T. 3114, 75 U.N.T.S. 31 (entered into force October 21, 1950); United Nations, Geneva Convention for the Amelioration of the Condition of the Wounded, Sick and Shipwrecked Members of Armed Forces at Sea, August 12, 1949, 6 U.S.T. 3217, 75 U.N.T.S. 85 (entered into force October 21, 1950); United Nations, Geneva Convention Relative to the Treatment of Prisoners of War, August 12, 1949, 6 U.S.T. 3316, 75 U.N.T.S. 135 (entered into force October 21, 1950); United Nations, Geneva Convention Relative to the Protection of Civilian Persons in Time of War, August 12, 1949, 6 U.S.T. 3516, 75 U.N.T.S. 287 (entered into force October 21, 1950).

10. T. G. Weiss, "Principles, Politics and Humanitarian Action," *Ethics and International Affairs* 13 (December 4, 1999): 1. Humanitarianism and War Project, Tufts University, http://hwproject.tufts.edu/publications/electronic/e_ppaha.html.

11. A. Donini, "The Future of Humanitarian Action."

12. Ibid., 11.

13. Ibid.

14. Megevand Roggo, "After the Kosovo Conflict, a Genuine Humanitarian Space."

15. Warner, "Politics of the Political/Humanitarian Divide."

16. For instance, in April 2003 Israeli troops took over UNRWA's Tulkarem Girls School for use over several days as a mass detention center for male residents of the Tulkarem refugee camp. Likewise, in September 2002 an armed Israeli special unit made an incursion into UNRWA's Qalqilya hospital, where it threatened staff and patients at gunpoint, beat five members of the hospital staff, including a female administrator and health official who had arrived at the scene to treat the wounded, and then arrested three other UNRWA staff members. Likewise, on May 23, 2003, Palestinian militants purporting to be members of the Al Aqsa Martyrs' Brigades broke into the Balata Camp Boys School and held a memorial ceremony attended by thousands of people, where political speeches were given and weapons were fired into the air.

17. Warner, "Politics of the Political/Humanitarian Divide."

18. Ibid.

19. Weiss, "Principles, Politics and Humanitarian Action," 12–13.

20. M. Anderson, "Reflecting on the Practice of Outside Assistance: Can We Know What Good We Do?" (handbook, Berghof Handbook for Conflict Transformation, Berlin, April 2001). See also M. Anderson, *Do No Harm: How Aid Can Support Peace or War* (Boulder, Colo.: Lynne Rienner, 1999).

21. See Anderson, "Reflecting on the Practice of Outside Assistance."

22. Ibid.

23. Michael Meyer, "Neutrality as a Fundamental Principle of the Red Cross," *International Review of the Red Cross* 315 (December 31, 1996): 627–630.

24. Ibid.

25. Anderson, "Reflecting on the Practice of Outside Assistance."

26. Ibid.

27. Article 103 of the UN Charter provides that "in the event of a conflict between the obligations under any other international agreement, the obligations of the present *Charter* shall prevail." Articles 104 and 105 of the UN Charter provide the general concepts of privileges and immunities of the United Nations upon which the 1946 Convention on the Privileges and Immunities of the United Nations is based, to which the State of Israel is a party.

28. Lincoln Chen, M.D., "Expanding Humanitarian Space: Challenge for Global Philanthropy" (paper, Humanitarian Interventions Today: New Issues, New Ideas, New Players conference sponsored by the Conrad Hilton Foundation, New York City, September 24, 2003, http://www.bettersaferworld.org/issues/lincoln_chen_article.

29. Ibid.

David Rieff, Humanitarian Action in a New Barbarian Age

Originally published in Kevin M. Cahill, M.D., ed., *Human Security for All* (New York: Fordham University Press, 2004), 52–59.

1. Raymond Aron, *Thinking Politically: A Liberal in an Age of Ideology* (New Brunswick, N.J.: Transaction Publishers, 1997).

Boutros Boutros-Ghali, The Challenges of Preventive Diplomacy: The Role of the United Nations and Its Secretary-General

Originally published in Kevin M. Cahill, M.D., ed., *Preventive Diplomacy: Stopping Wars Before They Start* (New York: Routledge, 2000), 189–204.

1. Johan Galtung and Daisaku Ikeda, *Choose Peace: A Dialogue between Johan Galtung and Daisaku Ikeda* (London: Pluto Press, 1995).

2. B. Boutros-Ghali, An Agenda for Peace, June 17, 1992, UN Document A/47277-S/24111.

Ed Tsui, Initial Response to Complex Emergencies and Natural Disasters

Originally published in Kevin M. Cahill, M.D., ed., *Emergency Relief Operations* (New York: Fordham University Press, 2003), 32–54.

Kofi A. Annan, The Peacekeeping Prescription

Originally published in Kevin M. Cahill, M.D., ed., *Preventive Diplomacy: Stopping Wars Before They Start* (New York: Routledge, 2000), 175–185.

Richard Falk, Reviving Global Civil Society After September 11

Originally published in Kevin M. Cahill, M.D., ed., *Traditions, Values, and Humanitarian Action* (New York: Fordham University Press, 2003), 344–367.

1. For amplification, see R. Falk, "Testing Patriotism and Citizenship in the Global Terror War," in *Worlds in Collision: Terror and the Future of Global Order*, ed. Ken Booth and Tim Dunne (New York: Palgrave Macmillan, 200), 325–335.

2. For a useful description of these dynamics, see Margaret E. Keck and Keck and Kathryn Sikkink, *Activists Beyond Border: Advocacy Networks in International Politics* (Ithaca, N.Y.: Cornell University Press, 1998).

3. This combination of chaos and complexity has reminded analysts of the contemporary world of the medieval period that preceded the emergence of a framework for world order that was based on the primacy of the sovereign state.

4. See R. Falk, "The First Normative Global Revolution: The Uncertain Future of Globalization," in *Globalization and Civilizations*, ed. Mehdi Mazaffari (London: Routledge, 2002), 51–76.

5. But see Michael Ignatieff, *Human Rights as Politics and Idolatry* (Princeton, N.J.: Princeton University Press, 2001), who challenges this assertion.

6. See George J. Andreopoulos, ed., *Concepts and Strategies in International Human Rights* (New York: Peter Lang, 2002), esp. 1–20, 213–220; see also Paul Gordon Lauren, *The Evolution of International Human Rights* (Philadelphia: University of Pennsylvania Press, 1999).

7. For overall assessments, see Thomas Risse, Stephen C. Ropp, and Kathryn Sikkink, eds., *The Power of Human Right: International Norms and Domestic Change* (Cambridge: Cambridge University Press, 1999).

8. For a convenient collection of the major human rights instruments, see Burns H. Weston, Richard A. Falk, and Hilary Charlesworth, eds., *Supplement of Basic Documents to International Law and World Order*, 3rd ed. (St. Paul, Minn.: West Group, 1997), 368–670.

9. See Thomas Franck, "The Emerging Right of Democratic Governance," *American Journal of International Law* 86, no. 1 (1992): 46; for a more skeptical and sophisticated view of democracy and human rights, see Susan Marks, *The Riddle of All Constitutions: International Law, Democracy and the Critique of Ideology* (Oxford: Oxford University Press, 2000).

10. There was a growing public appreciation that it was not only governments that were responsible for repressive practices. In the Indian context, cultural practices in defiance of the law, such as bride-burning or *suti*, were responsible for cruelty to individuals that departed from international human rights norms. The same pattern in associated with "honor killings" in the Middle East and "female circumcision" in Africa. Even in the United States, it is the citizenry that has exerted pressure on governmental institutions to reestablish capital punishment.

11. For a discussion of cases and principles pertaining to humanitarian intervention, see Nicholas J. Wheeler, *Saving Strangers: Humanitarian Intervention in International Society* (Oxford: Oxford University Press, 200); for a focus on a debate occasioned by the NATO intervention in Kosovo, see Independent International Commission on Kosovo, *Kosovo Report: Conflict, Response, Lessons Learned* (Oxford: Oxford University Press, 2001).

12. For a useful review of the debate, see Ken Booth, ed., *The Kosovo Tragedy: The Human Rights Dimensions* (London: Frank Cass, 2001); see also sources cited in note 11.

13. On Rwanda, see particularly Linda Melvern, *A People Betrayed: The Role of the West in Rwanda's Genocide* (New York: Zed, 2000); on Bosnia, see David Rieff, *Slaughterhouse* (New York: Simon & Schuster, 1995).

14. A perceptive overview of these developments can be found in Elazar Barkan, *The Guilt of Nations: Restitution and Negotiating Historical Injustices* (New York: Norton, 2000); for a philosophical inquiry into these issues, see Janna Thompson, *Taking Responsibility for the Past: Reparation and Historical Injustice* (Cambridge: Polity, 2002).

15. For an approach to justice and reconciliation for indigenous peoples, see Maivan Clêch Lam, *At the Edge of the State: Indigenous Peoples and Self-Determination* (Ardsley, N.Y.: Transnational Publishers, 2000).

16. Two excellent books examine the development. See Martha Minow, *Between Vengeance and Forgiveness: Facing History after Genocide and Hand of Violence* (Boston: Beacon Press, 1998); Gary Jonathan Bass, *Stay the Hand of Vengeance: The Politics of War Crimes Tribunals* (Princeton, N.J.: Princeton University Press, 2000).

17. For an attempt to provide national courts with a standardized framework with which to deal with these issues, see *The Princeton Principles on Universal Jurisdiction*, published by the Program in Law and Public Affairs, Princeton University, 2001.

18. Victors' justice is well depicted in Richard H. Minear, *Victors' Justice: The Tokyo War Crimes Tribunal* (Princeton, N.J.: Princeton University Press, 1971).

19. For a sense of the range and depth of concerns arising from this transnational peoples perspectives, see Robin Broad, ed., *Global Backlash: Citizen Initiatives for a Just World Economy* (Lanham, Md.: Rowman & Littlefield, 2002); *Alternatives to Economic Globalization: Another World is Possible*, Report of the International Forum on Globalization (San Francisco: Barrett-Koeler, 2000).

20. See George Soros, *George Soros on Globalization* (New York: Public Affairs, 2002); Joseph E. Stiglitz, *Globalization and Its Discontents* (New York: Norton, 2002).

21. See the cover story in *The Economist* bearing the caption "Is Torture Ever Justified?" *The Economist* (January 11–17, 2003), 18–20.

22. Such an issue is posed vividly by Michael Ignatieff, "The Burden," *New York Times Magazine* (January 5, 2003), 22–27, 50–54; for a far more skeptical rendering, see Alain Joxe, *Empire of Disorder* (Los Angeles: Semiotext[e], 2002).

Joseph A. O'Hare, S.J., The Academy and Humanitarian Action

Originally published in Kevin M. Cahill, M.D., ed., *Traditions, Values, and Humanitarian Action* (New York: Fordham University Press, 2003), 113–122

Peter Tarnoff, Government Responses to Foreign Policy Challenges

Originally published in Kevin M. Cahill, M.D., ed., *Traditions, Values, and Humanitarian Action* (New York: Fordham University Press, 2003), 328–343.

Jeremy Toye, Disasters and the Media

Originally published in Kevin M. Cahill, M.D., ed., *More with Less: Disasters in an Era of Diminishing Resources* (New York: Fordham University Press, 2012), 123–141.

1. For North America see the Audit Bureau of Circulations (ABC) website (http://www.accessabc.com) and the related ABC sites for other countries.

2. Pliny's account of the disaster makes clear warning signs that Vesuvius was about to erupt were ignored, and no help came. See Andrew Wallace-Hadrill, "Pompeii: Portents of Disaster," BBC.co.uk, last modified March 29, 2011, available at http://www.bbc.co.uk /history/ancient/romans/ Pompeii_portents 01.shtml.

3. News of the assassination in 1865 took its time to reach the rest of the world—a steamship voyage across the Atlantic. The laying of the first transatlantic cable and subsequent global network made information flow almost instantaneous.

4. See http://www.parliament.uk.

5. See "Issue Brief: Ethiopian Famine 25th Anniversary," One.org, available at http://one.org/c/us/issuebrief /3127/.

6. See the Museum of Broadcast Communications (http://www.museum.tv), an archive of TV footage that features news of Vietnam War.

7. The video won the George Polk award for videography in 2009. See Robert McFadden, "Times Reporter Held by Taliban Is among Polk Award Winners," *New York Times*, February 16, 2010.

8. Between August 6 and 10, 2011, several districts of London and provincial cities were hit by riots involving looting and arson, with the police seemingly unable or unwilling to intervene.

9. Copies of the video can be found on the web, but their distribution was condemned at the time.

10. Reporters without Borders (http://www.rsf.org) said sixty -seven journalists were killed in 2011 alone. See "2011: 67 Journalists Killed," Reporters without Borders, available at http://en.rsf.org/press-freedom-barometer-journalists-killed.html?annee=2011.

11. See http://www.rt.com and others.

12. "Television? The word is half Greek and half Latin. No good can come of it." Attributed to Scott by various sources, in slightly different forms.

13. Scottish Television's Roy Thomson, quoted by http://www.news.bbc.co.uk, available at http://news.bbc.co.uk/2/hi/entertainment/1229805.stm.

14. In a Mozambique community where I have worked on a tiny community support scheme, we sent a messenger on foot for several hours to deliver a phone SIM card to a village chief so he could discuss the next stage in building classrooms. See http://www.mandawilderness.org.

15. See http://www.guardian.co.uk/katine.

16. Conversation with the author, 2011.

17. Newspaper Death Watch (newspaperdeathwatch.com) listed fourteen U.S. metropolitan dailies that had closed by early 2012, including the *Rocky Mountain News* and the *Albuquerque Tribune*.

18. See report on online versus traditional advertising on readwriteweb.com.

19. See the *Huffington Post* (http://www.huffingtonpost.com) and others. The fact that more than 70 million people watched a thirty- minute video produced by the hitherto little-known charity Invisible Children provoked controversy, though it was unclear whether it would help or hinder the search for the leader of a ruthless band of killers operating in Central Africa.

20. There are surprisingly few truly international agencies: Associated Press, Reuters, Agence France Presse, and Kyodo are the main ones.

21. When I asked the Information Minister of Ethiopia why he never seemed to have any information to impart, he replied with a smirk that it was his job to collect information, not to hand it out to the likes of me.

22. I asked a government spokesman for an update on a bird flu outbreak: "Eighty percent of the poultry tested was unaffected," he said loftily. "So 20 percent had bird flu?" I said. "That is not an acceptable question," he railed. To be fair, it was a training session, and once he had calmed down, he accepted that it might have been better handled.

23. Bolton speaking on February 3, 1994. See "John Bolton in His Own Words: Bush's UN Ambassador Nominee Condemns United Nations," Democracy Now, last modified March 31, 2005, available at http://www.democracynow.org/2005/3/31/john bolton_in his own words.

24. It was originally the United Nations International Children's Emergency Fund.

25. See http://www.wfp.org/about/executive-director.

26. See http://www.unicef.org.

27. See http://www.wfp.com/molly.

28. The fashion chain Benetton courted further controversy when it showed images of such mutilations in a series of advertisements.

29. Journalists at a MediaTrain conference in Khartoum readily agreed that naming and showing the faces of child soldiers involved in a Justice and Equality Movement rebel attack could lead to reprisals against them and their families by both sides in the conflict.

30. One supposedly genuine NGO in East Africa repeatedly sends invitations to conferences that do not exist, working a scam that echoes the infamous e-mails from alleged Nigerians offering million-dollar payouts in return for bank account details.

31. See conservapedia.com/climategate.

32. The huge unused stocks of Tamiflu in some countries that were built up in response to the bird and swine flu scares are testimony to how that reaction can itself be excessive.

33. See Steven Ross, *Toward New Understandings: Journalists and Humanitarian Relief Coverages* (San Francisco: Fritz Institute, 2004). Available at http://www.fritzinstitute.org/PDFs/Case-Studies/Media studyexcSum.pdf.

34. See the Governance and Social Development Resource Center (http://www.gsdrc.org).

35. See "Burma's Aung San Suu Kyi Makes Landmark Campaign Speech," BBC.co.uk, last modified March 14, 2012, available at http://bbc.co.uk/news/world-asia-17363329.

36. See "Schindler's Factory in Krakow," Krakow-Info, available at http://www.krakow-info.com/schindler.htm.

Christopher Holshek, Humanitarian Civil-Military Coordination: Looking Beyond the "Latest and Greatest"

Originally published in Kevin M. Cahill, M.D., ed., *The Pulse of Humanitarian Assistance* (New York: Fordham University Press, 2007), 103–131.

1. From an informal paper provided at the start of "Humanitarian Roles in Insecure Environments: A Strategic Workshop," U.S. Institute of Peace, Washington D.C., January 13–14, 2005. Notes on the Workshop are available at http://www.usip.org.

2. The Challenges Project, *Challenges of Peace Operations: Into the 21st Century—Concluding Report* 1997–2002 (Stockholm: Elanders Gotab, 2002), 143, http://www.peacechallenges.net.

3. The *Code of Conduct for the International Red Cross and Red Crescent Movement and Non-Governmental Organisations (NGOs) in Disaster Relief* is available at http://www.sphereproject.org/handbook/hdbkpdf/hdbk_ann.pdf; *UNHCR and the Military – A Field Guide* is available at http://www.unhcr.org/refworld/pdfid/465702372.pdf; and the *Guidelines on The Use of Foreign Military and Civil Defence Assets in Disaster Relief* – "Oslo Guidelines," OCHA-Nov2006, Revision November 2007, is available at http://www.humanitarianinfo.org.

4. Karen Guttieri, "Civil-Military Relations in Peacebuilding," *Sicherheitspolitik und Friedensforschung* 2 (2004): 84.

5. Challenges Project, *Challenges of Peace Operations*, 143–144. Bullet points are paraphrased from the report.

6. Ibid., 144.

7. From an informal copy of the Agency Coordinating Body for Afghan Relief (ACBAR) bulletin obtained by the author on 27 December 2002.

8. Ibid.

9. Christopher J. Holshek, "The Operational Art of Civil-Military Operations: Promoting Unity of Effort," in *Lessons from Kosovo: The KFOR Experience*, ed. Larry Wentz, Command and Control Research Program, Department of Defense, Washington D.C., July 2002, 270-71, http://www.dodccrp.org.

10. Maj. Gen. Timothy Cross, "Military/NGO Interaction," in *Emergency Relief Operations*, ed. Kevin M. Cahill, M.D. (New York: Fordham University Press, 2003), 204.

11. Ibid., 205.

12. Fouzieh Melanie Alamir, "The Complex Security-Development Nexus – Practical Challenges for Development Cooperation and the Military," *Sicherheit und Frieden*, 2/2012, 72; http://www.sicherheit-und-frieden.nomos.de/fileadmin/suf/doc/Aufsatz_SuF_12_02.pdf.

13. Christopher J. Holshek, "Interdisciplinary Peace Operations Professional Development: Investing in Long-Term Peace Operations Success," in *Cornwallis Group VII: Analysis for Compliance and Peace Building*, ed. Alexander Edward Richard Woodcock and David F. Davis (Cornwallis Park, Nova Scotia: Pearson Peacekeeping Center, 2003), 53.

14. Robert M. Schoenhaus, "Training for Peace and Humanitarian Relief Operations," *Peaceworks* 43, United States Institute of Peace, Washington, D.C., April 2002, 7.

15. For more on this construct, see Christopher Holshek, "Thinking Globally, Acting Locally: Civil-Military Coordination in the 21st Century," in a forthcoming volume of papers from the 23-24 February 2012 Kennesaw State University – U.S. Army Strategic Studies Institute symposium, *Conflict Management and Peacebuilding: Pillars of a New American Grand Strategy*.

16. Cheryl Bernard, "Afghanistan without Doctors," *Wall Street Journal*, August 12, 2004.

17. Holshek, "Thinking Globally, Acting Locally."

18. Oliker, *Aid During Conflict*, 40–43.

19. Chris Seiple, *The U.S. Military/NGO Relationship in Humanitarian Interventions* (Carlisle, Pa.: U.S. Army Peacekeeping Institute, 1996), 187.

Especially in the past few years, a number of guidelines, references, and tools have emerged to promote civil-military coordination. Among the most important:

> OCHA's *Guidelines on The Use of Foreign Military and Civil Defence Assets in Disaster Relief*—"Oslo Guidelines," November 2007 (http://www.humanitarianinfo.org/iasc/page loader.aspx?page=content-products-products&sel=8); as well as Civil-Military Guidelines & Reference for Complex Emergencies, 2008 (http://reliefweb.int/node/24014).

> *UNHCR and the Military—A Field Guide*, UNHCR, March 2006 (http://www.unhcr.org/refworld/pdfid/465702372.pdf).

> The U.S. Institute of Peace's *Guide for Participants in Peace, Stability, and Relief Operations*, 2010 (http://www.usip.org/publications/guide-participants-in-peace-stability-and-relief-operations-web-version).

> The Sphere Handbook: *Humanitarian Charter and Minimum Standards in Disaster Response*, The Sphere Project, 2004 (http://www.sphereproject.org/handbook/index.htm).

> Web-based tools such as OCHA's Relief Web (http://www.reliefweb.int) and One Response (http://oneresponse.info/Pages/default.aspx), as well as the Sphere Project, *Humanitarian Charter, and Minimum Standards in Disaster Response* (http://www.sphereproject.org).

> Code of Conduct for the International Red Cross and Red Crescent Movement and Non-Governmental Organisations (NGOs) in Disaster Relief, 1994 (http://www.sphereproject.org/handbook/hdbkpdf/hdbk_ann.pdf).

20. Ibid., 11. Note that this was published in 1996.

Frederick M. Burkle Jr., M.D., Evidence-Based Health Assessment Process in Complex Emergencies

Originally published in Kevin M. Cahill, M.D., ed., *Emergency Relief Operations* (New York: Fordham University Press, 2003), 55–79.

1. S.W.A. Gunn, *Multilingual Dictionary of Disaster Medicine and International Relief* (Dordrecht, The Netherlands: Kluwer Academic Publishers, 1990), 7.

2. A. Zwi and A. Ugalde, "Political Violence in the Third World: A Public Health Issue," *Health Policy and Planning* 6, no. 3 (1991): 203–217.

3. M.J. Toole and R.J. Waldman, "The Public Health Aspects of Complex Emergencies and Refugee Situations," *Annual Review of Public Health* 18 (1997): 283–312.

4. M. J. Toole, "The Role of Rapid Assessment," in *Humanitarian Crises: The Medical and Public Health Response*, ed. Jennifer Leaning, M.D., et al. (Cambridge: Harvard University Press, 1999), 15–39.

5. R. Margolis et al., "Rapid Post-Disaster Community Needs Assessment: A Case Study of Guatemala After the Civil Strife of 1979–1983," *Disasters* 13, no. 4 (1987): 287–299.

6. Ibid.

7. Toole, "The Role of Rapid Assessment."

8. R. J. Brennan and F.M. Burkle, "Disaster Assessment for the Public Health Sector II: Risk Assessment and Rapid Health Assessment," in *Disaster Preparedness in Schools of Public Health: A Curriculum for a New Century*, ed. L. Landesman, (Washington, D.C.: Association of Schools of Public Health, and Atlanta: Centers for Disease Control and Prevention, 2000), 1–20.

9. Centers for Disease Control and Prevention, "Famine-Affected, Refugee and Displaced Populations: Recommendations for Public Health Issues," *Morbidity & Mortality Weekly Report (MWR)* 41 (1992): 1–76; M. J. Toole and R.J. Waldman, "Prevention of Excess Mortality in Refugee and Displaced Populations in Developing Countries," *Journal of the American Medical Association* 263 (1990): 3296–3302.

10. F. Davidoff, "In the Teeth of the Evidence: The Curious Case of Evidence-Based Medicine," *Mt. Sinai Journal of Medicine* 66 (1999): 75–83.

11. J. C. Desendos, D. Michel, F. Tholly, et al., "Mortality Trends Among Refugees in Honduras, 1984–1987," *International Journal of Epidemiology* 19, no. 2 (1990): 367–373.

12. F. M. Burkle, K. A. W. McGrady, S. L. Newett, et al., "Complex, Humanitarian Emergencies: III. Measures of Effectiveness." *Disaster Medicine* 10, no. 1 (1995): 48–56.

13. C. J. Elias, B. H. Alexander, and T. Soky, "Infectious Disease Control in a Long-Term Refugee Camp: The Role of Epidemiologic Surveillance and Investigation," *American Journal of Public Health* 80, no. 7 (1990): 824–828.

14. Toole and Waldman, "Public Health Aspects," 283–312; D. Guha-Sapir, "Rapid Assessment of Health Needs in Mass Emergencies: Review of Current Concepts and Methods," *World Health Statistical Quarterly* 44 (1991): 171–181.

15. P. A. Hakewill and A. Moren, "Monitoring and Evaluation of Relief Programs," *Tropical Doctor* 21(suppl. 1) (1991): 24–38.

16. Ibid.

17. UN High Commissioner for Refugees. *Handbook for Emergencies*, 2nd ed. (Geneva: UN High Commissioner for Refugees, 2002), 40–46.

18. Ibid.; Hakewill and Moren, "Monitoring and Evaluation," 24–38.

19. A. P. Davis, "Targeting the Vulnerable in Emergency Situations: Who Is Vulnerable?" *Lancet* 348 (September 28, 1996): 868–871.

20. UNHCR, *Handbook for Emergencies*, 40–46; *Public Health Guide for Emergencies* (Baltimore: Johns Hopkins School of Hygiene and Public Health, 2000).

21. F. M. Burkle, "Lessons Learnt and Future Expectations of Complex Emergencies," *BMJ* 319 (1999): 422–426.

22. Relief and Rehabilitation Network. Review of: Counting and Identification of Beneficiary Populations: Registration and Its Alternatives. http://www.ennonline.net/fex/03/rs6.html, accessed 2/22/2002.

23. Davidoff, "Teeth of the Evidence," 75–83; *Public Health Guide for Emergencies.*

24. Toole and Waldman, "Public Health Aspects," 283–312.

25. Toole and Waldman, "Prevention of Excess Mortality," 3296–3302.

26. Toole and Waldman, "Public Health Aspects," 283–312.

27. Ibid.

28. Desendos et al., "Mortality Trends Among Refugees," 367–373.

29. Davidoff, "Teeth of the Evidence," 75–83; Hakewill and Moren, "Monitoring and Evaluation," 24–38; Davis, "Who Is Vulnerable?" 868–871; M. Anker, "Epidemiological and Statistical Methods for Rapid Assessment: Introduction," *World Health Statistics Quarterly* 44, no. 3 (1991): 94–97.

30. P. T. Glaziou and V. T. Mackerras, "Vitamin A Supplementation in Infectious Diseases: A Meta-Analysis," *BMJ* 306 (1993): 366–370.

31. Organization for Economic Cooperation and Development, *Evaluation and Aid Effectiveness: Guidance for Evaluating Humanitarian Assistance in Complex Emergencies* (London: Development Assistance Committee/Overseas Development Institute, 1999), 13–14.

32. J. Cosgrave, "Refugee Density and Dependence: Practical Implications of Camp Size," *Disasters* 3 (September 20, 1996): 261–270.

33. WHO, *Health Assessment Protocols*; Sphere Project, *Minimum Standards*; Hakewill and Moren, "Monitoring and Evaluation," 24–38; Davis, "Who Is Vulnerable?" 868–871; *Public Health Guide for Emergencies*.

34. B. T. Burkholder and M. J. Toole, "Evolution of Complex Emergencies," *Lancet* 346 (1995): 1012–1015.

35. R. J. Brennan and B. T. Burkholder, Centers for Disease Control and Prevention, unpublished data (1997); P. B. Spiegel and P Salama, "War and Mortality in Kosovo, 1998–99: An Epidemiological Testimony," *Lancet* 357 (2000): 2204–2209.

36. L. P. Boss, M. J. Toole, and R. Yip, "Assessments of Mortality, Morbidity, and Nutritional Status in Somalia during the 1991–1992 Famine," *JAMA* 272, no. 5 (August 3, 1994): 371–376.

37. OECD, *Evaluation and Aid Effectiveness*, 13–14.

38. Burkle et al., "Measures of Effectiveness," 48–56.

39. Ibid.

40. Ibid.

41. Boss, Toole, and Yip, "Mortality, Morbidity, and Nutritional Status," 371–376; M. B. Gregg, *Field Epidemiology* (Oxford: Oxford University Press, 1996).

42. Boss, Toole, and Yip, "Mortality, Morbidity, and Nutritional Status," 371–376.

43. Ibid.

44. Gregg, *Field Epidemiology*.

45. F. M. Burkle, "Characteristics of Complex Emergencies That Affect Epidemiology," lecture for Combined Humanitarian Assistance and Response Training (CHART) course, Center of Excellence in Disaster Management and Humanitarian Assistance, Honolulu, 1997.

46. S. Hansch, "The Demography of Vulnerability: Somalia in the 1990s," Unpublished paper presented for the National Academy of Sciences Workshop on Mortality Patterns in Complex Emergencies; Washington, D.C., 18 November 1999, National Research Council.

47. V. Brown, G. Jacquier, D. Coulombier, et al., "Rapid Assessment of Population Size by Area Sampling in Disaster Situations," *Disasters* 25, no. 2 (2001): 164–171.

48. W. C. Robinson, M. K. Lee, and G. M. Burnham, "Mortality in North Korean Migrant Households: A Retrospective Study," *Lancet* 354, no. 9175 (July 24, 1999): 291–295.

49. Burkle, "Emergencies That Affect Epidemiology."

50. P. Spiegel, F. M. Burkle, C. C. Dey, and P. Salama, "Developing Public Health Indicators in Complex Emergency Response," *Prehospital & Disaster Medicine* 16, no. 4 (2001): 281–285.

Pamela Lupton-Bowers, Teamwork in Emergency Humanitarian Relief Situations

Originally published in Kevin M. Cahill, M.D., ed., *Basics of International Humanitarian Missions* (New York: Fordham University Press, 2003), 59–110.

Sam Rose, Education as a Survival Strategy: Sixty Years of Schooling for Palestinian Refugees

Originally published in Kevin M. Cahill, ed., M.D., *Even in Chaos: Education in Times of Emergency* (New York: Fordham University Press, 2010), 228–245.

1. Photo-story available at: http://electronicintifada.net/v2/article10223.shtml.

2. Convention on Certain Conventional Weapons, Protocol III—Protocol on Prohibitions or Restrictions on the Use of Incendiary Weapons, Geneva, 10 October 1980.

3. See UNRWA in figures, available at: http://www.unrwa.org/userfiles/20120317152850.pdf.

4. *Report of the Director of UNRWA* (Paris: UNRWA, 1951).

5. Maya Rosenfeld, "From Emergency Relief Assistance to Human Development and Back: UNRWA and the Palestinian Refugees, 1950–2009," *Refugee Studies Quarterly* (forthcoming).

6. *UNRWA: A Brief History, 1950–1982* (Vienna: UNRWA, n.d.).

7. Ibid.

8. B. Schiff, *Refugees Unto the Third Generation: UN Aid to Palestinians* (Syracuse, N.Y.: Syracuse University Press, 1995).

9. This approach finds voice in the "W" for works in UNRWA's name. The Economic Survey Mission, which led to UNRWA's establishment, estimated in 1949 that works projects could lead to the deletion of 100,000 names from UNRWA's ration rolls by mid-1951. The need to limit the Agency's relief budget was given added urgency by global flour shortages and the Korean War, which pushed up prices of nonfood items. See *Report of the Director of UNRWA.*

10. One of these projects involved the construction of a canal to divert water from the Suez Canal to the Sinai to support the economic development of the area and the resettlement of refugees. See http://untreaty.un.org/unts/1_60000/5/22/00009078.pdf. UNRWA also committed to advance US$83 million for the Aswan Dam project, although the initiative was eventually shelved.

11. *UNESCO Executive Board, Resolutions and Decisions Adopted By the Executive Board at Its 30th Session.* The statement was in response to a communiqué from UNRWA's Deputy Director that it would be unable to increase its budget for primary education, since this would not further the primary goal of making refugees economically independent.

12. This five-year plan included a proposal to establish a nine-year cycle of elementary and preparatory schooling, a system that continues to this day. See Friedhelm Ernst, "Problems of UNRWA School Education and Vocational Training," *Journal of Refugee Studies* 2, no. 1 (1989). It should also be noted that when the General Assembly extended UNRWA's mandate in 1959, it made explicit reference to the need for an expanded vocational training program.

13. *UNRWA Annual Report* 1960.

14. Ibid. In June 1963, Davis reported that these plans had been implemented successfully: the capacity of UNRWA's training centers had actually grown from around 600 to 4,000, while investment in general education programs had brought "educational opportunities available for refugee children almost up to the level of those which existed for the children of the local population in Jordan, Lebanon, the Syrian Arab Republic and the Gaza Strip." See *Yearbook of the United Nations*, 1963.

15. Rosenfeld, "From Emergency Relief Assistance to Human Development and Back."

16. See *Finding Means, UNRWA's Financial Crisis and Refugee Living Conditions* (New York: FAFO, 2003).

17. Schiff, *Refugees Unto the Third Generation.*

18. *Report of the Director of UNRWA.*

19. *UNRWA Annual Report,* 1950; Rosenfeld, "From Emergency Relief Assistance to Human Development and Back."

20. *UNRWA Annual Report,* 1950–1951; Nabil A. Badran, "The Means of Survival: Education and the Palestinian Community, 1948–1967," *Journal of Palestine Studies* 9, no. 4 (Summer 1980). By comparison, an estimated 97 percent of Jewish children in Mandate Palestine were in school by 1944. See Rosemary Sayigh, "Palestinian Education—Escape Route or Strait-Jacket?" *Journal of Palestine Studies* 14, no. 3 (Spring 1985).

21. Ernst, "Problems of UNRWA School Education and Vocational Training."

22. From UNRWA's perspective, investment in education programs also had tactical motivations. Perennially straitjacketed by resource constraints, the Agency saw education and training programs as a way to support refugee self-sufficiency and reduce dependency on monthly food rations.

23. Muhammad Hallaj, "The Mission of Palestinian Higher Education," *Journal of Palestine Studies* 9, no. 4 (Summer 1980).

24. For a detailed exposition of the concept of education as a "family project," see Maya Rosenfeld, *Confronting the Occupation* (Stanford: Stanford University Press, 2004).

25. Hallaj, "Mission of Palestinian Higher Education"; Sayigh, "Palestinian Education."

26. Hallaj, "Mission of Palestinian Higher Education." This arrangement continues to this day, in all fields except Lebanon.

27. *UNRWA: A Brief History,* 1950–1982.

28. *UNRWA Medium Term Plan,* 2004–2009.

29. Schiff, *Refugees Unto the Third Generation.*

30. *Memorandum submitted by UNRWA to the UK Treasury,* February 2006.

31. See *UNRWA Annual Reports,* 1967–1980.

32. To help counter the loss of educational services, UNRWA produced and distributed self-learning materials and audiovisual aids. Requests to Israel to permit the extension of the school year were often rejected, although the agency argued that such moves might reduce Intifada violence. See *UNRWA Annual Reports,* 1988–1993; B. Schiff, *Refugees Unto the Third Generation.*

33. This system had been a permanent feature of life for Palestinians in the occupied territories since the 1980s, with closures typically tightened or relaxed in response to political or security-related considerations.

34. See Bir Zeit University Right to Education Campaign, http://right2edu.birzeit.edu.

35. Palestinian National Early Recovery and Reconstruction Plan for Gaza, March 2009.

36. Much of the criticism of Palestinian textbooks has been based on research published by the Center for Monitoring the Impact of the Peace (CMIP), now known as the Institute for Monitoring Peace and Cultural Tolerance in School Education (http://www.impact-se.org). In response to the allegations made by CMIP, a number of other studies have been commissioned, including by the U.S. Consulate in Jerusalem. Those involved in these studies include the Israel/Palestine Center for Research and Information (IPCRI), the Georg Eckert Institute and the Harry S. Truman Institute for the Advancement of Peace at the Hebrew University in Jerusalem. Nathan Brown, professor of political science at George Washington University, has also published extensively on this subject. His analysis of the controversy is available at http://www.geocities.com/nathanbrown1/Adam_Institute_Palestinian_textbooks.htm.

37. The reintroduction of school feeding programs, a staple in UNRWA schools in earlier decades, in Gaza in 2008 is a sign of the socioeconomic regression that plagues the territory.

38. See *West Bank and Gaza Education Sector Analysis: Impressive Achievements Under Harsh Conditions and the Way Forward to Consolidate a Quality Education System* (New York: World Bank, 2006).

39. I am grateful to Rema Hammami of the Institute of Women's Studies at Bir Zeit University for this analysis, and also for the insights of Penny Johnson.

40. Likewise, during the first Intifada, requests from UNRWA to Israel to permit the extension of the school year were often rejected, although the agency argued that such moves might reduce violence. See *UNRWA Annual Reports*, 1988–1993.

41. See *EFA Global Monitoring Report 2010–Reaching the Marginalized* (UNESCO/OUP, London 2011)

42. These plans were conceived as part of programwide reforms.

Margareta Wahlstrom, What Can Modern Society Learn from Indigenous Resiliency?

Originally published in Kevin M. Cahill, M.D. ed., *More with Less: Disasters in an Era of Diminishing Resources* (New York: Fordham University Press, 2012), 70–77.

1. National Information Center of Earthquake Engineering of India, *Guidelines for Earth-quake Resistant Non-Engineered Construction* (Kanpur: Indian Institute of Technology, 2004). Available at http://www.traditional-is-modern.net/LIBRARY/GUIDELINES/1986IAEE-Non-EngBldgs/1986GuidelinesNon-Eng(ALL).pdf.

Kevin M. Cahill, M.D., To Bind Our Wounds: A One-Year Post-9/11 Address

Originally published in Kevin M. Cahill, M.D., ed., *To Bear Witness: a Journey of Healing and Solidarity* (New York: Fordham University Press, 2005), 115–123.

Richard Ryscavage, S.J., The Transition from Conflict to Peace

Originally published in Kevin M. Cahill, M.D., ed., *Emergency Relief Operations* (New York: Fordham University Press, 2003), 284–294.

1. P. Weiss-Fagen, "The Challenges of Rebuilding War-Torn Societies: A Bibliographic Essay," War-Torn Societies Project, UN Research Institute for Social Development, Geneva, 1995.

2. John Galtung, "Three Approaches to Peace: Peacekeeping, Peacemaking and Peacebuilding," in *Peace, War and Defense: Essays in Peace Research* (Copenhagen: Christian Eljers, 1976), 2:297–304.

3. K. Hewitt, ed., *Interpretation of Calamity from the Viewpoint of Human Ecology* (London: Allen and Unwin, 1983).

4. For more about the "contract culture" and humanitarian relief, cf. Graham Hancock, *Lords of Poverty* (London: Macmillan, 1989).

5. Joanna Macrae, "Aid under Fire: Redefining Relief and Development Assistance in Unstable Situations," background discussion paper, Dept. of Human Affairs Seminar, ActionAid, Overseas Development Institute, Wilton Park, U.K., April 7–9, 1995.

6. Mark Duffield, "Complex Emergencies and the Crisis of Developmentalism," *Institute of Development Studies Bulletin* 25, no. 3 (U. of Sussex).

7. NORDSAMFN, *Nordic Peacekeeping Handbook,* Nordic UN Standby Forces (Helsingfors: Tryckericentralen AB, 1993), 28.

8. Cf. General Assembly, "Report of the Secretary-General on the Work of the Organization," UN Document A/49/1, Sept 2, 1994.

9. See the work of Nobel Prize winning economist Amartya Sen and also Catholic Social Teaching, especially the social encyclicals of Pope Paul VI, "Populorum Progressio" (1967), and Pope Benedict XVI, "Caritas in Veritate" (2007).

10. Cf. F. Cuny, *Disasters and Development* (New York: Oxford University Press, 1983).

11. R. Gorman, *Refugee Aid and Development: Theory and Practice* (Westport, Conn.: Greenwood Press, 1983).

12. For definitions of conflict resolution, mediation, peacekeeping, peace research, etc., cf. Graham Evans and J. Newnham, eds., *The Penguin Dictionary of International Relations* (London: Penguin Books, 1998).

13. Herbert Kelman, "The Interactive Problem-Solving Approach," in *Managing Global Chaos* (Washington, D.C.: U.S. Institute of Peace, 1996), 501–520.

14. E. Voutira and Shaun Brown, "Conflict Resolution: A Cautionary Tale," Report No. 4, Refugee Studies Program, University of Oxford, 1995.

15. Marina Ottaway and Thomas Carothers, eds., *Funding Virtue: Civil Society Aid and the Promotion of Democracy* (Washington, D.C.: Carnegie Endowment for International Peace, 2000).

16. For descriptions of various peacemaking projects of NGOs, cf. David Smock, ed., *Private Peacemaking,* Paperworks #20, U.S. Institute for Peace, 1998.

17. For a summary view of the relationship problems between NGOs and the military, cf. T. Lanzer, B. Harrell-Bond, and R. Ryscavage, "The Role of the Military in Humanitarian Emergencies," Conference Report, Refugee Studies Program, Oxford, U.K., October 29–31, 1995.

18. As an example of how complex the process can become: In the run-up to the Iraq war, when it was clear the U.S. government planned to attack the Hussein regime, I chaired a series of meetings between key U.S. nongovernmental organizations (NGOs) and the U.S. Department of Defense planners. It was obvious that the U.S. military was operating on the assumption that after the collapse of the Iraqi government hundreds of civilian NGOs and UN agencies quickly could enter the country and start the relief and rehabilitation process. In fact, extreme postwar violence prevented the normal civilian relief process from developing. Further complicating these discussions was the fact that most of the NGOs distrusted working with the military and opposed the invasion in the first place.

19. Adam Roberts, "Humanitarian Action in War," Adelphi Paper No. 305 (London: International Institute for Strategic Studies, 1996).

20. For example, Guus Van Der Veer, *Counseling and Therapy with Refugees and Victims of Trauma: Psychological Problems of Victims of War, Torture and Repression* (New York: John Wiley & Sons, 1998).

21. Cf. "Forgiveness in Conflict Resolution: Reality and Utility," Conference Report, Woodstock Theological Center, Washington D.C., December 9, 1996.

22. Anne-Marie Smith, *Advances in Understanding International Peacemaking* (Washington, D.C.: U.S. Institute of Peace); John Clark, *Democratizing Development: The Role of Voluntary Organizations* (London: Earthscan, 1991).

23. Larry Diamon, Juan Linz, and Seymour Lipset, *Democracy in Developing Countries,* 3 vols. (Boulder, Colo.: Lynne Rienner, 1989); and Guillermo O'Connell, Philippe Schmitter, and L. Whitehead, *Transitions from Authoritarian Rule: Prospects for Democracy,* 4 vols. (Baltimore: Johns Hopkins University Press, 1986).

24. Gary Dempsey with Roger Fontaine, *Fool's Errands: America's Recent Encounters with Nation Building* (Washington, D.C.: Cato Institute, 2001).

25. Paul F. Diehl, J. Reifschneider, and Paul Hensel, "United Nations Intervention and Recurring Conflict," *International Organization* 50, no. 4 (autumn, 1996).

26. Lawrence Harrington and Samuel Huntington, eds., *Culture Matters* (New York: Basic Books, 2000).

Ghassan Salamé, Humanitarianism's Age of Reason

Originally published in Kevin M. Cahill, M.D., ed., *Human Security for All* (New York: Fordham University Press, 2004), 81–98.

1. Arend Lijphart, *Democracy in Plural Societies* (New Haven, Conn.: Yale University Press, 1977); Arend Lijphart, *Democracies: Patterns of Majoritarian and Consensus Government in Twenty-One Countries* (New Haven, Conn.: Yale University Press, 1984); Theodor Hanf, *Coexistence in Wartime Lebanon* (London: I. B. Taurus, 1993); Theodor Hanf, Heribert Weiland, and Gerda Vierlag, *South Africa: The Prospects for Peaceful Change* (Bloomington: Indiana University Press, 1981).

Richard J. Goldstone, Healing with a Single History

Originally published in Kevin M. Cahill, M.D., ed., *Human Security for All* (New York: Fordham University Press, 2004), 215–228.

1. A. V. Dicey, *Law of the Constitution* (London: Macmillan, 1895).

2. A. Cox, *The Court and the Constitution,* 10th ed. (Boston: Houghton Mifflin, 1987), 202.

3. The Geneva Conventions of 1949; the 1973 Convention, which declared Apartheid to be a crime against humanity; the 1984 Torture Convention; and some sixteen United Nations Conventions dealing with acts of terrorism all recognized universal jurisdiction.

4. "Assessing the New Normal" (paper, Human Rights Watch, New York, September 2003).

5. Ibid.

6. "International Terrorism: Legal Challenges and Responses" (paper, International Bar Association, Ardsley, New York, September 2003).

Kevin M. Cahill, M.D., The Evolution of a Tropicalist

Originally published in Kevin M. Cahill, M.D., *Tropical Medicine: A Clinical Text, Eigth (Jubilee) Edition,* (New York: Fordham University Press, 2011), 278–285.

Contributors

Valerie Amos is the Under-Secretary-General and Emergency Relief Coordinator for OHCA. She had previously served as a Minister in the British Government, and has been active on the promotion of human rights, social justice, and equality on the African continent. She is Chair of Royal African Society, a member of the Fulbright Commission, and Fellow at the Center for Corporate Reputation.

Kofi A. Annan served as Secretary-General of the United Nations for two terms. In 2001, Annan and the UN were co-recipients of the Nobel Peace Prize. In 2012, he was the UN-Arab League Envoy to Syria.

Judy A. Benjamin served as the gender advisor to USAID in Kabul, Afghanistan. She is trained as an anthropologist and international health consultant, with a focus on the impact of conflict on civilian populations.

Boutros Boutros-Ghali was Secretary-General of the United Nations. He was Professor of International Law and International Relations at Cairo University, and Deputy Prime Minister for Foreign Affairs of Egypt. He was also Secretary-General of the Francophonie. He is a Director of the CIHC.

Frederick M. Burkle Jr., M.D., is a Senior Fellow at the Harvard School of Public Health. He was Visiting Professor at the Center for International Emergency, Disaster, and Refugee Studies at Johns Hopkins University and had also been Deputy Assistant Administrator at the Bureau for Global Health, USAID. He is a member of the Institute of Medicine of the National Academy of Sciences.

Kevin M. Cahill, M.D., is University Professor and Director of the IIHA at Fordham University and President of the CIHC. He is the Senior Advisor on Academic Affairs for the United Nations Alliance of Civilizations. He has served as the Chief Advisor on Humanitarian and Public Health Issues to three Presidents of the UN General Assembly. He is the Chief Medical Advisor on Counterterrorism for the NYPD, Director of the Tropical Disease Center of Lenox Hill Hospital, and Professor of Clinical Tropical Medicine at NYU.

Francis Deng is the UN Ambassador and Deputy Minister of Foreign Affairs of South Sudan. He has served as Special Adviser to the UN Secretary General for the Prevention of Genocide and UN Special Representative for IDPs. Other past positions include Ambassador and Minister of State for Foreign Affairs of Sudan, and Senior Fellow at the Brookings Institution.

Alain Destexhe, M.D., is a Senator in the Belgian Parliament and a Senior Advisor of the International Crisis Group. He was Secretary General of *Médecins sans Frontières.* He was awarded the Prize of Liberty by Nova Civitas. He is the author of *Rwanda and Genocide in the Twentieth Century.*

Sir Francis Drake enjoyed a long career at sea, with duties that ranged from being a privateer to serving in the British Admiralty. In 1579 he circumnavigated the earth, later dying of dysentery off Panama.

Richard Falk is Albert G. Milbank Emeritus Professor of International Law and Practice, Princeton University; He is also Visiting Distinguished Professor at the University of California, Santa Barbara. He is a member of the editorial boards of *The Nation* and *The Progressive,* and is Chair of the Board of the Nuclear Age Peace Foundation.

Richard J. Goldstone is Retired Justice of the Constitutional Court of South Africa and Former Chief Prosecutor of the International Criminal Tribunal for the former Yugoslavia and Rwanda. In 2009, he was the first to be granted the title "The Hague Peace Philosopher." He is Visiting Professor of International Politics at Fordham University and is a Director of the CIHC.

Paul Grossrieder was the Director-General of the ICRC. After retiring, he accepted the Presidency of Voice, a network of some 100 European NGOs. He also held the position of Advisor to the Ministry of Foreign Affairs of the Vatican.

Peter Hansen is a Diplomat-in-Residence at Fordham University's IIHA. He was Commissioner-General of UNRWA, and a former Under Secretary General for Humanitarian Affairs. He is a Director of the CIHC.

Timothy W. Harding, M.D., is Emeritus Professor of forensic medicine at the University of Geneva. He has also worked as Visiting Professor at the University of Kobe, Japan. He founded and was the first director of the Centre for Education and Research in Humanitarian Action in Geneva.

Larry Hollingworth is Visiting Professor of Humanitarian Studies at the IIHA and the Humanitarian Programs Director for the CIHC. He was UNHCR Chief of

Operations in Sarajevo during the Balkan Conflict. He has served as Humanitarian Coordinator on CIHC-sponsored missions for the UN in Iraq, Lebanon, Palestine, Pakistan, and East Timor.

Christopher Holshek is a strategic analyst with Wikistrat, focusing on civil-military training and education. He commanded the first U.S. Army Civil Affairs battalion to deploy in support of Operation Iraqi Freedom.

Irene Khan is the Chancellor of the University of Salford and Director-General of the IDLO. She was Secretary General of Amnesty International and a member of the Charity Commission of England and Wales.

Pamela Lupton-Bowers has led team-building programs for the CIHC and IIHA for many years. She was Head of Training and Development at the IFRC in Geneva, Switzerland. She has worked extensively in management development and team building in Africa, Asia, and Europe.

Joseph A. O'Hare, S.J., is the former President of Fordham University, New York, and former Editor in Chief of *America* magazine. He was also Chairman of the Association of Jesuit Colleges and Universities (AJCU) and the Association of Catholic Colleges and Universities (ACCU). He is a Director of the CIHC.

Lord David Owen was Minister of Foreign Affairs, Health and the Navy in the United Kingdom. He was also Chancellor at the University of Liverpool. He is a Director of the CIHC.

David Rieff is an author and journalist whose books include *Slaughterhouse: Bosnia and the Failure of the West,* and *A Bed for the Night: Humanitarianism in Crisis.* He is the co-editor, with Roy Gutman, of *Crimes of War: What the Public Should Know* and is a contributing author to the *New York Times Magazine.*

Sam Rose is a humanitarian adviser working for the UK Department for International Development. Previously, he was the humanitarian coordinator for UNRWA.

Richard Ryscavage, S.J., is a Professor at Fairfield University. He served as Country Director of the Jesuit Refugee Service/U.S.A. and as the National Secretary for Jesuit Social and Internal Ministries. He was the first Pedro Arrupe Tutor at Oxford University's Refugee Studies Centre in Great Britain.

Ghassan Salamé is the Dean of the Paris School of International Affairs. He was Senior Political Adviser to the United Nations Special Representative of the Secretary-General for Iraq. He currently sits on the Boards of the International Crisis Group, the International Peace Institute and the Open Society Foundations.

Nicola Smith has had major field operational experience in conflict and disaster zones around the world.

Peter Tarnoff is former U.S. Undersecretary of State for Political Affairs, and former President of the Council on Foreign Relations. He is a Director of the CIHC.

Jeremy Toye is a Founding Member of MediaTrain. He was a Reuters correspondent and international manager, for twenty-eight years, working in some sixty counties.

Ed Tsui has had extensive experience in the fields of social and economic development and humanitarian affairs. His prior positions include Chief of Staff for the UN Undersecretary General and Director of Policy in the Department of Humanitarian Affairs and OCHA.

Michel Veuthey is Professor at the International Institute of Humanitarian Law. He is also a Board Member of MSF-Switzerland and the Geneva Fund. He served for thirty years with the ICRC in many positions including Assistant to the President. He was the Geneva Representative and Academic Director of the CIHC.

Margareta Wahlstrom is the Special Representative of the Secretary-General for Disaster Risk Reduction for the UN and Head of the UN International Strategy for Disaster Reduction (UNISDR). She has served as Deputy Emergency Relief Coordinator and Assistant Secretary-General for Humanitarian Affairs, OCHA.

Alec Wargo is responsible for Asia, the Middle East and North Africa in the Office of the UN Under Secretary-General for Children and Armed Conflict. He has worked in Bosnia, Rwanda, East Timor, Guinea, and the Democratic Republic of Congo.

The Center for International Humanitarian Cooperation and the Institute of International Humanitarian Affairs

The Center for International Humanitarian Cooperation (CIHC) was founded in 1992 to promote healing and peace in countries shattered by natural disasters, armed conflicts, and ethnic violence. The Center employs its resources and unique personal contacts to stimulate interest in humanitarian issues and to promote innovative educational programs and training models. The CIHC has sponsored symposia, exhibits, and published books, including *Silent Witnesses, A Directory of Somali Professionals*, and *Clearing the Fields: Solutions to the Global Land Mine Crisis*, as well as the International Humanitarian Book Series of Fordham University Press.

The CIHC has collaborated with Fordham University to foster close links between academia and humanitarian field operations, creating an Institute of International Humanitarian Affairs (IIHA). Its flagship course is the International Diploma in Humanitarian Assistance (IDHA). The IIHA offers a graduate masters degree in International Humanitarian Action (MIHA) and an undergraduate International Humanitarian Affairs minor program. The IIHA also offers specialized training courses for humanitarian negotiators, international human rights lawyers, and mental health workers in war zones. Short (one- to two-week) courses in forced migration, humanitarian law, mental health in complex emergencies, civil-military cooperation, among others, are presented in countries around the world. In the past few academic years, courses were offered in fourteen countries across five continents. The IIHA also issues Occasional Papers on timely issues as diverse as a ban on cluster munitions, to reports from Gaza, Sudan, Somalia, and the role of the university in humanitarian crises. For more information, visit www.fordham.edu/iiha.

The Directors of the CIHC serve as the Advisory Board of the IIHA. The President of the CIHC is the University Professor and Director of the Institute; the CIHC Humanitarian Programs Director is Visiting Professor at the IIHA; other CIHC Directors are Diplomats in Residence at Fordham University.

Directors

Kevin M. Cahill, M.D., President

Nassir Abdulaziz al-Nasser

Boutros Boutros-Ghali

Francis Deng

Richard J. Goldstone

Helen Hamlyn

Peter Hansen

Eoin O'Brien, M.D.

Joseph A. O'Hare, S.J.

David Owen

Peter Tarnoff

Index

environmental health
assessment, 296
epidemiological-based definition
of complex emergency,
296–99
Ericsson, 50–51
ethics, emergency ethic, 55
ethnic conflict, 210
EU (European Union),
solidarity, 249
Europe, Convention for the
Protection of Human Rights
and Fundamental Freedoms,
78–79
*Even in Chaos: Education in
Times of Emergency* (Cahill,
ed.), 4
evidence-based health
assessment in complex
emergencies, 288–302
evil adversaries, 246–47

Facebook, 45
feedback, teamwork and, 316
food distribution: exchange for
sex, 85; gender and, 84–85
force *versus* violence, 99–100
Fordham University: IDHA,
307–9; IIHA, 5, 6
foreign policy: American,
immediate past, 244;
American, terrorism and,
232; Bush Doctrine, 245–46;
creating in democracies,
252–54; doctrinaire,
244–46; EU solidarity,
249; evil adversaries,
246–47; fence-mending,
250–52; humanitarian
interventionism (Clinton),
245; Monroe Doctrine and,
244; new world order, 245;
Obama administration,
246; outcast regimes, 249;
sanctions, 250–52; threatened
governments and, 248–49;
Truman Doctrine, 245
funding: for emergency
response, 203; UNRWA,
327–28

GDACS (Global Disaster Alert
and Coordination System), 46

gender: food distribution and,
84–85; humanitarian aid and,
85–87; POP analysis and, 87;
refugees and, 85–86; as social
construct, 85; vulnerability
and, 89
gender-based violence, 88–95
Geneva Conventions, 8; articles
of First Convention, 29; ICRC
and, 20; ICRC Commentary,
29; IHL mechanisms,
33–34; ratification, 29; Red
Cross and, 55–56; Refugee
Conventions, 20
genocide: definition, 61–62; IHL
and, 31; neutrality and, 61–65
global civil society, 230–31
global economy, humanitarian
action progress and, 172–73
global justice, society and,
228–29
Global Platform on Disaster Risk
Reduction, 335
Global Pulse (UN), 46
global security: human rights
and, 112–21; war on terror,
115–16
global society, normative
revolution, 224–31
Golden Rule, spiritual origins of
humanitarian standards, 27
Good Offices Mission,
preventive diplomacy and, 180
Grassroots Mapping Project,
43–44
Greeks humanization of war,
14–15
group survival, origins of
humanitarian standards,
26–27
Guantanamo Bay, 73
guerilla-style conflicts, Red
Cross and, 58
Guiding Principles on Internal
Displacement, 138
Gupta, Rakesh: terrorism
definition, 98; terrorists *versus*
rebels, 102

Hague Peace Conference (1899),
Martens Clause, 39
Hague Regulations, 28–29
Hezbollah, Israel and, 109–11

HFA (Hyogo Framework for
Action), 335
High Commissioner for Human
Rights, 225–26
history: of conflict, resolution
and, 357–58; violence and,
371–72
HPTs (high performing teams),
305–6
Human Right to Food, 32
Human Right to Health, 32
Human Right to Peace, 32
human rights: in armed
conflicts, 28; development,
372–75; global security and,
112–21; globalization, 120–21;
humanitarian intervention
and, 226; instruments,
30–31; international, NGOs and,
225–26; international, past
crimes, 227–28; mechanisms,
34–35; NGO activism and,
224; NGOs and world policy,
225; Solidarity Human Rights,
31; UDHR and, 224; violation
allegations and government
reputation, 225
*Human Security for All: A
Tribute to Sergio Vieira de
Mello* (Cahill, ed.), 2
humanitarian action: liberation
movements and, 20–21;
limits of, 64–65; military, 23;
period between World Wars,
18–19; politicization of, 22–23;
progress, 169–76; September
11th and paradigm shift,
23–24; World War I, 18
humanitarian aid: distribution
effects, 161; gender analysis,
85–87; manipulation, 62–64;
neutrality and, 54–55; phases,
347–50
humanitarian crises, 9–10
humanitarian interventionism
(Clinton), 245
humanitarian interventions. *See*
interventions
humanitarian law, 28
humanitarian operations, early,
17
humanitarian placebo, 211
humanitarian space: Anderson,

437

United States: contributions to suffering, 233; as empire, 232–33; foreign policy, terrorism and, 232; international law and, 375–76
universality of IHL, 29–30
universities, 235–36; education internationalization, 237–38; humanitarian discipline, 10–11; intercultural understanding and, 238–39; international terrorism and, 236–37; interreligious dialogue, 239–41
UNJLC (UN Joint Logistics Centers), 202
UNOSOM II, 213
UNPREDEP (United Nations Preventive Deployment Operation), 213
UNPROFOR (UN Protection Force): Bosnia and, 59–60, 212–13; Yugoslav Republic of Macedonia, 213
UNRRA (United Nations Relief and Rehabilitation Agency), 7
UNRWA (United Nations Relief and Works Agency for Palestine Refugees in the Near East): deterioration, 328–29; education program challenges, 327–29; education program success, 324–27; education programs early history, 321–24; emergencies, 329; funding shortfalls, 327–28; humanitarian space, 156–68; OPT (Occupied Palestinian Territory) and,

166–68; RAO (Refugee Affairs Officer), 166
U.S. Army, terrorism definition, 98
U.S. Department of State: State Sponsors of Terrorism list, 103; terrorism definition, 98

values, renaissance of fundamental humanitarian values, 35–39
video communication, 45
Vietnam War, international law codification and, 29
violence: cultural relativism, 90–91; cycle, 100; *versus* force, 99–100; gender-based, 88–90; gender-based, international response, 93; history and, 371–72; IHL (International Humanitarian Law), 28–29; International Criminal Tribunals, 373; limiting and group survival, 26–27; of oppressed, 100; rape as dehumanizer, 88–89; religious behavior and, 15; short-term coping and, 88; St. Thomas Aquinas, 99; terrorism, 99–100. *See also* sexual violence
Violence (Ellul), 99
Virtual OSOCC (On-Site Operations Coordination Centre), 46
Vodafone Foundation, 50
vulnerability, gender and, 89

war: Cold War, 20–21; conflicts on the periphery, 21–22;

Greeks' humanization, 14–15; international law codification and, 28–29; on terror, global security and, 115–16; against terrorism, 24; from total war to total humanitarianism, 60–61. *See also* World War I; World War II
warning systems, 43–44
waterboarding, 73
WFP (World Food Programme), electronic cash transfer and, 49
women: CEDAW, 92–93; food distribution and, 84–85; mobility of refugees, 89; refugee reintegration, 93–94; refugee repatriation, 93–94; refugees, 84; skills training, 92; vulnerability, 89. *See also* gender
workers, realism and, 10
World Bank, Mapping for Results, 44
World War I, ICRC, 18
World War II: ICRC and, 19; international law codification and, 28; postwar associations formed, 19–20; "Quarantine the Aggressors" (FDR), 220–21

Yugoslav Republic of Macedonia, UNPROFOR in, 213

Zhare Dasht (yellow desert), 40–41